Migration, Ethnicity, Race, and Health in Multicultural Societies

Migration, Ethnicity, Race, and Health in Multicultural Societies

SECOND EDITION

Raj S. Bhopal **CBE, DSc (Honorary), MD, MBChB, BSc (Hons), MPH, FFPH, FRCP(E)**

Bruce and John Usher Professor of Public Health,
University of Edinburgh and Honorary Consultant in Public Health,
NHS Lothian

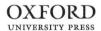

OXFORD
UNIVERSITY PRESS

OXFORD
UNIVERSITY PRESS

Great Clarendon Street, Oxford, OX2 6DP,
United Kingdom

Oxford University Press is a department of the University of Oxford.
It furthers the University's objective of excellence in research, scholarship,
and education by publishing worldwide. Oxford is a registered trade mark of
Oxford University Press in the UK and in certain other countries

First Edition published in 2007

Second Edition published in 2014

Impression: 1

Published in the United States of America by Oxford University Press
198 Madison Avenue, New York, NY 10016, United States of America

British Library Cataloguing in Publication Data
Data available

Library of Congress Control Number: 2013945067

ISBN 978-0-19-966786-4

Printed and bound in Great Britain by
Clays Ltd, St Ives plc

I dedicate this book: to my parents-in-law, Mr Subash and
Mrs Anjani Mazumdar, for raising my loving and beautiful wife Roma;
to Roma for her unstinting support; and to my sons Sunil (and his wife and my
daughter-in-law Hannah), Vijay, Anand, and Rajan for making me such a proud
father by their excellent contributions to our multi-ethnic world.

Preface

Much of the world now comprises multi-ethnic, multicultural societies, i.e. people from widely varying ancestry, cultures, languages, and beliefs. With globalization of trade, increasing international travel, and migration the whole world is destined to become multi-ethnic, probably within the next 20 to 30 years. This poses huge challenges for medical and social scientists, doctors, nurses, public health practitioners, health-care managers, and policy-makers. They have to meet social, ethical, legal, and policy obligations to deliver evidence-based health care of equal quality and effectiveness to all. To achieve this, they need a solid understanding of the concepts of race and ethnicity and how these are applied to achieve robust and meaningful health statistics, workable health policies, effective health-care systems, and better health for all. They also need to have a high level of awareness of how things can go wrong; particularly taking into account the history of racism that permeates many societies to this day. This book lays the foundation for those wishing to acquire this knowledge.

This book provides a conceptual framework, explores reasons for the incomplete success of past approaches, and offers alternatives for the future. The purpose of this book is to help readers use the concepts of race and ethnicity for population-based research and practice, particularly in the setting of epidemiology, clinical services, and public health. Readers are encouraged to consider these concepts in policy-making, health service planning, and health promotion. The book emphasizes theory, ideas, and principles and hopes to counter the study and use of ethnicity and race in an a theoretical, ahistorical, and routine way.

The book will be of interest to students of medical, science, social science, public health, and epidemiology, and also to practitioners and researchers interested in migration, race, and ethnicity. Health service managers and policy-makers may find this book a source of insights that they need to confront the legal, policy, and organizational challenges they face.

This book shows how the study of health by migration status, race, and ethnicity can benefit the whole population, not just minorities, particularly by setting a new and demanding vision based upon the best demonstrable health status. It rejects the time-honoured but narrow perspective of setting the majority population as the standard for minorities to aspire to. It asks us to grasp the vast opportunities for knowledge that are in our hands in multicultural, multi-ethnic societies.

Book authors—especially solo ones—need to be brave, perhaps even foolhardy, especially when they tackle broad and controversial issues such as migration, race, ethnicity, and multiculturalism. The first edition of this book was well received, and even won a couple of prizes. I am grateful to readers and book reviewers who have sent constructive, mostly positive, feedback. The time for a second edition has come because there has been enormous change since 2007. My recent thinking, and hence the new emphases in this edition, is:

1. The field of research and practice on the topic here is growing fast, but splintering. Splintering is occurring for many reasons, some of which we can resolve. Words and concepts, for example, are important and agreement is difficult but surely achievable. In some countries it is not socially and politically acceptable to talk of colour, ethnicity, or race but it is fine to talk of migrants or indigenous groups. In others, the opposite applies. Whatever words we use, we will find that the underlying issues are the same,

i.e. of subgroups arising from differences in ancestry, migration status, language, culture, and social standing. The needs of indigenous (aboriginal) groups are also similar, though the challenges are even greater. The same applies to undocumented migrants. The new title of the book—including migration—and the retitled chapters, including migration and race/racial, reflect my new stance. Previously, I promoted the concept of ethnicity, which I still think is an excellent one because of its breadth and flexibility. I have, however, learnt that the goal is more important that the route (indeed, vocabulary) to it. If some find the goal is better reached by country of birth, migration status, or race rather than ethnic group—excellent! I have also contextualized the subject as best placed within the broader inequalities/inequities/social determinants agenda.

2. A cursory glance at 'state-of-the-art' reviews or policy documents internationally shows the commonality of the issues facing multicultural societies. While retaining a strong UK foundation, I have built on the international perspectives in the first edition, to illustrate more clearly how similar the challenges are. Just because people are called South Asians (UK), Asian Indians (US), or Hindus (The Netherlands) and may be thought of as ethnic/racial/migrant minorities or even aliens does not mean their needs are greatly different. In addition to strengthening the international, comparative perspective, I have pulled together good practice from across the world, and drawn on WHO initiatives of 2008 and 2010.

3. I have long-emphasized that attending to the needs of minorities improves matters for the whole population. After all, migration status, ethnicity, and race provide variables that portray important and sizeable inequalities (largely unparalleled by other variables). Such portrayals are important in the public health goals of understanding causes of variations in population and reducing and eradicating inequality.

4. In addition, readers will also find the following alterations:

   a) simplification of language;
   b) pruning, especially of the reference lists, to make space for the new ideas;
   c) updating of all aspects of the book, including the implications of the Human Genome Project on the biology underlying racial and ethnic differences;
   d) substantial new material, especially on migration, various groups of migrants, and special groups including indigenous (aboriginal) minorities and the Roma (Gypsy) populations.

In the time-honoured way, if you like the book tell others, if you don't (or have ideas for improvement) tell me! I would be glad to hear from you at raj.bhopal@ed.ac.uk.

R. S. Bhopal

13 May 2013

Foreword

In the early phase of the Han dynasty (206 BC to AD 220) in China the idea of being Chinese equated with the adoption of specific cultural and political practices, rather than a person's ethnic origin. In due course, 'Han' was synonymous with Chinese and others were 'non-Han'. The Han dynasty was an exceptionally long period in Chinese history and is associated with stability, prosperity, and the creation of a central nation state.

So the original fluidity of defining a person's identity was gradually replaced by a concept based on ethnicity, national borders, and many other things.

This book covers one of the most complex aspects of the human condition. Depth of scholarship is not common, but it is not rare either. Texts that give the reader deep and thought-provoking insights are not encountered every day nor are they plentiful in bookshops and bookshelves around the world. Academic books that grip the reader and make them want to read on, rather than dip and dive into the text only occasionally, are seldom encountered.

To open Raj Bhopal's book is to find all three: impressive scholarship from a career-long interest, insights that keep you thinking days after you have read them, and accessibility. Historical perspectives on race and ethnicity, concepts, principles, methodology, research, and politics are all distilled into a work of great power.

Raj Bhopal is one of relatively few with a background in public health worldwide who has been writing, researching, teaching, and thinking about ethnicity, race, migration, and health. As such he is the perfect guide for those seeking to understand, those who want to learn, and those in search of a moral compass in their practice, their policy-making, or their leadership.

The chapter on policy and strategy to improve health and health care is of particular practical value and covers experience in the UK (Scotland in particular), the United States, and other parts of the world.

One of Raj Bhopal's trademarks is his use of clear learning objectives and exercises. Always good practice, but essential in such a complex area.

Going into this, its second edition, with a new title, *Migration, Ethnicity, Race, and Health in Multicultural* Societies, it remains a towering work that illuminates a complex field of thought in science and practice.

The controversial Irish politician, historian, and sage Conor Cruise O'Brien, once said 'anti-Semitism is a very light sleeper'* Insert the word 'racism' for 'anti-Semitism' and it becomes universally applicable to one of the evils of society and global affairs that Raj Bhopal's book (amongst many other aims) seeks to dispel through enlightenment.

Liam J. Donaldson
Chair in Health Policy, Imperial College, London

---

* Runnymede Commission (1994) *A Very Light Sleeper: the persistence and dangers of antisemitism.* London: Runnymede Trust.

Acknowledgements (first and second editions)

A book writer performs the task with the help of far too many people to name, and even to remember. My thanks go to the people who helped me but are not specifically listed. Among these are the thousands of people whose papers, books, lectures, and conversations have taught and inspired me. I hope you recognize your influence. I have recorded the contributions of co-authors separately.

The idea of writing this kind of book was Liam Donaldson's. He optimistically suggested in the early 1990s that I should be able to draft the book in a couple of weeks! Work started in earnest in 2004 when Helen Liepman of OUP guided my proposal through OUP's demanding peer review and committee stages. I thank her and her successor Georgia Pinteau and other staff at OUP for their unstinting help. I thank the OUP's referees for helpful feedback. Nicola Wilson at OUP instigated and, with her colleague Caroline Smith, guided the second edition.

I was privileged in having four excellent readers of drafts for the first edition. My research assistant Taslin Rahemtulla exemplified my target audience, so her carefully prepared constructive criticism together with the delivery of missing information was invaluable. Sonja Hunt's pointed and honest feedback was of immeasurable value—all writers need critics who are on their side. Aziz Sheikh is one of the busiest (and most productive) people I know, so it was an honour when he volunteered precious time to read my drafts. I did not want to ask Gina Netto to read drafts for me even although I thought she was perfect for the task—but she volunteered, and even read some of the manuscript in the early hours. Surprisingly, she did not find it to be a cure for insomnia!

Needless to say, while the people who are acknowledged here may rightly share in any praise that may be due they take no responsibility for my errors, misjudgements, or biases.

Normally book writers report that they occupied all the flat surfaces of their homes, forcing their families into a corner. I have behaved this way in the past but this book was prepared in the quiet of my study and my office at the University of Edinburgh. In the modern research-active university medical school, books of this kind are seen as a luxury—best left to the years before or after retirement. As I did not do this I record my gratitude to my university, department, and colleagues who supported me, uttering not one word of complaint even when there may have been neglect of other duties (though I hope this did not occur).

I am grateful for the dedicated and expert assistance of secretaries who worked with me on these editions, principally Tori Hastie, Robyn Arsenault, Helen Christie, and Anne Houghton.

Delivery of the first edition has some resemblance to giving birth. It was a job that needed passion, knowledge, drive, partnership, sacrifices, pain, and labour but it ultimately gave a sense of fulfilment. The second edition has been more akin to looking after a grandchild—a challenging but rewarding duty. My wife Roma gave birth to my four wonderful children (Sunil, Vijay, Anand, and Rajan). I could not understand the drives that made her do this (but I supported her and have been the beneficiary). She has no drive for writing but she has supported me unquestioningly. I cannot find the words to thank her, but after the first edition dinner, flowers, and champagne conveyed the message, though a Caribbean cruise would have been fairer recompense. So, for the second edition, a Caribbean cruise it must be!

Contents

Abbreviations

BMI	Body mass index
CDC	[US] Centers for Disease Control
CHD	Coronary heart disease
CLAS	Culturally and Linguistically Appropriate Services
CRE	Council for Racial Equality
EU	European Union
GP	General practitioner
HDL	High-density lipoprotein
HNA	Health needs assessment
ICD	International Classification of Diseases
IOM	International Organization for Migration
ISD	Information Services (Division)
LDL	Low-density lipoprotein
NCMHD	National Center on Minority Health and Health Disparities

NHS	National Health Service
NIH	National Institutes for Health
NRCEMH	National Resource Centre for Ethnic Minority Health
OGTT	Oral glucose tolerance test
OMB	Office of Management and Budget
REACH	Racial and Ethnic Approaches to Community Health
SHELS	Scottish Health and Ethnicity Linkage Study
SMR	Standard mortality (or morbidity) ratio
SRR	Standardized registration ratio
UN	United Nations
UNESCO	United Nations Educational, Scientific and Cultural Organization
WHO	World Health Organization
WHR	Waist to hip ratio

Chapter 1

Introduction: the concepts of ethnicity and race in health and their implications in the context of international migration

Objectives

After reading this chapter you should be able to:

- Understand both the historical and current basis of the concepts of race and ethnicity in the context of historical, recent, and predictable patterns of human international migration.
- Understand the overlaps and distinctions between these two and other closely related concepts.
- Define these two concepts in relation to other related concepts such as nationality or country of birth.
- Analyse your own background and identity using the concepts of race and ethnicity.
- Appreciate the potential problems in using these and related concepts in health and health care.
- Appreciate the potential benefits of these concepts in the health context.

1.1 **Introduction**

Despite all their splendid variety in skin colour, facial features, and of course behaviour, individual humans and human societies are actually most remarkable for their genetic similarity, itself a reflection of the unity of our species, as emphasized by Steve Jones in his 1991 Reith Lectures. He pointed out that the genetic differences between the snail populations of two Pyrenean valleys are much greater than those between Australian aboriginals and other humans. Amusingly, he reflected that if one was a snail it would make good biological sense to be a racist, but that humans are rather uniform, so by inference being a racist doesn't make sense (Jones 1991).

This similarity goes beyond obvious and physical features such as general body shape (but not skin colour) and posture and applies to emotions, culture, and behaviour. Social scientists have defined hundreds of attributes possessed by all human societies studied thus far. As Pinker (2002) discusses, in 1991 Donald Brown published a list of human universals—attributes possessed by all human societies as observed by ethnographers—comprising several hundred items. Among these universals are the following: insulting, leaders, music, play, poetry, the husband older than the wife on average, taxonomy, trade, and empathy. The list is being added to. Some of these similarities are extremely surprising, and many of them are relevant to the subject of this book. You may wish to reflect on other potential universals, with particular emphasis on those that might lead humans to place emphasis on differentiating themselves, both as individuals and as groups. Before reading on, reflect on Exercise 1.1.

Exercise 1.1 Human universals and social subgrouping

◆ If every aspect of human life was a universal would there be any (a) ethnic or (b) racial subgrouping?

◆ Reflect on some characteristics of human societies that you think are universals which might underpin a human tendency to subgroup populations.

◆ Reflect on some characteristics that are not universals that might promote subgrouping.

If every aspect of human life was a universal there would be little or no way of differentiating human groups and societies, although individual differences would remain. Differences between individuals would not only be in physique, e.g. height, but also in psychology, e.g. temperament. Such differences would, however, by the law of averages be distributed evenly between societies, making them indistinguishable.

Several of the human universals, however, indicate both a capacity for and emphasis on differentiating people, both individually and as groups, from others. For example, the universals include: classification, ethnocentrism, collective identity, recognition of individuals by face, formation of social structures, judging others, making comparisons, and awareness of self-image, including a concern for what others think. Colour terms, including white and black, are also universals. Golby et al. (2001) carried out brain function studies and reported that recognition memory was superior for same-race versus other-race faces. More recent studies indicate that differing perceptions of people from different race groups starts in infancy, certainly by 6 months, and perhaps earlier.

Alongside these universals there are many specific differences between human societies, e.g. dress codes, marriage customs, and behaviours in relation to the use of drugs such as alcohol and tobacco. Humans are skilled at distinguishing both obvious (different dress codes) and subtle (nuances in the accent) differences between themselves and others, both as individuals and as members of social groups. These differences have permitted the subgrouping, or stratification, of human populations.

One of the most fundamental questions is whether humans comprise one or more species; this was a contentious question in Europe in the 18th and 19th centuries, but not necessarily at other times or in other parts of the world. Reflect on Exercise 1.2 before reading on.

Exercise 1.2 Human species

◆ What is a species?

◆ Do humans comprise one or more species?

◆ If one, what are the prospects of evolving into more than one?

◆ If more than one, what are the prospects of evolving into one?

In biology, a species is a class of animals or plants having certain permanent characteristics which clearly distinguish it from other animals or plants. One of the most important of these characteristics is the capacity to produce fertile offspring from sexual unions in natural circumstances. All living human groups meet this characteristic and, therefore, belong to one species, i.e. *Homo sapiens sapiens*. This has now been agreed, and has been reinforced by modern genetics, although the debate is reopened periodically. Having said this, science has not satisfactorily explained why and how modern human populations developed such different physical characteristics (such as skin colour and facial features) over the last 50 000 to 100 000 years. It is not surprising, perhaps, that in the early days of global exploration there was fierce debate about whether humans were one (monogenic) or several (polygenic) species—after all, outwardly, people in different continents looked very different and they also dressed and behaved differently (and still do).

There have been many other human species that have now become extinct. There is a great deal of evidence that some tens of thousands of years ago three or even more human species coexisted: *Homo sapiens, Homo floresiensis* and *Homo neanderthalensis*, the latter two species now being extinct. Since physical or social separation, preventing interbreeding within a species, is a driver for the formation of new species, it seems unlikely that modern humans will ever form separate species.

Surprisingly, all dogs belong to one species, that of wolves, *Canis lupus*. Within this species, there are clearly differences of varying importance, both physical and temperamental. Humans have found it useful to differentiate different kinds of dogs, such as Alsatian, Labrador, spaniel, etc. Using the apparent differences between dogs, biologists and other scientists, breeders, farmers, and the general public have tried to define subgroups, or more scientifically, subspecies, of dogs.

Humans have also tried to differentiate different kinds of their own species using the concept of race, but this practice has not been universally useful and the following quotation from Richard Cooper exemplifies a powerful view shared by most scientists (that we will discuss in due course):

> *Use of the category of race in epidemiologic research presupposes scientific validity for a system that divides man into subspecies. Although the significance of race may be clear-cut in many practical situations, an adequate theoretical construct based on biologic principles does not exist.*
>
> Cooper (1984, p. 715)

There are, clearly, variants of *Homo sapiens*. Furthermore, humans place emphasis on differences relating to factors such as sex, age, height, weight, attractiveness, apparent social status, clothing, language, skin colour, facial features, and hair type. These are among the characteristics which can be, and have been, used to create social subgroups. These differences are captured in a number of concepts (complex and interrelated ideas) which are used to create classifications comprising a set of labels that are agreed as potentially useful.

Traditionally, differences relating to factors that define culture are clustered under the concept of ethnicity, and those relating to physical features under the concept of race. This is an extreme simplification of two very complex and contentious concepts of great importance to human societies, and this simplification will be subjected to analysis and development.

The division of people in any way, but particularly on the basis of race and ethnicity, raises questions about human values, because the consequences of such divisions have been, and continue to be, great. Neither local nor international ethical codes have prevented the disastrous consequences of racism and racial prejudice. Population growth, travel, and increasing global communications are requiring a radical shift in values in relation to ethnicity and race and a stronger application of humanitarian ethics in the 21st century than in the 20th. A renewed understanding of the risks and benefits associated with promoting these concepts in the 21st century is an essential step. Before discussing migration—the driving force behind human ethnic and racial diversity—I introduce the perspective that permeates this book.

1.2 **Epidemiology and public health—the author's professional perspective in relation to ethnicity, race, and related variables**

This book is about improving health using race and ethnicity in multidisciplinary, multicultural settings. It is not about the epidemiology of race and ethnicity. Nonetheless, I come to race and ethnicity as a medical, public health epidemiologist, and personal and professional perspectives have a major influence on a person's stance. The epidemiological and public health perspective of this book both reflects my interests and the importance of race and ethnicity within my professional discipline. Epidemiology is one of the major and growing scientific disciplines underpinning public health and clinical medicine, and guides priorities in health-care policy and delivery. Chapters 3, 5, 7, 8, and 9 are particularly influenced by my epidemiological viewpoint, and by the approach to the subject in my textbook *Concepts of Epidemiology* (Bhopal 2008) (the central strategy is introduced below, and principles and methods are given as required throughout the text). My expectation is that the principles derived from this epidemiological viewpoint are widely shared and applicable, particularly in other quantitative health sciences.

Epidemiology is the study of the patterns of disease and the factors that influence the emergence, propagation, and frequency of disease in populations, with particular reference to causal understanding and prevention. Its major strategy, particularly for investigating the causes of disease, is to compare populations with different exposures to potential causes. These are known as exposure variables, in the sense that a change in exposure might alter disease incidence. Usually, the qualifying word exposure is dropped and epidemiologists refer simply to variables. Comparison lies at the heart of scientific reasoning: hypotheses are both generated and tested using the differences found. Similarities give less leverage for understanding health problems (and are also less interesting).

Epidemiological exposure variables are measures which aid the analysis of disease patterns within and between populations, e.g. sex, age, occupation, social class, health behaviours, etc. Most variables used in epidemiology indicate underlying phenomena of interest which cannot be measured easily, if at all. For example, social (occupational) class is a proxy indicator of various differences between populations including income, education, and styles of consumption. Even apparently simple variables may reflect complex differences; e.g. sex may act as a proxy for genetic, hormonal, psychological, lifestyle, or social status in different studies. These variables may be used to define the distribution of disease and plan for service provision, or to generate hypotheses about the causes of disease. Such observations do not, in themselves, explain disease processes, and hypotheses generated need to be tested.

Ethnicity and race (and related concepts such as migration status) are potentially valuable exposure variables and are, therefore, used to subdivide populations. Differences by ethnicity and race in both the characteristics of populations and their disease experience have been easy to describe, and the scientific literature on ethnicity and health is large and growing. We will discuss the strengths and weaknesses of these variables throughout the book, but particularly in relation to research in Chapter 9.

Based on these general principles, and the questions in Exercise 1.3, reflect further on the potential value of ethnicity and race in epidemiology before reading on.

Exercise 1.3 The epidemiological exposure variable

- What qualities should the exposure variables of race and ethnicity have to make them worth using in epidemiology?
- How do the purposes and uses of epidemiology help us to assess the potential value of the race and ethnicity variables?

According to Senior and Bhopal (1994) a good epidemiological variable should:

- be an important factor in health and disease in individuals and populations,
- be measurable accurately,
- differentiate populations in their experience of disease or health,
- differentiate populations in some underlying characteristic relevant to health, e.g. income, childhood circumstances, hormonal status, genetic inheritance, or behaviour relevant to health,
- generate testable hypotheses on the causes of ill-health or disease and/or,
- help in developing health policy and/or,
- help plan and deliver health care and/or,
- help prevent and control disease.

These attributes of epidemiological variables are closely related to the purposes of epidemiology. Ethnicity and race, and related concepts, lead to contested and controversial variables in epidemiology and public health, and yet they are of central and growing interest. South Africa is a place where categorization by race and population was deeply abused in the era of apartheid (1948–94) but scholars cannot agree whether the country should abandon or continue with race-based categorization. It is crucial for us to understand the strengths and weaknesses of these variables. Try Exercise 1.4 before reading on.

Exercise 1.4 Ethnicity and race as epidemiological variables

- Do ethnicity and race have an impact on health?
- Are ethnicity and race good at showing population differences in experience of disease?
- What underlying differences between people do ethnicity and race reflect?
- How can these differences be used to advance understanding of disease causation, health policy, or health-care planning?
- Are ethnicity and race easily and accurately measured?

There are many dangers of gas as a fuel, particularly explosions, but we can nevertheless make use of it. The fuel of epidemiology, and some other quantitative social and medical sciences, is the analysis of differences in the pattern of ill-health and disease in populations. Ethnicity and race are rich epidemiological fuels, providing a myriad of differences that are challenging to explain. Directly or indirectly, race and ethnicity have a major impact on populations' health patterns. This book has a selection of examples, including the finding of huge variations in stroke rates, as shown in Table 1.1.

Table 1.1 Mortality for stroke given as standardized mortality ratios (SMR; 95% confidence interval) in Bangladeshi-born men and women living in England and Wales compared with the standard population (England and Wales)

	Standard population	Bangladeshi men	Standard population	Bangladeshi women
SMR for stroke 1981 (ICD 9, 430–8)[1]	100	267 (229–319)	100	139 (87–210)
SMR for stroke 1991 (ICD 9, 430–8)[2]	100	281 (232–337)	100	151 (95–229)
SMR for stroke 2001 (ICD 10, 160–9)[3]	100	249 (213–92)	100	207 (164–258)

Source: Data from (1) Balarajan R et al, Mortality among immigrants in England and Wales, 1979–83 in Britton M (ed.) *Mortality and Geography*, London: HMSO, pp. 103–121, Copyright © 1990; (2) Gill PS et al, Black and Minority Ethnic Groups, in Raftery J (ed.), *Health Care Needs Assessment: The Epidemiologically Based Needs Assessment Reviews: Third Series*, Radcliffe Medical Press Ltd, Copyright © 2006; and (3) Wild S et al, Cross-sectional analysis of mortality by country of birth in England and Wales, 1970–1992, *British Medical Journal*, Issue 314, pp. 705–10, Copyright © 1997

Blood pressure is the single most important known risk factor for stroke. Bangladeshi men, however, have comparatively low blood pressure yet their stroke mortality is very high. This unexpected paradox forces the reappraisal of the causes of stroke, not just in this population but more generally, as discussed by Bhopal et al. (2005). This is one example of how ethnicity-related work contributes to causal thinking.

Public health policy is often founded upon such data, particularly where differences are inequitable, in the sense of being unjust. The central question that analysis by ethnicity or race leads to is this: why is a disease more or less common in one racial or ethnic group of people than in another? For example, why in comparison to the British population as a whole is diabetes so common in people who originated in India but live in Britain, and yet why is colorectal cancer relatively uncommon in those same people? Answers to these questions would help us to understand better the causes of disease, and would bring benefit to all populations. Epidemiologists are quickly intrigued by ethnicity and health research, and particularly the questions of why differences in disease occur. Although differences are easy to describe, the mysteries behind the myriad of differences are not easily solved. The causes of differences in general will be discussed in Chapter 6, and the research challenges in Chapter 9. Chapters 5 and 8 will focus on appropriate policy, health-care, and public health responses to findings of such research.

Unfortunately, among many other difficulties that we will discuss, ethnicity and race are very difficult to assess accurately. Furthermore, there is little consensus on appropriate terms for use in the scientific study of health by ethnicity and race, and published guidelines on how to use these concepts are yet to be widely adopted. In view of the importance of terminology and classification, this matter will be discussed in Chapter 2.

In Table 1.2 race and ethnicity are reviewed in the context of other similar variables in epidemiology, showing why they are of interest and, in brief, how one would like to measure them in an ideal world and how one does so in practice. The point is this: ethnicity and race (and related variables) are no different from other variables in their measurement challenges.

Table 1.3 summarizes the characteristics of a good exposure variable and analyses ethnicity in relation to these. An analysis for race, country of birth, nationality, or indeed any other variable, would need to follow similar principles.

An emphasis on disease differences, so appropriate to the analysis required in the sciences, is also deeply influential in the arena of health policy and management, where it is sometimes, but

Table 1.2 Reasons for interest in, and measurement of, some important variables in epidemiology, including race and ethnicity

Variable	Underlying epidemiological interest	Ideal assessment/ measurement	Practical assessment/ measurement
Age	Most diseases are strongly influenced by age, presumably through a combination of biological ageing factors and accumulating environmental exposures	There is no reliable test for biological age (the ideal), so age is chronological, and not biological. The ideal is for chronological age to be extracted from accurate administrative records, e.g. birth certificate	Self-report at interview or self-completed questionnaire. Humans are good at assessing age. In clinical situations where it cannot be ascertained, e.g. the patient is unconscious or there is a language barrier, observer-assessed age is likely to be reasonably accurate
Sex	The incidence of many diseases varies markedly by sex, presumably resulting from one or more of genetic, hormonal, lifestyle, and environmental factors	There is a reliable biological test for sex (chromosomal analysis) but it is rarely used	Self-report at interview or self-completion questionnaire; or extract from administrative records, e.g. birth certificate or passport. Humans are good at assessing sex. In clinical situations where it cannot be ascertained, e.g. the patient is unconscious or there is a language barrier, observer-assessed sex is likely to be extremely accurate
Education	Generally, the well-educated have better health than the uneducated	Testing of academic ability in the context of epidemiological studies would be the correct assessment of education, but it is not done	Self-report data are usually used, with categories such as—none, primary school, secondary school, further education, and university education. Examination of objective records of educational achievement is unusual
Social class/ socio-economic status	Individuals with higher social and economic standing in society have, with a few exceptions, better health than those of lower standing	Ideally, social class would be measured by a combination of assessment of social standing and economic worth, including wealth and income	Usually measured by indicators such as occupation, or location of residence, or educational status, or ownership of durable goods
Race	Individuals belonging to different groups on the basis of physical, biologically determined features have different disease patterns	The biological (genetic) basis of the varying physical features would be measured with DNA analysis	Historical racial groupings underlie current classifications and these have mostly been based on assessors' observations, with some modern-day consultation with populations so defined. Using these classifications people are asked to self-report (in the recent past they were assigned to a group by the assessor)

(Continued)

Table 1.2 (Continued)

Variable	Underlying epidemiological interest	Ideal assessment/ measurement	Practical assessment/ measurement
Ethnicity	Individuals belonging to different groups on the basis of both physical and cultural characteristics have different disease patterns	Both biological and cultural characteristics would be measured and used, singly or in combination, to form human groups	Pragmatic classifications based upon a combination of external assessors' ideas and consultation with the populations to be defined. People are asked to self-report, choosing from classifications

Table 1.3 Ethnicity (or race or country of birth) as an epidemiological variable

Criteria for a good epidemiological variable	Criteria in relation to ethnicity (or race or country of birth)
Impacts on health in individuals and populations	Ethnicity is a powerful associated influence on health
Accurately measurable	In most populations ethnicity is difficult to assess (not true for country of birth)
Differentiates populations in their experience of disease or health	Huge differences by ethnicity are seen for many diseases, health problems, and for factors which cause health problems
Differentiates populations in some underlying characteristic relevant to health, e.g. income, childhood circumstance, hormonal status, genetic inheritance, or behaviour relevant to health	Differences in disease patterns in different ethnic groups reflect a rich mix of environmental factors and may also reflect population changes in genetic factors, particularly in populations where migration has been high
Generates testable aetiological hypotheses, and/or helps in developing health policy, and/or helps plan and deliver health care, and/or helps prevent and control disease	It is hard to test specific hypotheses because there are so many underlying differences between populations of different ethnicity Ethnic differences in disease patterns profoundly affect health policy Knowing the ethnic structure of a population is critical to good decision-making By understanding the ethnic distribution of diseases and risk, preventative and control programmes can be targeted at appropriate ethnic groups

by no means always, inappropriate (as will be discussed in Chapter 5). Since interest in, and the influence of, research on ethnicity and race and related variables is increasing, it is important that the conceptual basis of the work is sound. As we will discuss throughout this book, the concepts are currently mostly inadequately defined and used and require further development. The starting point is an understanding of one's own and others' perceptions of race and ethnicity and that, in turn, is informed by an understanding of migration.

1.3 **Migration**

In Chapter 4 I discuss migration in relation to health and health care from a historical perspective, with examples from several countries. Given the centrality of migration to ethnicity and race, a brief introduction on the phenomenon of migration and its consequences is important.

Homo sapiens is a relative newcomer to the Earth, evolving in East Africa about 150 000 years ago. At some times during this short history, the number of humans plummeted. Modern-day humans can trace their genetic history to a very small number of ancestors, and this is the reason for the surprising genetic similarity among all humans. From their origin in East Africa humans have migrated across the entire globe, successful emigrations having been dated to about 70 000 years ago. In those days there were other *Homo* species but none have survived to the present, for reasons that are unclear. No other primate (humans belong to this order of mammals) has a population size approaching that of humans, and none has lived in all continents. With a population of more than 7 billion, humans have greatly exceeded the predicted population total for a primate of our body size (perhaps by a factor of 7000–70 000). The capacity to survive and thrive after migration is a central factor in this success. Humans have been migrants throughout history, and in terms of absolute numbers of people moving, now more than ever. An estimated 215 million or more people were living outside the country of their birth in 2010. If all such emigrants were in one country it would be the 5th most populous country after China, India, the United States, and Indonesia. These emigrants have children, so this figure might be doubled, and they have been preceded by other emigrants. So, perhaps 10% of the world's population either were born outside their country of residence or have a parent born outside. In addition to international migration we also have movement from the countryside to cities (urbanization) and regional movement. When we add short-term travel for study or work experience (including volunteering) and, of course, vacations we see the full dimension of intermingling of people internationally.

1.3.1 **Health challenges prior to migration**

The process of migration is stressful, costly, and needs careful administration and organization. Visas, passports, and tickets need to be organized and purchased, and residences sold or otherwise secured. Migration requires uprooting in many respects. The recipient country may require health checks prior to issuing a visa and also further checks at the port of arrival. For these, and related, reasons most immigrants are not a random sample of people from the donor country. They are a selected sample and people with essential resources whether financial or social. The result, for the purposes here, is that we generally have a 'healthy migrant effect', i.e. migrants may be surprisingly healthy both compared with the populations they leave behind and those they join. The main exception to this principle is the asylum-seeking population, which is discussed in Section 1.3.5.

1.3.2 **The act of migration**

Until air travel became common in the 1950s migration was a testing time, with a long journey both overland and by sea being normal. Such journeys were hazardous and further selected the fittest among the migrants. One extreme example of such selection that reverberates to this day is the enforced emigration of slaves from Africa via perilous transatlantic journeys in chained, cramped, unhygienic quarters in the holds of ships. Modern-day migration has comparatively minor hazards, with the main exception of undocumented migration.

1.3.3 **After migration**

Assuming they clear passport control, immigrants will arrive to pre-arranged destinations and homes, whether with acquaintances, friends, family, or strangers. They will need to find long-term accommodation, employment, and learn how their new society and its institutions work. In particular, they need to know how to access, utilize, and benefit from the health-care system. This is obviously a major issue for consideration here, especially for Chapters 4–8. The problem is that living conditions for many are likely to be tough with a shortage of resources. Accommodation may be crowded and nutrition poor. Even with pre-existing good health, immigrants may succumb to both physical disorders, including serious infections such as tuberculosis, and mental disorders, including anxiety and depression. Over time, as immigrants settle in, they may acquire the lifestyles and health-risk factors of the local population, e.g. less physical activity, high-fat, calorie-dense food, and acquire local health problems, e.g. becoming overweight and in due course developing diabetes. This process of acculturation is not, of course, one-way—it may also bring many beneficial changes. The key issue for us, however, is a rapid transition towards the disease patterns of the recipient population, and this will be discussed in detail in Chapters 5, 6, and 9.

1.3.4 **Across the generations**

The children of migrants are not, of course, themselves migrants. They should not, therefore, be either called or thought of as second-generation (or third-, fourth-, etc.) migrants. This phrase, and its short-hand variant (second generation), which is more acceptable, are commonplace. Children of immigrants are not always seen as part of the normal population but part of the immigrant population. This is particularly so for countries where nationality is not automatically associated with birthplace but is dependent on ancestry. This is a greater issue for offspring who look different from the majority recipient population, but it is still relevant for those who do not, for there may be other distinguishing features, e.g. their name, dietary requirements, language spoken at home, etc.

It is not good to pretend there are no differences, because there are—and they are important to societies. The concepts of race and ethnicity potentially hold the key here. It could be valuable to think of migrant groups as being integral components of ethnic or racial subgroups—rather than just immigrants. We shall consider this proposition throughout the book. In some countries and studies parental and even grandparental place of birth is used as the primary marker for ethnicity or race in the absence of other data. This pragmatic action should not, however, be allowed to perpetuate immigrant status on children or grandchildren.

One question of importance is whether migration status, ethnicity, and race will continue to matter across the generations. Clearly, and hopefully, the answer should be yes, but much less so. Across the generations, acculturation will mean a convergence of language, living standard, lifestyles, and many other factors. Patterns of health-care utilization should, largely, become similar. What about disease patterns or health-related behaviours? In many instances these too will converge. Three kinds of difference will not, however, converge rapidly. Firstly, differences that are deep-rooted parts of culture and possibly ordained by religion, e.g. the taboo against smoking and alcohol in many immigrant groups of women. These change slowly. Secondly, differences that are a result of complex gene/environment variations, e.g. birth weight, or risk of type 2 diabetes. Third, those that arrive from deep-rooted social factors, e.g. discrimination against those with dark skins, unfamiliar names, or a religion that is not that of the majority. For some children (e.g. Irish children in England) these factors will be less important than for others (e.g. African children in The Netherlands). The point of emphasis here is that social factors are as important as biological ones, both for immigrants and for their descendants.

That the issues are lasting is easily seen by examining health by ethnic or racial group status in countries where multi-ethnic societies are hundreds of years old, e.g. the United States. The issues are as important as ever—something we will return to.

1.3.5 Asylum seekers and refugees

The provision of a safe haven to persecuted strangers is a time-honoured ancient custom that is now an internationally accepted legal obligation under the United Nations (UN) Convention. There are many grounds for seeking a safe haven but most commonly it is based on a serious threat to human rights, e.g. freedom to pursue a religion, hold a political belief, and live free from the threat of torture. People requesting this safe haven are asylum seekers. All nations are obliged under UN laws to follow due process in handling asylum applications. Where a request is upheld the asylum seeker becomes a refugee, with rights of residence and generally all rights related to this. When asylum is not granted and if appeals are rejected the asylum seeker has no further right to stay. This system is a vital part of civilization but it has become extremely controversial, not least because of media-led adverse publicity and an increasing lack of public support. Several factors are particularly important from a health perspective. Asylum seekers and refugees (when genuine) are involuntary migrants. Some of them have endured long-term serious persecution including mental and physical torture. They have often been torn away from their friends and families. The health consequences are evident, and it may take many years of skilled care to rehabilitate some of them.

Those whose applications fail may not be willing to return to the country of origin. Some will be forcibly repatriated at considerable financial, health and well-being, and social costs. Others will become irregular migrants as discussed in Section 1.3.6.

1.3.6 Illegal, irregular, undocumented migrants

Commonly, and certainly in the generally antagonistic mass media, migrants with no formal right of residence are called illegal migrants. This extremely negative description, however, over-simplifies a complex situation. Understanding some of these complexities is essential in the health-care context, because health care is often the focal point for controversy. To soften the tone for more even and fairer discussion, the phrases irregular or undocumented migrant are preferable and will be used henceforth.

Some irregular migrants have, undoubtedly, taken pains and paid large amounts of money to enter a country illegally. Journeys of this kind are often dangerous, with high mortality, e.g. being squashed onto boats or in secret compartments of lorries. These risks are, in themselves, a matter of public health investigation and action. While sympathy is often in short supply in recipient countries we should reflect on the forces that lead people, often with children, to such extreme action. There must be hunger, fear, despair, loneliness, or destitution that drives this behaviour. Alternatively, people may be lured or duped into this behaviour. Perhaps it would be appropriate to reflect on similar forces that in the past afflicted the currently rich countries and led to the same behaviour among their citizens, whether fleeing from famine in Ireland or the Nazi persecution in Germany. (These migrants too were resisted by potential recipient countries.) Other irregular migrants have been smuggled in against their will—these are trafficked people who are then used by prostitution rings or for other manual roles in conditions of enslavement. The mental and physical health problems of such unfortunate people are a grave concern for health professionals.

There are people who come to a country temporarily—perhaps to visit, or study, take a temporary job, or seek asylum—who do not leave. They may like their new country or may see no viable alternative. Having been in the country for some time they are likely to have contacts and networks that they rely on for work, income, accommodation, etc. Their health care is, however, a matter of controversy, as discussed in Chapters 5 and 8.

To survive, irregular migrants need to have support, particularly financial. There are employ-ers—both individuals and companies—who benefit from employing irregular migrants. These benefits may be as simple as lower wages and fewer statutory obligations or the availability of people to do jobs that others will not readily do (au-pairs, housekeeping, fruit picking, restaurant work, etc.). A collusion of interests is required, including, at times, the non-interference of gov-ernment to allow the system to proceed. In recognition of the value of irregular migrants, and the inability to effect change, it is the practice for governments to periodically offer amnesty to those who wish to become regular migrants. Irregular migrants play an important role in the economy, including keeping costs down, and may well pay taxes. Given this, it is rightful that they also ben-efit from the economy, including health care.

Migrants of all kinds will join the support networks and functions of their own ethnic or racial groups and are likely to blend in to minority communities. We now return to consider ethnicity and race in this context of a rapidly diversifying multi-ethnic, multiracial world.

1.4 Migration status, ethnicity and race: self- and others' perception

1.4.1 Migration status

There are so many different kinds of migrants, and their status is so dependent on the era and circumstances, that it is very hard to discuss self and others' perceptions. Furthermore, these perceptions are likely to be dominated by race and ethnicity so that considering migration status independently is difficult.

Migrant status is more a matter of fact (you are or you are not a migrant—there are only two categories) than of perception. Nonetheless, other factors come into play. In many countries migrants have rights based on their ancestral and geographical origins. So, a person whose par-ents or grandparents were born in country X but who has never resided in country X is likely to have rights of residence there. The self-perception, and others' perception too, of such a per-son going to country X may be more that of someone 'coming home' rather than that towards a migrant. This kind of affiliation is likely to be accompanied by commonality in race and/or ethnic-ity, especially (but not necessarily) if there have been visits to the ancestral country in earlier life. A good example of this is Russian Germans migrating to the reunified Germany. Similarly, but to a lesser degree, there may be affiliations when migrants are from a colony of country X, especially when they have been educated in that country's language and educational methods (and possibly curriculum). Indonesians going to The Netherlands and Indians to the UK are good examples. For many if not most immigrants such ties will not exist. All immigrants are likely to perceive themselves as such, even if they migrated as children. One reason for this is that they will be constantly reminded of their migration status by their documents and by bureaucracy, as country of birth of self (and less so of parents) is one of the commonest questions to be asked, whether completing papers at birth, death, census, and for schooling, banking, travelling, and many other aspects of everyday life. Human curiosity means that conversation, whether with strangers or friends, revolves around country of origin/birth. Humans find such conversations interesting. So, the identity 'migrant' is not one that can be shrugged off. This is especially so when the migrant is different from most people in the recipient country whether in terms of looks, language, religion, or even accent.

Others' perception of a migrant, or migrants in general, is also extremely variable but as a generalization many studies show that some suspicion, concern, or even hostility is commonplace. The reaction is at least in part related to worries about increased competition for resources, especially jobs, houses, and schooling. Beyond this there are often deeper issues that relate to worries that are sometimes based on myths and stereotypes about other groups. A recent book by Joanne Nagel (2003) explores, as an example, how important sexual matters have played a dominant role in ethnic and race relations, whether it be ideas about virility, sexually transmitted diseases, fertility, competition for mates, or prejudice about mixed race relationships and children.

Migrants' social status is not entirely comfortable. For this reason, it is not right to perpetuate such status on those who are not migrants, i.e. the children of migrants. Such children may soon become indistinguishable from the general population. They may, however, remain different for many generations for reasons of biology and/or culture so the migration status of their forebears may have lasting effects.

1.4.2 Race

The word race has a multiplicity of meanings and interpretations. Using the biological concept of race, your race is the group you belong to and/or that you are perceived to belong to by other people in the light of a limited but important range of physical factors. This type of race concept is deeply ingrained in human societies, and can be traced back to the roots of history, including in the writings of the great Greek physician Hippocrates some 2000 years ago. Hippocrates (as translated by, e.g., Chadwick and Mann) contrasted the feebleness of the Asiatic races to the hardiness of the Europeans. His concept of race was of human groups shaped by their ancestry in different geographical environments, especially emphasizing climate. Race has played a major role in the way societies work and interact and, unfortunately, the concept has been abused in the past to justify atrocities, e.g. in slavery, colonialism, apartheid, and the Nazis' attempt to exterminate Jews.

The still dominant, though still deeply contested, idea of race is biological. Race in the biological sciences means one of the divisions of humankind based on physical characteristics. Race was studied intensively by many scientists and scholars, particularly in the disciplines of anthropology and biology in the 19th century, with the development of classifications to provide a framework for understanding evolution and examining variation. The strategy for developing classifications was based upon the measurement of physical features. Many physical features were studied, but emphasis was placed upon some obvious ones including skin colour, hair type, eye colour, shape of the head and face, and shape of specific features such as nose and lips, etc. However, the search for difference was intensive, with few aspects of anthropometry (the measurement of the body's form) left unstudied.

Such classifications were not created in a social or political vacuum. Societies were already divided and distinguished on the basis of physical features. For example, this was apparent even within northern European populations, e.g. descriptions of 'criminal features' and the subdivisions of Europeans as Nordic, Alpine, and Mediterranean. There were forces in place to take political or economic advantage of observations that could demonstrate the superiority of northern, Nordic European populations which, in an era of colonization, was important to establishing the moral authority for this. While physical differences between human populations were quite obvious, there was a deeper question underlying this work: were these human populations also different in relation to innate human capacities of overriding importance such as intelligence? If so, this would provide a scientific rationale for contested behaviours, e.g. slave owning, control of immigration, and colonization. A hierarchy of human races could be used to justify such policies, as reflected in the words of Ashley Montagu:

> It is a fact worth remarking that throughout the nineteenth century hardly more than a handful of scientific voices were raised against the notion of a hierarchy of races. Anthropology, biology, psychology, medicine, and sociology became instruments for the 'proof' of the inferiority of various races as compared with the white race. What H. G. Wells called 'professional barbarity and braggart race-imperialism' played a major role in the rationalization justifying the disenfranchisement and segregation of 'inferior races, and thus prepared the way for the maintenance of racial thinking and exploitation of 'native' peoples, and the unspeakable atrocities of the nineteenth and twentieth centuries.
>
> Montagu (1997, p. 80), reproduced with permission of AltaMira Press.

Describing human variation by racial group ought, in theory, to help clarify the genetic and environmental basis of disease. Physical characteristics such as face shape and colour that were the primary features used to distinguish races, however, result from a small number of genes that are not associated with the deeper human traits around intelligence, behaviours, attitudes, and decision-making processes. In practice, geographical variation in gene frequency is great, and however races are defined, large numbers of populations straddle boundaries. No race possesses a discrete package of genetic characteristics. Genetic diseases are not confined to specific racial groups, although the risk varies by region of ancestral origin. There is a great deal of genetic variation within races (indeed about ten times more than between them). Modern genetics has undermined the traditional scientific concept of race by showing that there are no clearly genetically definable subgroups (subspecies) in the human species. Differentiation is, however, possible at the continental level using DNA analysis, and this reflects ancestry. In the 21st century it has become possible to do DNA analysis at the whole genome level. This new work has reopened controversies about race, as discussed in Chapter 9, and has both undermined and bolstered the biological basis of race depending on who is interpreting it.

The massive effort over 150 years to classify races scientifically has largely failed, though we still use crude classifications which are based on continental groupings and which trace their heritage to Linnaeus, the great biologist who devised a classification of all living things. His grouping of humans had four categories, giving us the division of populations as follows: *Homo afer* (later synonyms, Black, African origin, Negro, Negroid), *Homo europaeus* (later synonyms, White, European origin, Caucasian, Caucasoid), *Homo asiaticus* (later synonyms include Mongoloid, Asian), and *Homo americanus* (later synonyms include American Indian, North American Indian, Native American). This work was developed by Blumenbach (1865) who added a fifth category, and most scholars trace current race classifications to his work. Variants of these classifications have a grouping for Australian Aborigines. Blumenbach emphasized that humans were one species and differences were gradual across geographical territory and that his divisions were arbitrary and over-simplified. He argued that all human subgroups were equal.

Most complex classifications have been forgotten, along with the idea that *Homo sapiens* evolved in several places independently, although these kinds of ideas have been published very recently, e.g. Carleton Coon published over several decades in the 20th century including a major volume as late as 1962. For example, the previous division of White European populations as Nordic, Alpine, or Mediterranean has become a relic of history. Though none of the numerous racial classifications have stood the test of time, there are echoes of them in current classifications. As we will see in Chapter 2 when we examine terminology and classifications, race remains important in modern thinking, though increasingly it reflects geographical, social, and class divisions rather than biological ones, notwithstanding the contributions of DNA analysis.

Before reading on try Exercise 1.5.

Exercise 1.5 Race as a social category

◆ Reflect on whether there is truth to the view that races and ethnic groups are socially constructed, artificial ways of categorizing human beings.

Irrespective of the quality of the science, the idea of race as a marker of biological differences between human subgroups was destroyed by international outrage at the abuses of the concept of race, particularly by the Nazis (see Chapter 6). With the defeat of the Nazis at the end of the Second World War, and the ensuing international debate on the dangers of the race concept, under the leadership of the United Nations Educational, Scientific and Cultural Organization (UNESCO) it was widely promoted that humans are one species, races are not biologically distinct, there is little variation in genetic composition between geographically separated groups, and the physical characteristics distinguishing races result from a small number of genes which do not relate closely to either behaviours or disease. Nonetheless, many individuals and governments (especially those using the race concept as part of institutions of government, such as South Africa and Rhodesia (now Zimbabwe) operating apartheid) resisted these ideas. Ashley Montagu was the most vociferous 20th-century opponent of the concept of race, and the following quotation from his landmark publication *Man's Most Dangerous Myth–the fallacy of race* testifies to the persistence of the concept:

> More than half a century has passed since this book was first published in 1942, and more than a generation has gone by since the fifth edition was published in 1974. In spite of those five new editions, each larger than the one before, the race problem, like a malady that will not go away, seems to have grown more troubling than ever. . . .
>
> I have never before put what is wrong with the idea of 'race' in the form of a formula. Let me do so here. What the formula shows, in simplified form, is what racists, and others who are not necessarily 'conscious' racists, believe to be the three genetically inseparable links which constitute 'race:' The first is the phenotype or physical appearance of the individual, the second is the intelligence of the individual, and the third is the ability of the group to which the individual belongs to achieve a high civilization. Together these three ideas constitute the concept of 'race.' This is the structure of the current conception of 'race' to which most people subscribe. Nothing could be more unsound, for there is no genetic linkage whatever between these three variables.
>
> Montagu (1997, p. 31), reproduced with permission of AltaMira Press.

Many scholars, at least in the social sciences, have concluded that race is a social, rather than biological, construction. If so, it follows that racial categories are also socially constructed, i.e. created from popular social perceptions and without sound biological foundation (see Chapter 9 for current views based on DNA analysis). The fact that so often racial categorization has been judged and imposed by observers is of interest in this debate, as will be discussed in Chapter 2. It is self-evident, however, than even a social concept of race is ultimately based on physical and hence biological factors. As we have already discussed in relation to Exercise 1.1, if every aspect of human life was a universal, including physical appearance, we would have no biological concept of race.

People often find genetic explanations for differences in health by race more interesting and attractive than social ones. Conclusions about genetic or biological factors as causes may be wrongly drawn from research showing health differences without proper consideration of factors that may equally, or more likely, be associated with ill-health, including poor housing, racism, low income, or poor nutrition.

The continued use of race classifications has legitimized them as acceptable descriptive labels for both populations, and individuals. In medicine using such labels as 'Asian', 'Black', 'Chinese', etc. is common and seen by some clinicians as important to diagnosis and treatment of disease. The custom of beginning the medical case history with a racial label—this patient is a 43-year-old White/Black/Asian—has often been questioned on scientific, medical, and ethical grounds but the practice continues. Such labels are also important in social discourse and self-identification.

The biological concept of race is of use in attempting to explain population variations in a small number of diseases, or other biological traits. Examples of diseases which illustrate this are mainly found in particular population groups, e.g. sickle cell disease in people of African origin (although not all African populations have a high prevalence of this trait, and many other populations evolving in places where malaria occurs do have it) or cystic fibrosis in those of European origin (with the same limitations as for sickle cell trait, e.g. it is uncommon in Finnish people). Usually, however, apparently racial differences in disease reflect differences in environmental and economic circumstances and not biology. Obviously, studies ought to indicate accurately the relative importance of genetic and environmental factors, but this does not happen because of a combination of conceptual and technical limitations of current research.

In retrospect, the biological concept of races as subspecies was ill-defined, poorly understood, and invalid. The science based on it needed sharper criticism. Race should be used with caution for its history is one of misuse and injustice. There is a strong argument that these injustices still need to be reversed, and to do this we require the very concept that led to them, i.e. race. Most societies have not discarded the race concept, and increasingly we see the adoption of the concept of ethnicity, mainly as a more acceptable synonym for race. A clear understanding of the race concept is, therefore, essential to understand modern societies and the related concept of ethnicity.

1.4.3 **Ethnicity**

In their 1936 book *We Europeans* Huxley and Haddon recommended that race be replaced by ethnic type, an idea now enjoying increasing support despite some criticism. The word ethnicity comes from the Greek word *ethnos*, meaning a nation, people, or tribe. Ethnicity is a multifaceted quality that refers to the group to which people belong, and/or are perceived to belong, as a result of certain shared characteristics, including geographical and ancestral origins, but with particular emphasis on cultural traditions and languages. The characteristics which underpin ethnicity are not fixed or easily measured, so ethnicity is a complex and fluid concept. Table 1.2 shows that complexity and fluidity are characteristic of other important variables, and in themselves are not problems. Ethnicity differs from race, nationality, religion, and migrant status, sometimes in subtle ways, but may include facets of these other concepts.

The concept of ethnicity implies, according to most accounts, one or more of the following:

- ◆ shared origins or social background
- ◆ shared culture and traditions which are distinctive, maintained between generations, and lead to a sense of identity and group-ness, and
- ◆ a common language or religious tradition.

Shared origins is also an essential part of race. These component factors open the way to group identity. Investigators who wish to study ethnicity should collect data on underlying factors, especially language, religion, and family origins, but often they do not. This need for further data will be discussed in Chapter 9.

While group allegiance is mainly dependent on culture it also encompasses physical features, particularly facial features, as in race. This is particularly important for migrants. For example, there are many ethnic groups in Punjab, India but they are not distinguished by their colour or other facial features. They may be distinguished by their clothing, e.g. the turban of the Sikh. When living in Europe or North America, however, their brown colour becomes an important factor in group-ness and identity.

In multi-ethnic societies ethnic groups may remain distinct while becoming different from the original migrant group that they descended from. So Sikhs abroad are often considered simply as part of the ethnic group of Indians (or South Asians). Sikh Indians in the UK are likely to be different from their counterparts in India.

For practical and theoretical reasons, the current preference is for self-assessment of ethnicity. (The alternatives include skin colour, birthplace of self or ancestors, ancestry, names, language, geographical origins, or a mix of such factors.) Self-assignment poses problems to offset its advantages, not least that some people may change their assignment over time, as is their prerogative. In a study following the 1991 British census 12% of 'Blacks' altered their ethnic group, 22% of the 'other' category did so, but only 1% of White and South Asian groups did so. The self-assignment changes in the United States are greater still (see Chapter 2).

While race and ethnicity are conceptually different, they are overlapping concepts that are often used synonymously, a trend which is being fostered by the increasing use, particularly in the United States, of the compound word race/ethnicity or variants. This trend reflects both the conceptual and practical problems of separating the two concepts, and also the strong traditions of race-based analysis in the United States. It also reflects the data collection guidance in the United States and particular needs of Hispanic (Latino) populations (see Chapter 2). In contrast, in Europe, where the Nazis' abuses of race are still remembered and perceived as both shameful and dangerous, race is being abandoned in favour of ethnicity. However, ethnicity too has a shared history of abuse alongside race in Europe, and remains a problem in some European countries, including Germany.

Whatever terms authors use, the underlying concepts ought to be discussed. In practice, a clear definition of what is meant by the terms ethnicity and race is often lacking making it difficult to compare studies, particularly internationally. This is not wholly surprising as race and ethnicity are complex, multidimensional concepts changing with time and therefore subject to varying interpretations. The study of ethnicity, race, and health has, however, been weakened by the diverse and inconsistent use of terms and concepts.

This theme is developed in more detail in Chapter 2. Before closing, however, it is important to underline a change in view from the first edition of this book, which strongly promoted ethnicity over race, and over alternative proxy measures such as country of birth. This edition takes a more relaxed approach, recognizing that the underlying concepts matter more than how they are operationalized. Choices of words will depend on historical and social context.

1.5 Some general problems in using migration status, race, and ethnicity concepts in epidemiology and other quantitative health sciences

Senior and Bhopal (1994) identified four major categories of problems with the concept of ethnicity in epidemiology, which are equally applicable to race and migration status, and in other quantitative health disciplines. These were measurement difficulties, heterogeneity of populations, ethnocentricity and ambiguity about the purpose of using these variables.

Other variables used in population sciences may be subject to some of the same problems. However, Senior and Bhopal proposed that ethnicity is unusual because it has the additional complexities of cross-cultural research. The difficulties of measurement will be discussed in Chapters 2 and 3, and the remaining issues will be introduced here and referred to throughout the text.

1.5.1 The problem of heterogeneous populations

The populations identified by current methods of defining migration status, race, or ethnicity are often too diverse to provide useful information. With migration status the key variable used is country of birth. Although it is occasionally used, it is obvious that analysis of foreign versus local born people leads to comparison of two very diverse populations and is unlikely to lead to anything other than more questions. Even the (improbable) finding of no difference would not be trustworthy as subgroups within these populations may well differ. When country of birth is specific, it is more valuable but even then we worry about heterogeneity. The Surinamese living in The Netherlands are an important subpopulation. They come from a small South American country, Suriname. In The Netherlands the country of birth of the person and parents is used to classify ethnic group. This does not work well for even this small group because it comprises two quite culturally distinct populations known as Creole (a mixture of African and European origins) and Hindus (of Indian subcontinent origin). In the United States official statistics are often published in six race/ethnicity categories—White, Hispanic or Latino, Black or African American, Asian, Native Hawaiian or other Pacific Islander, Native American and Alaska Natives. These are extremely broad categories, especially Asian, which comprises the countries east of Istanbul in Turkey through to Japan—that includes about 50% of the world's population. The need for more specific statistics (an idea captured by the word 'granularity') is increasingly recognized in the United States. In the UK also, ethnic group categories include White, Indian, and Pakistani, which have massive within-group heterogeneity. Such heterogeneity diminishes the value of migrant status, and racial/ethnic categorization as tools for delivering culturally appropriate health care and in understanding the causes of variations in disease.

Even within one Indian-origin Hindu community in Dar es Salaam, Tanzania, substantial variations in risk factors and disease prevalences have been demonstrated (Ramaiya et al. 1991). The term 'Asian' has been very popular in both North America and the UK but it is extremely broad and masks important variations by country of origin, religion, language, diet, and other factors relevant to health and disease. Exactly the same criticism applies to categories such as Latino or Hispanic, Chinese, Black, and African. A study postulating a causal role for diet in the aetiology of coronary artery disease which compared the risks of Indians and non-Indians would give only limited insights since 'Indian' diets are extremely diverse. By contrast, the findings of a study on first-generation Punjabi Muslims, compared with another ethnic group of like age and sex, though more limited in its scope would surely be more valuable. The importance of social class variations within groups also needs to be considered. Furthermore, there is also heterogeneity across generations and countries. An observation of, say, high cancer rates in an ethnic group of interest in one country may not apply in another country because of differences that include social and economic circumstances, acculturation, generation, and of course the selection of different people at the time of migration. Heterogeneity of ethnic minority populations may cause misleading conclusions to be drawn. Studies on broad, heterogeneous migrant, racial, or ethnic groups, however, have value as exploratory or pilot studies; as a first step to generating questions and research that will lead to deeper understanding.

1.5.2 **Ambiguity about the purpose of the research**

There has been a tension between the needs of causal research, which relies on detailed information and focuses on measures such as relative risks, and health and health-care needs research, which relies primarily on absolute risks, i.e. actual numbers and rates and not relative risks. These ideas will be discussed in some detail in Chapter 5 and 7.

Research data cannot easily be collected and presented to achieve simultaneously the needs of causal enquiry and health needs assessment and care planning. Most researchers on ethnicity and health have emphasized the potential to illuminate causal enquiry rather than develop health policies and services. There is no doubt that causal enquiry is stimulated by examining variations by migrant status, race, and ethnic group. The process of moving from observation of variation to understanding variation is extremely difficult, and progress is slow for the reasons discussed in Chapter 9. By contrast, the same kinds of observations can provide evidence and be rapidly applied in policy, health care, and health promotion. Migration status, race, and ethnic group can be key variables for formulating and implementing health policy, e.g. given the extremely high rates of tuberculosis in South Asian immigrants we see the need to identify, for the purpose of BCG immunization, children of Indian subcontinent birth or ancestry (other examples are considered in Chapter 5 and 8). They can be identified by a mixture of variables including their own, their parents', or their grandparents' birthplace, self-reported race or ethnic group, and in the absence of such information by clinical observation of the person. Other obvious clues may come from religion or name. Generally, researchers tend to emphasize causal advances, rather than service or policy advances. One possible reason for this is ethnocentricity, which is discussed below.

1.5.3 **The problem of ethnocentricity**

Ethnocentricity is the inherent tendency to view one's own culture as the standard against which others are judged. This has implications for all aspects of research on migration, race, ethnicity, and health. It will impinge on the design, aims, and methods of studies and the presentation and interpretation of results. Ethnocentricity makes 'value-free' observation impossible. The impact of researchers' values on the presentation and interpretation of results is illustrated in Table 1.4, which contains data originally presented by Marmot et al. (1984) in their landmark report 'Immigrant mortality in England and Wales 1970–78'.

The standardized mortality ratio (SMR) is the summary outcome of a statistical method for taking account of differences in the age (and sometimes simultaneously sex) structure of the compared populations, and the SMR allows a fair comparison of the mortality in the population of interest relative to a standard population, which gets an SMR of 100 by definition, the result being interpreted like a percentage. In Table 1.4 SMRs for the Indian subcontinent-born population, relative to the population of England and Wales, provided the crux of the tables (presenting disease ranking by SMR) and text of the report by Marmot et al. The left-hand column ranks diseases by their relative frequency based on the SMR, as done by Marmot et al., the right-hand column (prepared by me) shows diseases among the same men ranked by the number of deaths.

In the rank-order presentation of data a very different impression of the importance of various diseases amongst Indian men emerges, shifting the emphasis away from the diseases which are common relative to the comparison population to those which are common independently of any such comparison. The primary perspective of Marmot et al., in common with most epidemiology then and now, was to compare and contrast the performance of immigrant and some limited ethnic groups with that of the majority, England and Wales born, population. This is the standard approach in migration, race, and ethnicity health research. The approach picks out conditions that

Table 1.4 Deaths and standardized mortality ratios (SMRs)* in male immigrants from the Indian subcontinent (aged 20 and over; total deaths = 4352)

By rank order of SMR				By rank order of number of deaths			
Cause	SMR	No. of deaths	% of total (4352)	Cause	SMR	No. of deaths	% of total (4352)
Homicide	341	21	0.5	Ischaemic heart disease	115	1533	35.2
Liver and intrahepatic bile duct neoplasm	338	19	0.4	Cerebrovascular disease	108	438	10.1
Tuberculosis	315	64	1.5	Bronchitis, emphysema, and asthma	77	223	5.1
Diabetes mellitus	188	55	1.3	Neoplasm of the trachea, bronchus, and lung	53	218	5.0
Neoplasm of buccal cavity and pharynx	178	28	0.6	Other non-viral pneumonia	100	214	4.9
Total	—	187	4.3		—	2626	60.3

*SMRs comparing with the male population of England and Wales which was by definition 100.

Reproduced from Senior P and Bhopal RS, Ethnicity as a variable in epidemiological research, *British Medical Journal*, Volume 309, pp. 327–330, Copyright © 2004 with permission from the BMJ Publishing Group Ltd.

are commoner in the minority than in the majority. Less emphasis is given to diseases where the standard population has an excess in relation to the minority population and still less to conditions which show no difference. The perspective of Senior and Bhopal (1994) was to consider the main problems of the Indian-origin ethnic groups, without concern for excesses or deficits but to find the common health problems confronting these groups. Both perspectives are based on valid research values but they lead to different emphases and interpretations of the same data. Researchers' and data interpreters' values are relevant in the collection, analysis, presentation, and interpretation of data (see Chapter 10).

There is increasing awareness that European and North American normal values may not apply across ethnic groups, e.g. for the oral glucose tolerance test (OGTT), waist cut-offs, and body mass index (BMI). There have been both propositions and empirical demonstrations that the group with the best health status for a particular condition should provide the standard, wherever the numbers are sufficient to provide precision. There is a slow realization that the majority population may be the greatest beneficiary of ethnic group comparisons, e.g. learning from the low rates of cardiovascular risk factors and outcomes in the Chinese in Scotland, and both high rates and low survival after heart attack in White Scottish populations. Ethnicity, race, and migration status are increasingly seen as variables that benefit the entire population, not just apparently disadvantaged minorities. As this perspective gains sway, ethnocentrism ought to decline.

1.6 Race, ethnicity, migrant status, and social harm and benefits

Migrant status, race, and ethnicity are not harmless concepts and variables, and it is worth reflecting on the potential dangers, as suggested in Exercise 1.6.

Exercise 1.6 Race, social abuses, and ethnicity

◆ List and reflect upon abuses of the concept of race, both historically and currently.

◆ Reflect upon the role of science in such abuses.

◆ Why do you think scientists and health professionals participated in such abuses?

◆ In what way might migrant status, race, and ethnicity give rise to similar abuses?

In the 19th century, in particular, differences among races as then defined were usually assumed to be innate and irreversible biological features, interpreted to show superiority of White races and used to justify policies which subordinated non-White groups. In other words, differences underpinned racism, a topic which is discussed in Chapter 6. Briefly, racism results from the belief that some races are superior to others, which is used to devise and justify actions which foster inequality among (socially created and often imposed) racial groups. It is self-evident that it requires power to implement such policies. In the absence of power it is difficult to put prejudices into action. Emphasis on differences is a prerequisite for racism.

Research focusing on problems that are more common in minority groups (whether defined by migrant status, race, or ethnicity), combined with data presentation techniques designed to high-light differences in comparison with the majority population, and a bias towards emphasizing an excess of a problem, so easily portrays the minorities as disadvantaged and weaker. When research implies genetic factors rather than environmental ones as the cause of such differences in health, minorities may be perceived as biologically weaker in an unchangeable way.

Science that implied and emphasized such weakness helped justify policies in favour of slavery, social inequality, eugenics, immigration control, and racist practice of medicine. Race-specific 'diseases' such as drapetomania (the irrational and pathological desire of slaves to run away) were invented. John Down's theory of 'mongolism' (trisomy 21 or Down syndrome) was that such infants were births from an inferior, Mongoloid, race:

> A very large number of congenital idiots are typical Mongols.... The face is flat and broad, and destitute of prominence. The cheeks are roundish, and extended laterally. The eyes are obliquely placed, and the internal canthi more than normally distant from one another....
>
> The boy's aspect is such, that it is difficult to realize that he is the child of Europeans; but so frequently are these characters presented, that there can be no doubt that these ethnic features are the result of degeneration....
>
> These examples of the result of degeneracy among the mankind appear to me to furnish some argument in favour of the unity of the human species.

Down (1867; reprinted 1995, pp. 55–6)

This view gives some insights into the thinking of scientifically well-educated people in the 19th century—they associated non-European 'races' (here Mongols) with inferiority and degeneracy.

The Tuskegee syphilis study in Alabama, lead by the US Public Health Service from 1932 to 1972, deceived and bribed 600 Black subjects into cooperating with research which examined the progression of syphilis without treatment, even once penicillin (a cure) was available. In May 1997 President Clinton apologized on behalf of the United States to the survivors of this experiment:

> The people who ran the study at Tuskegee diminished the stature of man by abandoning the most basic ethical precepts. They forgot their pledge to heal and repair. They had the power to heal the survivors and all the others and they did not. Today, all we can do is apologize. But you have the power, for only

you—Mr Shaw, the others who are here, the family members who are with us in Tuskegee—only you have the power to forgive. Your presence here shows us that you have chosen a better path than your govern-ment did so long ago. You have not withheld the power to forgive. I hope today and tomorrow every American will remember your lesson and live by it.

Clinton (1997), reproduced under Creative Commons Attribution 3.0

Tuskegee was not a unique racist research project. In their review, Osborne and Feit (1992) con-cluded that much American health research on race and ethnicity contributes to the idea that some human groups are inferior.

The division of people on the basis of race and ethnicity raises important questions about human values, for the consequences of such divisions have been great. Studies of ethnic and racial variations in disease pose a challenge to the maintenance of high ethical standards in health research, themes I discuss in Chapters 8–10. Racial prejudice is fuelled by research portraying ethnic minorities as different, these differences being interpreted as showing their inferiority. Objectively, there is substantial evidence showing that minorities are advantaged in many features of social life and behaviour that relate to better health, as demonstrated by a 'healthy migrant effect'. Infectious diseases, population growth, and culture are, however, common foci for adverse publicity. Following the release of statistics on the ethnicity of single mothers, the *Sunday Express*, a popular UK newspaper, ran the headline 'The ethnic time bomb' (13 August 1996) even though in some ethnic groups being a single mother was rare. Researchers cannot be responsible for media reporting, but must be aware of the attractions of their work to the media and of the poten-tial and usually adverse impact of their work on race relations. Immigrants are in an awkward situation, for their failures may be portrayed as a drain on national resources while their successes may be seen as being at the expense of the local population.

Race and ethnicity are variables that show, dramatically and unequivocally, the importance of historical, political, and social awareness among health researchers. Although the term is rarely used, ethnicism, the idea that some ethnic groups are superior to others, is as much a danger as racism. Recent immigrants are vulnerable to such social prejudice which may compound their own challenges in the resettlement process.

Table 1.5 identifies a few of the potential benefits and problems of ethnicity and race as concepts in the health sciences.

One important psychological barrier is in separating out the modest effects of biology, seen as central to the concepts of race and ethnicity by professionals and public alike, from the huge effects of environment. Differences due to the environment are sometimes perceived as transitory and therefore unimportant, indeed possibly even unrelated to race or ethnicity, while biological differences are perceived as permanent and fundamental to race and ethnicity. This perception of permanence may lead to undue prominence. From a public health perspective, factors that can be controlled and changed deserve prominence. Reflect on Exercise 1.7.

Exercise 1.7 The impact of similar environments on ethnicity and race

◆ Imagine, for any broadly defined ethnic group, e.g. Indian, Native American, African-Caribbean, that following birth everything in the social and physical environment, defined as every non-genetic influence, was held constant.

◆ Would the health/disease outcomes be the same for all ethnic groups?

◆ Outcomes you may wish to consider include diabetes, lung cancer, coronary heart disease, and schizophrenia.

Table 1.5 Potential problems and benefits of ethnicity and race in the health sciences

Issue	Potential problems	Potential benefits
Credibility	Gives backing to scientifically difficult concepts that have been abused previously	Utilizing concepts in health sciences will lead to their development and improvement and to health improvement
Division of society	Reducing social cohesion, by an emphasis on differences, and the creation of a sense of inferiority and superiority	Helping heal existing social divisions by acknowledging and working on differences, as well as demonstrating similarities
Racism	Provides information that can be abused by those who wish to demonstrate inferiority and superiority of particular groups	Information can combat past injustices, and guide future actions to prevent such racism
Ethnocentricity	Sets a standard usually based on the majority population that may be inappropriate for a particular ethnic group	By demonstrating that in some respects ethnic minority populations have better health, more challenging standards can be set for the population, including the majority, e.g. the standard is the population with the best health
Emphasis on problems	Stigmatizing and stereotyping minority populations by focusing on conditions where their health is worst	By showing that in some respects their health is better or no worse than the majority's research can counteract existing stigmas and stereotypes about minorities
Scientific advances	As in the past, science might be led into unsound inferences, and unethical practices	If the causal dividend of studying race and ethnicity can be realized, important advances in population health could be achieved
Development of health services	Either as a result of faulty information or interpretation health services may veer away from true needs	With the appropriate data services might adapt to meet needs better
Individual clinical care	Clinicians might be misled by generalities, stereotypes, and misleading research and scholarship	Armed with an understanding of ethnicity and race clinical care might become more effective
Attitudes to immigration	Adverse data on health status or health-care utilisation may create/ perpetuate negative attitudes to immigration	By showing immigrants' contributions to health-care delivery or the health of the nation the benefits of immigration may be clearer

This thought exercise is not actually feasible, as cultural factors, especially those linked to religion or tradition, are not controllable. The thought experiment, nonetheless, is helpful to our understanding. Even in identical environments health is going to vary between groups, although much less so than under normal circumstances, where there are huge differences in the environment. The result will differ by disease. Obviously, genetic factors are relevant, though mostly modest, and over generations will remain largely unchanged until altered by interracial and interethnic group marriage. Non-genetic factors can also, however, be transmitted across generations. Diabetes is a disorder where the interaction between genetic and environmental factors is particularly strong. Diabetes is also influenced by the fetal environment, i.e. the health (not the genes) of the mother, and quite likely the grandmother and possibly even generations before her. Given identical environments, group variations will remain, though these will decline over generations depending on outcome. Lung cancer is largely an environmentally acquired disease so, given identical environments, especially identical smoking patterns, we would anticipate very little variation. This is also so for coronary heart disease (CHD), where the genetic influence is relatively small and diffuse. The causes of schizophrenia are poorly understood and the answer to the question posed in the exercise is unclear. While schizophrenia may well have a strong biological, indeed genetic, component, there will be an essential interaction with the environment. Given equivalent environments, racial and ethnic variations in schizophrenia are likely to reduce very greatly. For a genetic disorder such as cystic fibrosis or sickle cell disease we would expect little change over a few generations.

This exercise does, however, point to convergence of health status outcomes in the immigrant/minority populations towards that of the recipient populations, itself resulting from adopting its physical, social, and behavioural circumstances Where the convergence is beneficial (e.g. tuberculosis or infant mortality rate) this is a process to be hastened. Where the convergence is damaging, e.g. the chronic diseases, especially diabetes, cardiovascular disorders, and most non-infection based cancers, there need to be strenuous efforts to resist the convergence. Rather, the aim should be to move the majority population to the rates of the minority.

1.7 Race and ethnicity in relation to ancestry, nationality, country of birth, and religion

Before reading on you may wish to reflect on Exercise 1.8.

Exercise 1.8 Ethnicity and race in relation to nationality, religion, and similar variables

Where are the overlaps and the similarities between ethnicity and race and:

◆ ancestry

◆ parental country of birth

◆ country of birth

◆ migration status

◆ nationality

◆ citizenship

◆ religion

◆ language?

Race and ethnicity are both closely related to ancestry. The biological concept of race relates to ancestry because the features it is based on are inherited. (The social concept of race also emphasizes lineage, because it impacts on both identity and cultural and political heritage.) These features are retained across many generations. Where ancestry is from a mix of racial/ethnic groups the relation between self-assigned or other perceived or assigned race and ancestry becomes complex, and undermines the concepts of race and ethnicity.

Many of the factors underlying ethnicity are also inherited, although not biologically, e.g. religion, taboos on behaviours, dietary preferences, etc. Such factors are changeable yet tend to linger through generations. Factors that maintain identification with a particular group include physical features (though weakly so); so biology also contributes to ethnic identity.

Country of birth is related to race and ethnicity when international migration into the particular country of birth under consideration is uncommon. Country of birth in high-immigration places, say the United States or New Zealand, is not a good marker of ethnicity or race.

Country of parental, or grandparental, birth may provide important additional information to add to or substitute for self-reported ethnicity or race but is not an exact substitute. For example, it may be that a person who is born in India, and whose parents were all born there, is not ethnically Indian, and perceives his/her ethnicity as, say, English. This situation is one outcome of colonization, church activity, international diplomatic services, and globalization.

Ethnicity should not be, but sometimes is, confused with nationality (usually associated with passport) or with migrant status. For example, immigrants from the Indian subcontinent may be Canadian nationals but members of a particular ethnic group, say Sikh Punjabis. Their children, born in Canada, are members of their parents' ethnic group, but may perceive themselves also part of a larger ethnic group such as Indians, Asians, or even (usually politically) Blacks. They may also perceive themselves to have an additional ethnic identity relating to the host community, e.g. Canadian, North American, etc. This is particularly likely when people have the right of residence in the country and to a passport. This additional ethnic identity, e.g. Canadian Indian, may help people to signal their citizenship and allegiance to the country of residence. While ethnicity, race, ancestry, country of birth, country of parental birth, nationality, and citizenship are conceptually distinct, some countries link ease of acquisition of nationality and citizenship to race or ethnicity. This is an abuse of the concepts of race and ethnicity that creates a sense of injustice, especially if privileges and rights are linked to citizenship and nationality rather than period of residence. This is what happened after German reunification. Russian immigrants of German descent found it easy to get citizenship whereas long-term Turkish and Moroccan immigrants did not.

Religion is of no relevance to the biological concept of race. It is, however, often a vital aspect of ethnicity, providing a strong sense of cultural and social identity, and governing important aspects of lifestyle and even language. Language is similar to religion in being of little importance to biological concepts of race, but is often vital to ethnicity. Table 1.6 shows the association between some characteristics of humans and the concept of race and ethnicity.

Table 1.6 Relationship between some attributes of humans and ethnicity and race

Relating mainly to biological concept of race	Relating mainly to concept of ethnicity	Sometimes related to ethnicity or race
Skin colour	Ancestry	Nationality
Other physical features such as hair texture and facial features	Language	Citizenship
Ancestral origin	Religion	Name
	Diet	Migration history
	Family origin	Country of birth
	Sense of group identity	Country of birth of parents or grandparents

1.8 **Analyse your own background and identity using the concepts of race and ethnicity**

A good way for readers to reflect on ethnicity and race, particularly to contrast them and the related concepts discussed in Section 1.7, is to mull over the self-descriptions of ethnicity first given by the author and close colleagues in the step-by-step guide by Mackintosh et al. (1998), and do this for themselves. Labelling of racial or ethnic groups can sometimes utilize terms relating to religion and language, not least because there is a link between territory or origin, ancestry, race, ethnicity, religion, and language. The following text extracts are adapted from Mackintosh et al. (2008) *Step-by-step Guide to Epidemiological Health Needs Assessment for Ethnic Minority Groups* with permission of the authors.

1.8.1 **Raj Bhopal on ethnicity**

I am of Indian birth (Moga, Punjab), raised in Scotland (Glasgow), and enjoy the benefits of two cultures. I think others see me as an Indian, Pakistani, or an Asian. I am a member of the Sikh religion by birth and practice. My first language is Punjabi, in the sense that this was the language I learned first, but I am much more fluent in English. In England I perceive myself as a British Indian, in Scotland as a Scottish Indian, at my parental home as a Punjabi Sikh, and when in India as a Punjabi. My behaviour, such as food eating and alcohol consumption, is context-dependent. My religion strongly forbids tobacco consumption. I may wear a turban or traditional Indian dress on symbolic occasions such as weddings. The census classification of Indian does not do justice to my complex self-image, but when forced to choose I am happy to pick the ethnic group category Indian (in the Scottish census, Scottish Indian is available).

1.8.2 **Raj Bhopal on race**

I do not know what race people think I belong to. They probably think I am Indian, although that is not a racial category. I am Indian born, to Indian parents. I have brown skin and black eyes and hair (sadly greying fast!). If forced to fit into the long-established racial catego-ries (see Chapter 2) I'd choose Caucasian (but not White) which I know will cause surprise because that word has been so closely linked to European or White but it was designed for a much bigger group including North Africans and North Indians. On the whole I believe I do not fit easily into a racial category. For sure, my race is *not* Asian. Others may see me as Asian. If I lived in the United States I would be classified as a member of the Asian race. That seems very odd.

1.8.3 **Joan Mackintosh on race and ethnicity**

I am British-born and I am classified by the census definition as 'White'. I am of Scottish ancestry (as far back as I know and before that almost certainly a mix of various others, e.g. Celt, Norman and who knows what else) and consider myself to be British, though when in Scotland I am seen as English and when in England I am seen as being from the north-east. My first language is English. I was brought up to respect the traditions of the Christian church both at home and at school. I was baptized in a Methodist chapel and was married in a Presbyterian church. I do not consider myself particularly religious. I attend church on ceremonial occasions and my children are members of church youth groups. If asked to describe myself, I would say 'British' and if asked to define my religion from within certain recognized groups, will either tick the box 'Christian' or if further definition is required 'Church of England' because it is easier than describing 'other'. I am certainly aware that a person's social class has an enormous bearing on the type of health care they will receive—particularly in terms of patient–practitioner interaction—which is why I believe that class and ethnicity are inextricably linked. Prior to starting this work I had never really given much consideration to the issue of ethnicity and self-defined ethnicity in particular (which probably speaks volumes). I found this quite a difficult exercise to undertake.

1.8.4 **Nigel Unwin on race and ethnicity**

This is very difficult. My ethnicity depends very much on the context. Within a British context I am north of England, lower middle to middle class background, brought up within the traditions of the Church of England (although I wouldn't describe myself as a Christian). You'll notice from the above that I think at least for me, and probably for many people, class and 'ethnicity' are inseparable in some contexts.

Within a broader context, such as Europe or elsewhere in the world, I like to see myself as 'British'. This is a pretty vague notion, but for me hints at the diversity of cultures (over many centuries up to the present) in Britain and the creative public face of Britain, linked together with threads of common underlying values such as a tolerance, or at best a celebration, of diversity alongside an instinct for social justice. I don't like describing myself as 'English' because to me this smacks of the opposite of what I've described as 'British': of establishment, stuffiness, conservatism, and colonial history and I don't see my background as being from that. However, I know that in certain contexts, particularly in North America or in some parts of Ireland, being labelled as 'English' is something I can't escape. Accent and body language, if nothing else, all attract this label and the connotations that go with it.

In some contexts I think of myself as 'north European'. This is also a very vague notion, but like the sense of 'British' is based on a sense of common threads of culture and values in north European societies.

I haven't really seen myself in terms of race. Interestingly this is one of the criticisms sometimes levelled at White people—that they see themselves as 'raceless', race being an attribute of others (non-White people). If pushed I would say I'm of European ancestry (but probably for all I know a mixture of Celtic, Anglo-Saxon, Roman, Norman, and maybe other 'tribes' or 'peoples') and clearly within the context of a racist society, where people are pre-judged on the basis of skin colour and appearance, I am 'White'. Certainly when travelling in Africa or the Caribbean I'm aware of often being seen as being of a different race, i.e. 'White' or 'European' and I'm often referred to in those terms.

1.8.5 **Naseer Ahmad on race and ethnicity**

I do not see myself as British, or Pakistani, as I am not fully accepted by both. I'm too different to be Pakistani and too different to be British, i.e. I don't speak the language and don't look the part, in both cultures.

A long time of growing up being called 'Paki' and 'coconut' and being beaten up for being Muslim, all left scars. The 'culture clash' which many people my age are facing leads some to go to extremes, i.e. deny their origin and see themselves as white through and through, or the other extreme where they love their origin and hate Britain. I do not ascribe to either of these views as extremism is not in my nature.

I describe myself as Muslim. That's it. I go further and describe myself as a Muslim living in Britain as opposed to a 'British Muslim', as I am not sure what British Muslim means and after speaking to those who describe themselves as British Muslim I know that they also do not know what British Muslim means. The reason for this is that the idea of artificial borders separating people, i.e. those created by humans, and then labelling those different based on these borders is just wrong, and dangerous. Rwanda and Bosnia show the dangers of labelling. It can be argued that separating based on religion, i.e. Muslim–Kafir, Jew–Gentile, etc., are the same thing, but in the end I feel there is a deep-rooted need for a man (and woman) to belong to something, and belonging to a thing that traverses colour, country, and background and categorizing based on the actual person, i.e. their thoughts, feelings, is somehow more just and more right, especially when it is emphasized that the 'others' have rights which must be respected, e.g. the right to justice and to practise their religion.

However, if I had to choose, and have to be pushed to do this, I am a 'Pakistani' as this is my origin, but it has to be realized that I do not see myself as Pakistani. I am British by passport and if anything Britain is my home (I don't feel that any other country is my home, even the 'Muslim' countries, as my family is in Britain) but I do not see myself as British, especially not English (for the same reasons that Nigel Unwin describes); however, British has the same connotation for me, i.e. British colonial rule etc.

The only label I feel comfortable with is Muslim. This is after a long, long time of being uncomfortable with myself. But, if I had to describe myself as anything, in Britain I am a Pakistani, and in Pakistan I am British. For statistics purposes, I am Pakistani, but it must be realized that I am uncomfortable with being described as British or Pakistani as I am neither!

1.8.6 Complexity of race and ethnicity as shown in the vignettes and an invitation to readers

Ethnicity and race are such complex ideas, as the vignettes above show, that they ought to raise questions about the reliability of making assumptions that a person may (or may not) possess a particular behaviour or health characteristic on the grounds that they are a member of a particular ethnic or racial group. The limited usefulness of recording a patient's ethnic (or racial) origin, using a simple label such as Indian, White, or Chinese, without taking account of other factors, has to be fully acknowledged. The vignettes show the importance of religion. Religions straddle ethnic and racial groups. Like Muslims (see Section 1.8.5), the Jewish people originate from many countries and cultures and have a range of religious practices but may identify themselves as Jewish. Thus, on a census which had a category Jewish, some would choose it over Black, Indian, White, etc. In addition to the complexity which is shown in the vignettes, within every ethnic group there are significant variations in social class, culture, and customs.

Now, reader, it is your turn to describe your race, ethnicity, and the related characteristics shown in Exercise 1.9.

Exercise 1.9 Self-analysis

Analyse your own perceived (1) racial and (2) ethnic group

- How would your close associates, and perhaps new acquaintances, see your race and ethnicity? Would their own race or ethnicity influence their perceptions?
- How do your race and ethnicity, in your mind, link to your nationality, and your and your parents' country of birth and religion?

1.9 **Realizing potential benefits of migration status, race, and ethnicity in the health context**

Studying migrant status, ethnic, and racial variations in health can, at least potentially, help us to understand the causes of disease, tackle inequalities, assess needs, make better health plans, and direct resource allocation. The use of country of birth, ethnic group, and race as variables in the health literature is increasing in recognition of this potential. The focus of this work tends to be on those populations with comparatively adverse health outcomes. Clearly, it is not only non-White ethnic groups which are in this position, so the White population may also benefit.

To improve health policy-making and health planning, give new insights into the causation of disease, and help the clinician in the differential diagnosis of disease we need to ensure that, as a minimum:

- Researchers, policy-makers and professionals in the field of race, ethnicity, and health should understand the ignoble history of race science, and be aware of the perils of its return.

- Ethnicity is perceived as different from race and is not merely used as a synonym for the latter.

- The complex and fluid nature of ethnicity is widely understood.

- The limitations of all current means for classifying migrant status, race, and ethnicity be acknowledged, and the approach to categorization be made explicit. Definitions of key concepts and terms may need to be devised to suit the needs of the particular project.

- As ethnicity and migration are fluid, dynamic phenomena and research findings may rapidly become out of date, results should be generalized across time periods, generations, and populations with different migration histories only with great caution.

- Investigators recognize the potential influence of their values, including ethnocentricity, on scientific research and policy-making.

- The importance of socio-economic differences in explaining health differences between migrant, racial, and ethnic groups is considered at the same time and with at least equal weight as cultural or genetic factors.

- Research on methods for classification of migrant, racial, and ethnic groups is given higher priority.

- Data from studies of migrant group, race, ethnicity, and health should, as a high priority, be analysed and applied to produce information of value in health-care policy and service development.

- Demonstrations of interesting disease variations should be followed by detailed examination of the relationship between environment, lifestyle, culture, and genes to assess the relative importance of these influences.

- In the absence of consensus on the nature of ethnicity and race, researchers need to state their understanding, describe the characteristics of both the study and comparison populations, and provide and justify the racial or ethnic coding.

- Editors must play a greater role in developing, with researchers, and then implementing a policy on the conduct and reporting of migration status, race, ethnicity, and health research.

- There should be wide recognition that migrant status, race, and ethnicity data, as for social class, have a key role in raising awareness of inequalities and stimulating policy and action.

Throughout this book we will be returning to these and other guidelines.

1.10 **Conclusions**

Humans are mentally equipped to differentiate between individuals and groups. Migrant status, race, and ethnicity are only three of many ways that humans differentiate and group themselves, and these have deep and lasting effects. They are of particular importance in multicultural societies, and especially to migrants in such places. Scientific disciplines have studied these concepts and attempted to utilize them to advance scientific understanding and help in the applications of science. The sheer complexity of the concepts has made this task difficult, and the misapplication of race and ethnicity has often done more harm than good. Nonetheless, migration status, race, and ethnicity are excellent means of differentiating the health and health-care status of subpopulations, and this property alone has given them central status in quantitative health sciences, and indirectly in public health and clinical care. The challenge now facing us is to ensure that the benefits of working with these variables far exceed the harms, and that our experience does not end in the same ignominious fate that met 19th-century research.

Purpose and context are the prime determinants of the way that the concepts of race and ethnicity are applied, classifications are devised and employed, and data are analysed and presented. Ethnic and racial labels and country of birth, as in national censuses, are no more than a first step to defining a person's ethnicity, and the remaining steps depend upon the purposes of data collection. Whatever the purpose, understanding the terminology we are using, and its origins, is vital to collecting the data. (This is the subject of Chapter 2. Some readers might find the historical and international background to the subject given in Chapter 4 useful preparation for reading Chapter 2.)

> In describing racial/ethnic groups, authors should use terminology that is not stigmatizing, does not reflect unscientific classification systems, and does not imply that race/ethnicity is an inherent, immutable attribute of an individual.
>
> Kaplan and Bennett (2003, p. 2713)

1.11 **Summary**

Humans comprise one species, and their global similarities, both genetic and behavioural, are remarkable. Nonetheless, humans also have, and place considerable emphasis on, their differences both between individuals and between human groups. Race and ethnicity are complex, intertwining, powerful, and lasting concepts that are used by individuals and societies to identify and evaluate social groups and individuals. Increasing international migration has made these concepts of great current importance. Traditionally, race focused around subgrouping humans based upon biological factors such as skin colour, facial shape, and hair type. Your race, based on this concept, is the group you belong to, or are perceived to belong to, in the light of such factors. Racial classifications based on biology have proven to be of modest scientific value and questionable validity, and have been open to social abuse, e.g. the Nazi final solution. This concept of race is changing to incorporate social factors, and a shared history, and hence it is converging with ethnicity. New genetic technologies are leading to a reappraisal of the biological concept of race.

Ethnicity is a concept that, in principle, uses cultural and social factors such as family origins, language, diet, and religion to divide people into subgroups. Your ethnicity, based on this concept, is the group you belong to, or are perceived to belong to, in the light of such factors. Family origin is based in ancestry, and that means in this respect ethnicity is akin to race. Ethnicity is the concept currently in vogue, particularly in Europe, partly due to the abuse of the concept of race in politics in both the 19th and 20th centuries. In practice, race and ethnicity are often used synonymously, with the compound term race/ethnicity becoming more common, especially in the United States. Both concepts are clearly related to, but separate from, nationality (the nation you belong to usually as identified by citizenship and/or passport) and country of birth. Both race and ethnicity are relevant to racism, the product of the view that some racial or ethnic groups are superior to others. Race and ethnicity are especially important components of identity in circumstances where people of different racial and ethnic groups mix, i.e. multi-ethnic, multiracial, multicultural societies, themselves resulting from rapid immigration. Reflecting on both one's own and others' perceptions of one's ethnic and racial group provides a route to understanding the strengths and weaknesses of the concepts.

Race and ethnicity are important in health and health care, particularly in demonstrating inequalities and inequities (called disparities in the United States). The analysis of such inequalities can lead to insights into the forces causing them, and hence point to the actions required to counter them. Such insights can add to scientific knowledge or stimulate new research.

Population health research, statistical analysis, and clinical work, ideally, require easy means of assessing, measuring, and classifying variables, but ethnicity and race are very complex. The related variable, country of birth, is easier but has other limitations.

While race and ethnicity are of value in clinical care, they can also lead to stereotyping, stigma, and racism. The potential value of ethnicity and race, and related variables, in modern multicultural societies will be achieved only if understanding and application of these concepts is advanced such that their advantages exceed their weaknesses. The first step towards this goal is the analysis of the terminology underlying these concepts and the classifications arising from it. This is the topic of Chapter 2.

References

Bhopal RS (2008) *Concepts of Epidemiology*. Oxford: Oxford University Press.

Bhopal R, Rahemtulla T, Sheikh A (2005) Persistent high stroke mortality in Bangladeshi populations. *British Medical Journal* 331: 1096–7.

Blumenbach JF (1865) *The Anthropological Treatises of Johann Friedrich Blumenbach*. London: Anthropological Society.

Clinton WJ (1997) *Remarks by the President in Apology for Study Done in Tuskegee*. Washington, DC: Office of the Press Secretary, The White House.

Cooper R (1984) A note on the biological concept of race and its application in epidemiological research. *Amercian Heart Journal* 108: 715–23.

Down JLH (1867) *Observations on an Ethnic Classification of Idiots*. Reprinted 1995 in: *Mental Retardation* 33: 54–7.

Golby AJ, Gabrieli JDE, Chiao JY, Eberhardt JL (2001) Differential responses in the fusiform region to same-race and other-race faces. *Nature Neuroscience* 4: 845–50.

Huxley JS, Haddon AC (1936) *We Europeans: a survey of 'racial' problems*. New York: Harper.

Jones S (1991) We are all cousins under the skin. *The Independent*, 12 December, p. 14. London.

Kaplan JB, Bennett T (2003) Use of race and ethnicity in biomedical publication. *Journal of the American Medical Association* 289: 2709–16.

Mackintosh J, Bhopal RS, Unwin N, Ahmad N (1998) *Step-by-step Guide to Epidemiological Health Needs Assessment for Ethnic Minority Groups*. Newcastle upon Tyne: Department of Epidemiology and Public Health, University of Newcastle upon Tyne.

Marmot MG, Adelstein AM, Bulusu L (1984) *Immigrant Mortality in England and Wales 1970–78*. London: HMSO.

Montagu A (1997) *Man's Most Dangerous Myth—the fallacy of race*. Lanham, MD: AltaMira Press.

Nagel J (2003) *Race, Ethnicity, and Sexuality: intimate intersections, forbidden frontiers*. New York: Oxford University Press.

Osborne NG and Feit MD (1992) The use of race in medical research. *Journal of the American Medical Association* **267**: 275–9.

Pinker S (2002) *The Blank Slate: the modern denial of human nature*. London: Penguin Press.

Ramaiya KL, Swai ABM, McLarty DG, Bhopal RS, Alberti KGMM (1991) Prevalence of diabetes and cardiovascular risk factors in Hindu Indian sub-communities in Tanzania. *British Medical Journal* **303**: 271–6.

Senior P and Bhopal RS (1994) Ethnicity as a variable in epidemiological research. *British Medical Journal* **309**: 327–9.

Other sources and further reading

Afshari R, Bhopal RS (2002) Changing pattern of use of 'ethnicity' and 'race' in scientific literature. *International Journal of Epidemiology* **31**: 1074–6.

Afshari R, Bhopal RS (2010) Ethnicity has overtaken race in medical science: MEDLINE-based comparison of trends in the USA and the rest of the world, 1965–2005. *International Journal of Epidemiology* **39**: 1682–3.

Bhatnagar D, Anand IS, Durrington PN, Patel DJ, Wander GS, Mackness MI, et al. (1995) Coronary risk factors in people from the Indian subcontinent living in West London and their siblings in India. *The Lancet* **345**: 405–9.

* Bhopal RS (1997a) Ethnicity. In Boyd KM et al. (eds) *The New Dictionary of Medical Ethics*, pp. 89–90. London: BMJ Books.

* Bhopal RS (1997b) Is research into ethnicity and health racist, unsound, or important science? *British Medical Journal* **314**: 1751–6.

* Bhopal RS (2001) Race and ethnicity as epidemiological variables: centrality of purpose and context. In Macbeth H (ed.) *Ethnicity and Health*, pp. 21–40. London: Taylor and Francis.

Bhopal R (2004) Glossary of terms relating to ethnicity and race: for reflection and debate. *Journal of Epidemiology and Community Health* **58**: 441–5.

Bulthoff I (2012) What gives a face its ethnicity. *Journal of Vision* **12**: 1282.

Cooper R, Rotimi C, Ataman S, McGee D, Osotimehin B, Kadiri S, et al. (1997) The prevalence of hypertension in seven populations of West African origin. *American Journal of Public Health* **87**: 160–8.

Ellison GTH, de Wet T, Ijsselmuiden CB, Richter LM (1996) Desegregating health statistics and health research in South Africa. *South African Medical Journal* **86**: 1257–62.

Hardimon MO (2013) Race concepts in medicine. *Journal of Medicine and Philosophy* **38**(1): 6–31.

Hinds DA, Stuve LL, Nilsen GB, Halperin E, Eskin E, Ballinger DG, et al. (2005) Whole-genome patterns of common DNA variation in three human populations. *Science* **18**: 1072–9.

Jackson FL (1992) Race and ethnicity as biological constructs. *Ethnicity and Disease*, **2**: 120–5.

Meier RJ (2012) A critique of race-based and genomic medicine. *Collegium Antropologicum* **36**(1): 5–10.

Morrison T (1993) *Beloved*. London: Chatto and Windus.

Rankin J and Bhopal RS (1999) Current census categories are not a good match for identity. *British Medical Journal* **318**: 1696.

Wild S and McKeigue P (1997) Cross-sectional analysis of mortality by country of birth in England and Wales, 1970–1992. *British Medical Journal* **314**: 705–10.

Winker MA (2004) Measuring race and ethnicity: why and how? *Journal of the American Medical Association* **292**: 1612–14.

Xiao WS, Xiao N, Quinn P, Anzures G, Lee K (2013) Development of face scanning for own- and other-race faces in infancy. *International Journal of Behavioral Development* **37**: 100–5.

Chapter 2

Terminology and classifications for migrant, ethnic, and racial groups: the centrality of census and population registers

Objectives

After reading this chapter you should be able to:

- Understand that the concepts of race and ethnicity, and migration status, are commonly used to create population groups, especially in censuses.
- Understand that the population groups created usually use one or a few aspects of the many that underpin migration, ethnicity, and race.
- Appreciate that the set of population groups created comprises a classification, but the classification is not itself the concept of race or ethnicity.
- See how such classifications permit the use of migration status, race, and ethnicity as epidemiological, public health, and clinical variables.
- Understand the difficulty of agreeing acceptable, precise, and lasting terminology to support such classifications.
- Understand that numerous classifications have been created but none have stood the test of time, and that this is both inevitable and the right result.
- Compare and contrast classifications of migration status, race, and ethnicity with others such as sex, age, social class, and education.
- Appreciate the underlying ideas, strengths, and weaknesses of some current classifications in Europe, North America, South America, and Africa.
- Balance the dangers of creating stigma and further inequity against the potential benefits of operationalizing migration status and the concepts of race and ethnicity through classifications.

2.1 Introduction: turning migration status and the concepts of ethnicity and race into classifications

Concepts are, by definition, complex ideas. Obviously, before they can be used they need to be defined in words that explain, simplify, and clarify the underlying complexities and allow the concept to be communicated easily. In this process the original, or underlying, meaning of the concepts may be altered, albeit in subtle ways. In particular, the interpretation of the concept may vary between time periods, places, disciplines, and individuals. For example, in the modern era many social and most public health scientists interpret race as a social or political concept where populations have been assigned by society (not nature) into racial groups, but most lay people and biomedical scientists see it as a biological concept. In the past, say 150 years ago, the biological basis of race and its use to create a hierarchy would rarely have been questioned, except by the brave, as indicated in the quotation by Ashley Montagu (see his p. 10 for the context of this quotation):

> ...hardly more than a handful of scientific voices were raised against the notion of a hierarchy of races. Anthropology, biology, psychology, medicine, and sociology became instruments for the 'proof' of the inferiority of various races as compared with the white race.
>
> Montagu (1997, p. 80), reproduced with permission of AltaMira Press.

The historical position on race as a biological concept is echoed in most contemporary dictionaries and encyclopaedias, although some change is now under way towards the social concept, though even this has been slowed by the new genetics. In 2012 a political scandal broke over a right-wing anti-Semitic Hungarian politician who underwent laboratory testing to show he had no Roma or Jewish genes and to demonstrate his racial purity. The controversy centres on whether scientific laboratories should lend credence to such ideas. Ironically, shortly afterwards, a leader of the same party discovered his parents were of Jewish origin and defended his anti-Semitic views on the basis that it was behaving like a Hungarian that mattered, not racial purity.

To use the concepts of race and ethnicity, whether in research or practice, we need to create population groupings which comprise a classification. The population groupings are not themselves the concept but are one way of putting them into operation. It is common to read or hear sweeping criticisms of classifications, and by inference the concepts of race and ethnicity. Rather, critics should seek to improve the way in which the concepts are put into operation. Before reading on reflect on Exercise 2.1.

Exercise 2.1 A society without racial, ethnic group, or migrant status classifications

- Imagine this society. In such a society it is likely that the use of the underlying concepts, themselves a consequence of observing differences statistically, would diminish but not disappear

- In such a society, how would we assess the dimension and consequences of factors such as varying physical features, behaviours, economic circumstances and racism?

- If you accept, even reluctantly, that some way of operationalizing the concepts is needed, what kind of terminology and structure would you like your classification to have, assuming you have health improvement in mind?

Given that the kinds of social observations of and responses to differences that underlie our concepts of interest (race and ethnicity) are human universals (see Chapter 1) these are not going to disappear. Equally, the consequences of such observations, could be good (hospitality to strangers) or bad (discrimination against the strange outsider). In a society that has no way to operationalize the concept, the effects will remain unmeasured. Is it better to remain ignorant of these effects or to attempt to inform ourselves about them?

In health and health care we need a terminology that not only describes the individual but also gives access, by association, to helpful information relating to the population from which the individual comes. For example, in medicine an ethnic or racial or migrant status label is only of value if it helps in diagnosis, management, or prediction of the prognosis of the illness under investigation. To describe a patient as White is unlikely to be helpful, but to specify that a person is White of Greek origin who has recently migrated into the country may be relevant, whether in terms of practical matters such as language support, or dietary advice, or assessing the likelihood of the social stresses of migration, or even of genetic haemoglobin disorders. This process of moving from concept to classification is pragmatic, although it should be developed upon both scientific and logical grounds as far as possible, and with a clear understanding of the purposes of the classification. There is a great deal of subjectivity in this process, with difficult choices needing to be made. The classification process will usually use only one or a few of the many facets of such complex matters as migration status, race, and ethnicity. For example, should the classification emphasize ancestry, language, religion, or skin colour? The choice of emphasis will determine the classification that arises. It is obvious that such classifications are socially constructed—but in this regard, race and ethnicity are by no means unique. Indeed, I cannot name any classification of any variable which is not. (It may well be that all classifications are socially constructed.) Even classification as male or female (sex) is nearly always a social construction, and in that regard is reflected in the increasing use of the word gender. To operationalize the variable of sex from a biological perspective would require chromosomal analysis. Even that can be fraught, as is sometimes seen in assessing the sex of athletes.

Each group in the classification needs to have a name (or label) that is, ideally, both meaningful and acceptable, both to those creating and using the classification and to the people who are so classified. In the past, too often those being classified had little say, as their race or ethnicity was assigned by the observer, usually the census enumerator or a professional gathering administrative data. Alternatively, the assessment would be done on other data, e.g. country of origin of both the person and parents. At present self-classification (usually from a choice based on a demonstrably acceptable classification) increasingly holds primacy. Nonetheless, the results of the classifications need to be, on the face of it, both valid and valuable, both to those being categorized and those examining and using the data. Achieving this ideal is extremely difficult. The value of the classification achieved, as opposed to the many alternatives, should be judged by whether it serves the purpose(s). As the purposes may be multiple and changing even this is not a simple matter. Some of these points are developed in Exercise 2.2, which you should do before reading on.

Exercise 2.2 Reflection on the word Asian as used in countries such as the UK and the United States

+ What do you understand by the word Asian as a label for a population group?
+ To which general and scientific purposes might the word Asian be put?
+ How might people described as Asians react?
+ Why might they be either annoyed or content with this label?
+ How might the meaning of this label be differently interpreted in different countries?
+ What are the disadvantages of such labelling in a scientific context such as epidemiology or in public health?
+ What can researchers do to overcome such disadvantages?

2.2 Reflections on the words Asian, Hispanic, Black, and similar labels

The concepts of race and ethnicity, and migration status, are widely used in society for many purposes including politics, everyday and intellectual discourse, education, research, service delivery, and entertainment. Each domain of activity may lead to a variety of labels to describe racial or ethnic subgroups. It is general knowledge that the word Asian means a person from the Asian continent, the largest continent on Earth that extends from Turkey to Siberia. We would expect a schoolchild to know that. It is rare, however, for that word to be used in this way because everyone knows it is too broad to be meaningful. Rather, the word is often used as an ethnic label, with a much more limited meaning and one that depends on geographical and social context. In the UK the label is usually applied to people of Indian subcontinental origins, who mostly came from India and Pakistan, with smaller numbers from Bangladesh and Sri Lanka. (Asian has a very different meaning in North America as we shall see later.) As a Punjabi-born Indian raised in Scotland I found the widespread use in the UK of the label Asian, particularly in the media, to describe people like me to be uninformed, simplistic, and irritating.

The label Asian appeals to the UK media, possibly because it encapsulates a large and heterogeneous population which may fit well with the perceptions of the majority White European community. Some people of Indian, Pakistani, and Bangladeshi origins also find this label quite acceptable, and describe themselves as Asian. This is particularly, but not exclusively, so amongst younger people whose upbringing is in the UK. A successful label must have meaning and value to the population so described, and this may be political, in the sense that it signals unity in an otherwise highly diverse population. Context is clearly important in relation to self-identification. Some ethnic minorities who would not perceive themselves in this way in everyday life might be agreeable to the label 'Black' as a political statement of solidarity but not necessarily reflecting their self-image or identity. Some qualitative research sheds light on the importance of such labels to communities, as indicated in this quotation from Campbell and McLean:

> Yet recent interviews we conducted with people who described themselves as African-Caribbean, Pakistani and White English suggested that beyond the world of academia, the discourse of ordinary people is replete with essentialist descriptions of their own and other ethnic groups. In this paper we examine such stereotypical representations. We will argue that they are very real in their effects—in so far as they play a key role in influencing the likelihood that people will participate in local community networks in the multi-ethnic communities which are increasingly a feature of multicultural Britain.
>
> Campbell and McLean (2002)

In 1984 I did my first research on ethnicity and health. I learned that the label Asian was embedded in the scientific literature too. In the UK, Asian was an ethnic group label restricted by common usage to people whose ancestral origins lay in the Indian subcontinent but who were living in the UK. Clearly, the world of research was reflecting a wider societal decision, almost certainly fostered by the majority population of White European origin. The origins of this term are certainly not scientific. There were warnings in the 1980s about the invalidity of such labels in the scientific setting, including that published in the influential *British Medical Journal* by Shaunak et al. (1986).

By contrast, the term currently preferred by population science researchers for the same large population, South Asian, is rarely used in political and everyday discourse or by the people who are described by this phrase. The word Asian illustrates how societies create racial and ethnic group labels to suit social purposes, and how researchers might utilize them. Which aspects of migration status, race, and ethnicity does this Asian label refer to that might interest researchers? The precise components/facets underlying the label are seldom specified. We can infer, however, that in the UK setting it definitely includes ancestral origin on the Indian subcontinent (relating to being an immigrant or child of immigrants), and probably includes a characteristic brown skin and dark hair of varying hue, a liking for a spicy cuisine, familiarity with one or more South Asian languages, and affiliation with the religions Sikhism, Hinduism, Buddhism, Jainism, or Islam.

The amount of information in the label is surprisingly high, but most is probabilistic not certain. A simple label based on complex concepts of race and ethnicity serves the purpose of allowing self- and other's identification, albeit in a partial, crude, and unscientific way.

Just as in the UK the word Asian is commonly used to describe a circumscribed population, so it is in the United States, where Asian mainly refers to Chinese, Japanese, and other Far Eastern peoples and excludes, at least in practice, those from the Indian subcontinent. The phrase Indian Asian is common in the United States, thus differentiating from American (Native) Indians.

In the UK the phrase Asian and Chinese is heard and seen, which distorts geography, but meets the need for popular ethnic labels. There are obvious problems for doing useful research using such labels. Such research will not be lasting, amenable to future interpretation, or generalizable beyond the location of the study. At the least, the writer needs to define the ethnic group terms.

In my early publications in the late 1980s I took the step of defining my use of Asian, e.g. 'For the purposes of this study, Asian refers to persons whose ancestry is from the Indian subcontinent'. I also tried italicizing the word Asian and putting it in quotations to alert the reader to the limited and specialized use of the word. In retrospect even these steps were insufficient. I followed general conventions used in the UK and, whenever appropriate, the terminology used by the original authors, and provided a statement on my use of terms. In recent work, I have provided an explanatory paragraph usually as an appendix, which some editors demoted to a footnote or merged with methods. A typical paragraph is as follows:

A note on terminology relating to ethnicity (or similar for migrant status or race)

As there is no consensus on the appropriate terms for the scientific study of health by ethnicity, and published guidelines are yet to be internationally adopted, I/we have followed general conventions used in the (name country or other place) and in referring to others' work, whenever appropriate, the terminology used by the original authors. For example, in the UK the term ethnic minority group usually refers to minority populations of non-European origin and characterized by their non-White status. The term South Asian refers to populations originating from the Indian subcontinent, effectively, India, Pakistan, Bangladesh, and Sri Lanka. White is the term currently used to describe people with European ancestral origins. By ethnicity we mean the group a person belongs to as a result of a mix of cultural factors including language, diet, religion, and ancestry. I/we use these terms in this way here.

In this way, writers make it easier for readers to understand what kind of populations they have studied. Unless authors are able to refer readers to an easily accessible glossary of terms—and use such a glossary—they should provide a statement like this one.

Popular terminology used to describe ethnic minority populations (Asians, Blacks, Chinese, etc.) may suffice for everyday conversation or political exchange but is too crude for scientific studies on the frequency and causes of diseases. Scientific studies are there to discover knowledge that is lasting over time and provide valuable information. The continuing use in the UK of the term 'Asian', to mean people from the Indian subcontinent but not Japanese, Mongolians, and Siberians, is unacceptable unless there is widespread, explicit agreement on such usage and when terms are carefully defined. Otherwise the dialogue becomes parochial. Loose terminology encourages inventions such as the description of an ethnic group as 'Urdus', as has been done and published in respectable journals. It also leads to phrases such as 'Asians and Chinese' being used incorrectly, both from a geographical sense and from the point of view of population sciences. Prior to the 2001 Scottish census there was a consultation, and I took the opportunity to point out that the separation in the 1991 census of Chinese from the Asian group and to have Chinese under other ethnic groups was illogical. I recommended that Chinese was included under the broad

Asian category. This was done in Scotland but not in 2001 in England (see Table 2.3). In 2011, however, this change was made. Logic prevailed, albeit slowly. (Amazingly, I recently discovered that this was the recommended approach for the 1981 census question that was developed but never used.)

Similar arguments have been made in relation to other terms including White, Black, Latino, and Hispanic, and no doubt apply to virtually all broad labels (Gimenez 1989). The issues raised go beyond semantics and are key to avoiding serious errors, such as reporting on cardiovascular disease in the United States using a broad Asian racial category. Within this category we have groups such as the Chinese with low rates of disease and Asian Indians (South Asians) with high rates. The data produced are wrong for both such groups separately, and not of value when aggregated.

This chapter is designed to give readers a thorough grounding in principles and past practice, so they can join in the quest for better terminology and classifications.

2.3 Facets of migration status, ethnicity, and race in classifications

It is easy to forget that categories are merely labels, and are no more than a first step to understanding and defining a person's migrant status, ethnicity, or race. Labels such as refugee, foreign-born, White, Asian, Latino, Afro-Caribbean, and Black need to be recognized as crude shorthand for potentially important information about a person. The ideal label would reflect important aspects of migration status, ethnicity, or race. Such labels might be long, e.g. an asylum seeker from Sri Lanka of Tamil origin gaining refugee status and given residence rights in 2003. Such a long label has its own problems, especially if it were to be used to provide summary statistics. It is worth reflecting on why the use of broad labels happens frequently. It may be a lack of insight into the importance of being specific. It may be optimism that the findings might be generalizable from a small population (say Gujeratis or Vietnamese) to a larger one (South Asians or Asians/East Asians). It may, however, also be designed to make the work seem more generalizable and hence important than it is. I have certainly been guilty of all these misdemeanours. In the interests of simplicity (perhaps the key motivator) labels usually reflect one aspect, e.g. colour, the country or region of birth or origin, language, and religion. The need for simplicity should be weighed against the dangers of stereotyping and inaccuracy. Authors should describe the specific populations they are referring to. The label 'South Asian' should not, for instance, be used if the population referred to is Bangladeshi. Bangladeshis are different from the other South Asian populations. For example, Bangladeshi men have an extremely high prevalence of smoking, while most South Asian groups of men (particularly Sikhs, but also Hindus) have a low prevalence, a vitally important fact lost by studies of smoking in 'South Asians' combined, and one that has led to misguided policies on smoking (see Table 3.1).

So, in developing a classification you need to start with a widely agreed definition of the underlying concept and an understanding of the context of the intended uses.

Most classifications put emphasis upon describing recent migrants, and ethnic and racial minority populations, mainly because of the perception that they require special attention. This perception is usually, but not always, correct, as sometimes the health of such minorities is better than that of the majority. A number of descriptions have been given to these groups, e.g. 'ethnic or racial minorities', 'ethnic or racial minority groups', or 'minority ethnic or racial groups'. Sometimes the simple phrase ethnic groups or racial groups is used, wrongly implying that only minority populations have an ethnicity or race. This shorthand is wrong, even though it is motivated by the wish to avoid the word minority which some people see as demeaning. The word minority relates to a numerical minority, nationally, even if not locally. The phrase minority groups is also in use, and is one I have sometimes used in this book as shorthand for migrant, racial, and ethnic minority groups.

The concepts of race and ethnicity are commonly put into operation in national censuses. Migrant status is one of the earliest and most consistently asked question in censuses worldwide. Rather than developing their own classifications, modern-day researchers have mostly used such administrative categories, even when these are acknowledged by those developing them as having no scientific or anthropological validity (as is the case for the US classification discussed below). I do not advocate a return to the 18th- and 19th-century approach when scientists developed apparently scientific classifications. However, population scientists could become more deeply involved in the development of categories for the censuses and other major surveys, and not simply be end-users. Scientists' classifications can be interpreted as an endorsement of their validity even when they do not believe this to be true. As a minimum, therefore, researchers should make clear their views on and understanding of the classification as they use it. These tasks are difficult, and readers should grapple with this matter directly by tackling Exercise 2.3 prior to considering the discussions of census classifications below. You may find the analysis of terms in current ethnicity, race, and health writings that is summarized in Table 2.1 of value in your work, and in the ensuing discussion.

Exercise 2.3 Creating and analysing a classification of migration status, ethnicity, or race

- ◆ What principles would guide you in drafting such classifications to meet the needs of population health research in your region?
- ◆ Develop your own labels that help describe the migration status, race, or ethnicity of population groups where you work.
- ◆ Compare your classification with those in the tables, and with that actually used in your country (you may need to find it).
- ◆ In what respect are these classifications, including your own, based upon migration status, race, and ethnicity?
- ◆ What do you perceive to be the strengths and weaknesses of these classifications?

2.4 **From concept, to category, to classification**

While concepts develop over time they have an inherent stability, so change is through refinements. Concepts are quite robust in the face of criticism, e.g. of race. Classifications, however, evolve over time and at a different pace in different places, reflecting the social and political circumstances, the pragmatic nature of the processes of their development, and the varying purposes for which they were designed. So in developing a classification you need to start with a widely agreed definition of the concept in your time and place and an understanding of the context where it is to be used, and of the potential uses in the longer term. Many classifications of race and ethnicity, of varying complexity, have been created over the last 200 years or so. In regard to race, only those relating to broad continental groupings e.g. African, European, etc., continue to hold influence internationally, although they have echoes in many current national systems. Both historically and at present, censuses are the most important and influential source of information

Table 2.1 An analysis of some of the terms currently in use in migration, ethnicity and race research

Term	Dictionary-derived meaning	Usual meaning in ethnicity and health research	Relationship to race or ethnicity	Strengths	Weaknesses	Comment and recommendation
Afro-/ African-Caribbean	No specific definition, but Caribbean relates to the territory comprising some West Indian islands	A person of African ancestral origins whose family settled in the Caribbean before emigrating and who self-identifies, or is identified, as African-/ Afro-Caribbean	See African	The label differentiates people of African origins coming from two distinct places, i.e. the continent of Africa and the West Indies	There is very considerable heterogeneity in the populations	Specification in more detail will be required, e.g. the island of origin, and the migration history
African	A person belonging to, or characteristic of a native or inhabitant of, Africa	A person with African ancestral origins who self-identifies, or is identified, as African, but excluding those of other ancestry, e.g. European and South Asian	This population approximates to the racial group known as Negroid or similar terms (see Black)	This term is the currently preferred description for more specific categories, as in, e.g., African American	In practice, northern Africans from Algeria, Morocco and such countries are excluded from this category (see also Black)	Specification in more detail will be required, e.g. the country of origin, and the migration history
Asian	A native of Asia, i.e. anyone originating from the Asian continent	In practice, this term is used in the UK to mean people with ancestry in the Indian subcontinent. In the United States, the term has broader meaning, but is mostly used to denote people of Far Eastern origins, e.g. Chinese, Japanese, and Filipinos	The racial term Malayan, coined by Blumenbach, is forgotten as purposeless, but approximates to this label	It appeals to the general public and the media, possibly because of its capacity to simplify complexity	Asians comprise more than 40% of the world's population, with tremendous cultural and substantial biological diversity	More specific terms should be used whenever possible

Asian Indian	Belonging to or relating to India; native to India	In North America the term is being used synonymously with South Asian with the qualification Asian for differentiating from the original inhabitants of America or the West Indies	The term defines a broad ethnic group. There is no clear-cut equivalent in terms of racial classifications, though historically northern Indians have been classified as Caucasian, and some Indian tribes as aboriginal	This term is being used in North America to distinguish the population from Native Americans, previously known as American Indians	A term currently used synonymously with South Asian (see later entry), but with the important limitation that major South Asian populations such as Pakistani and Bangladeshi may not identify with it	Users need to state which South Asian populations are included and excluded
Bangladeshi	A person whose ancestry lies in the Indian subcontinent who self-identifies, or is identified, as Bangladeshi (see also South Asian)	As per dictionary meaning	Defines an ethnic group relating to a nation. There is no clear-cut equivalent in terms of racial classifications, though historically northern Indians have been classified as Caucasian, and some Indian tribes as aboriginal	Between 1947 and 1971 the country known as Bangladesh was East Pakistan and before that India. The term approximates to territory	The recent political and geographical changes mean that identity with the country may be ill-defined	The term works reasonably well, notwithstanding its recency
Black	A person with African ancestral origins, who self-identifies, or is identified, as Black, African or Afro-Caribbean (see African and Afro-Caribbean)	People whose origins lie in sub-Saharan Africa, e.g. excluding northern Africans, and settlers. In some circumstances the word Black signifies all non-White minority populations, and in this usage serves political purposes	This use relates to race. The word is capitalized to signify its specific use in this way	Large numbers of people described by this label are content with it. It has a long history	The cultural, social, and genetic diversity captured by this term is vast	While this term was widely supported in the late 20th century, there are signs that such support is diminishing as people use more specific identities, e.g. African American

(Continued)

Table 2.1 (Continued)

Term	Dictionary-derived meaning	Usual meaning in ethnicity and health research	Relationship to race or ethnicity	Strengths	Weaknesses	Comment and recommendation
Caucasian	An Indo-European. Blumenbach's term (1800) for the White race of humankind which he derived from the Caucasus	Synonym for White	While often used in the context of ethnicity, it relates to race	Some relation to genetic composition. Defines populations by geographical origin in the distant past	Heterogeneous. Not geographically linked now. Not related to ethnicity	Means originating in the Caucasus region and refers to Indo-Europeans. Widely misunderstood. Widely used as synonym for 'White'. Being abandoned
Chinese	Of or pertaining to China. A native of China	A person with ancestral origins in China, who self-identifies, or is identified as Chinese	Usually used as an indicator of ethnic group. In terms of historical racial classifications, Chinese approximate to the group known as Mongolian or Mongoloid	Widespread appreciation of the grouping referred to	Massive heterogeneity	Combined with a description of the population under study, and possibly a qualification indicating population subgroup, this label seems to work
Ethnic minority group	Based upon the word ethnic, which has a number of meanings including a group of humans having a common national or cultural tradition	Usually, but not always, this phrase is used to refer to a non-White populations. Alternatively, it may be used to describe a specific identifiable group, e.g. Gypsy Travellers, (Roma) and less commonly, Irish in the UK	Although relating to ethnicity, it is often used synonymously with race	Widespread use. Used with surprisingly little misunderstanding and easy to say	Some people consider the phrase inaccurate and prefer minority ethnic group, but the two phrases are used synonymously	Over time, this phrase is likely to be replaced with minority ethnic group

Term	Definition				
European	A native of Europe	It is usually used as a prefix to the term White, e.g. White of European origin	Usually used in the context of ethnicity. Caucasian is a synonym used in the context of race	Signifies geographical origin. Purports to describe a culture (though some would dispute its validity)	Describes heterogeneous populations. Ancestral origin may be difficult to ascertain	Comparable, in breadth, to terms such as Chinese, South Asian. Useful for international studies comparing large areas
Europid	Not defined but denotes origins in Europe	Rarely used, but it is a synonym for European origin	As above	Clear geographical status. New term, no past associations	Describes heterogeneous populations. Ancestral origin may be difficult to ascertain	Unfamiliar term. Comparable, in breadth, to terms such as Chinese, South Asian.
General population	Not defined but the epidemiological meaning is everyone in population being studied	Usually refers to a predominantly White population that is a comparison	Relevant to ethnicity and health studies	Makes no assumptions about racial/ethnic origin. Truly a whole population	Inaccurate unless it is a truly representative population (sometimes ethnic minority populations are removed)	Excellent term for representative population samples
Hindu	A person from northern India; of, pertaining to, or characteristic of the Hindus or the religion; Indian	An old, now seldom used term, for Indians. Rarely used, but in some countries such as Holland the term is used to describe the ethnicity of Surinamese of Indian subcontinent ancestry	Refers to ethnicity	None, other than the fact that some Surinamese people identify with this term (South Asian or Indian Surinames would be more accurate)	The word describes a religion	Avoid unless referring to religion

(Continued)

Table 2.1 (Continued)

Term	Dictionary-derived meaning	Usual meaning in ethnicity and health research	Relationship to race or ethnicity	Strengths	Weaknesses	Comment and recommendation
Hispanic	Pertaining to Spain or its people	A person of Latin American descent (with some degree of Spanish or Portuguese ancestral origins), who self-identifies, or is identified, as Hispanic irrespective of other racial or ethnic considerations	In the United States this term, often used interchangeably with Latino, is considered an indicator of ethnic origin	Widely accepted and used. Links heterogeneous populations	Massive heterogeneity	Needs a rigorous reappraisal, particularly with the intent of adding in detail
Indian	Belonging to or relating to India; native to India, with the prefix Asian in differentiating from the original inhabitants of America or the West Indies	A person whose ancestry lies in the Indian subcontinent who identifies, or is identified, as Indian (see South Asian)	Ethnicity	Widely accepted term that links heterogeneous populations	Major changes to India's geographical boundaries took place in 1947 when Pakistan was created. Massive heterogeneity	Qualify and describe the groups under study, e.g. Indian Gujaratis
Indigenous	Native or belonging naturally to a place. Pertaining to natives, aborigines	Various, but usually referring to the inhabitants prior to colonization or to non-migrants	Unclear	Links internationally to a wide variety of peoples across the world who have become displaced by colonization and migration in their own country	Imprecise. Conflates concepts of place of birth, residence, and ancestry	Some in the non-minority groups are not indigenous; some in the minority groups are. Abandon except when referring to original inhabitants of a place who have become a small minority, e.g. Australian Aborigine

Term					
Irish	The inhabitants of Ireland, or their descendants, especially those of Celtic countries	A person whose ancestry lies in Ireland who self-identifies as Irish but generally restricted to the White population (see, White)	Ethnicity	Meaning is self-evident, although a prefix such as White may be needed	As Ireland becomes a multi-ethnic society, the term will lose its specificity	The term works reasonably well
Other race or ethnic group	Self-evident	Groups not already included within the specific categories offered	Both	This term makes the classification inclusive in that either people excluded, or those who perceive themselves to be excluded, can offer a (usually free text) response	The 'Other' group is usually so heterogeneous that interpretation of statistical data is not possible. Alternatively, data may not be analysed for this group	While it is important to develop classifications that minimize the use of this phrase, it is likely to remain a vital component of any classification
Mixed race or ethnic group	The offspring of a couple from different races or ethnic groups	The term is relatively infrequently discussed, but its meaning is as per the dictionary one	Relevant to both	The increasing acceptance of sexual unions that cross ethnic and racial boundaries requires meaningful data for these groups	The way to categorize mixed race people is unclear. Current approaches are inadequate, partly because the number of potential categories is huge	The increasing importance of the category mixed (ethnicity or race) is self-evident. One solution is to offer space for free-text responses for individuals to identify themselves. These responses, however, need to be coded, analysed, and published
Mulatto	A person of mixed White or Black parents	Mixed race (slightly pejorative)	Race	Acknowledges the important mixed population	There is non-specificity if used generally, and a narrowness if used as in the dictionary way	Although still in use (e.g. in Brazil) it is better to think of specific mixed race or ethnicity

(Continued)

Table 2.1 (Continued)

Term	Dictionary-derived meaning	Usual meaning in ethnicity and health research	Relationship to race or ethnicity	Strengths	Weaknesses	Comment and recommendation
Native	One born in a place. Also, one belonging to a non-European and imperfectly civilized or savage race	Used to define minority groups that originally populated the land, e.g. Native Americans, or to differentiate the long-settled population from recent migrants, e.g. Native Dutch	The term relates to ethnicity and migration status rather than race	Links to land and birthplace, and perhaps most important to minorities such as Native Americans in establishing their rights (see Indigenous)	Historical connotations of being non-European. Conflates concepts of place of birth, residence and ancestry	Similar to, and often used synonymously with, indigenous and has similar value (see Indigenous)
Non-Asian/non-Chinese etc.	Not defined but implies those not belonging to the group named	The meaning is self-evident	The term may fit either race or ethnicity	Logically correct	Extremely broad and imprecise	Avoid if possible
Occidental	A native or inhabitant of the Occident (where the sun sets, the West)	Rarely used, but usually a synonym for White or European	Either race or ethnicity	Geographically based	Heterogeneous	Abandon
Oriental	A term meaning a native or inhabitant of the Orient (East).	Most usually used to indicate Far Eastern populations, e.g. Chinese, Japanese	Either race or ethnicity	Geographically based	Heterogeneous, and unnecessary as better terms are available	It is too general to be useful

Term	Definition					
Pakistani	A person whose ancestry lies in the Indian subcontinent who identifies, or is identified, as Pakistani (see South Asian).	This is usually used as a term of identity even for those born before the creation of Pakistan in 1947, i.e. those born in the Indian land that became Pakistan	It is a term of nationhood and ethnicity, and not race	Some Pakistanis may have birth or ancestral roots in the current territory of India but identify with Pakistan, a country created in 1947	Hitherto, the considerable heterogeneity within the Pakistani population has been largely overlooked, but it should not be	This term is sometimes used as a form of abuse in the UK, usually in the abbreviated form 'Paki'. This said, Pakistani is the correct term for populations who perceive themselves as Pakistani
Reference/control/ comparison	The standard against which a population that is being studied can be compared	In practice, this usually denotes a majority White, European origin population or a general population	Either depending on context	Neutral terms. Recognizes purpose of the non-minority group in the research. Forces writer to describe population and clarify terminology of study or review	The nature of the reference/control population is not-self-evident. Could be misunderstood to mean closer matching than is actually carried out	Prefer these terms
South Asian	A person whose ancestry is in the countries of the Indian subcontinent, including India, Pakistan, Bangladesh, and Sri Lanka	In practice, often used to describe populations from anywhere on the Indian subcontinent, and equally frequently confined to India, Pakistan, and Bangladesh	Refers to ethnicity and nationhood	In terms of racial classifications, most people in this group probably fit best into Caucasian or Caucasoid but this is confusing and is not recommended	This is a good label, particularly when the population is truly from a mix of South Asian regions, when it should be qualified by a clear description	This label is usually assigned, for individuals rarely identify with it. (See also Indian, Indian Asian, Asian, Pakistani, Bangladeshi)

(Continued)

Table 2.1 (Continued)

Term	Dictionary-derived meaning	Usual meaning in ethnicity and health research	Relationship to race or ethnicity	Strengths	Weaknesses	Comment and recommendation
Western	Of or pertaining to the Western or European countries or races, as distinguished from the Eastern or Oriental	Usually it is a synonym for White or European	Refers to geography, ethnicity, and sometimes race	Refers to a culture and places	Not geographically specific. Describes heterogeneous populations	Abandon as a term of popular culture too diffuse for research
White	Applied to those races of humans (chiefly European or of European extraction) characterized by light complexion	The most commonly used term in race, ethnicity, and health research for European origin populations	Ethnicity and race (as a synonym for Caucasian)	Used in census. Socially recognized, widely acceptable and historically lasting concept. Antithesis of the term Black	Heterogeneous populations. Geographical links are historical, i.e. Europe	In practice refers to people of European origin not necessarily of pale complexion. If used in the context of a reference/control population, use that terminology and describe the population

relevant to migration status, ethnicity, and health. The use of censuses in health settings will be discussed in Chapter 3. The primary, historical purposes of censuses include their use by governments for control of immigration and collection of taxes. In some countries, including The Netherlands, the census has been stopped and data come from a population register (linked to other databases). In such countries the classification in population registries becomes of paramount importance.

Table 2.2 provides summary information on the development of selected ethnic labels in censuses in seven different countries on five continents. Try Exercises 2.4, 2.5, and 2.6 before reading on.

Exercise 2.4 Tracing the evolution of the description of African-origin Americans in the United States

♦ Examine the column relating to African origin populations in Table 2.2. Why do you think the terminology varies between countries and changes over time within countries?

♦ Why do you think the basis of data collection changed in 1960 from assessment by the enumerator (the person collecting the data) to self-assessment by the person(s) on whom data are collected?

Exercise 2.5 Facets of ethnic labels

♦ Examine each of the labels in the current census classifications of the UK, the United States, and New Zealand and your own country if different and note the underlying facets of either ethnicity or race that the label is emphasizing. (Do the same for other countries if you want to.)

Exercise 2.6 Sustaining and adapting terminology over time

♦ Look at the classifications in the UK, the United States, New Zealand, and your own country. What future limitations can you predict, knowing about the changing demography and social circumstances of these countries? (Do the same for other countries if you want to.)

♦ What ideas do you have for changing these classifications for the better?

Table 2.2 alone proves that numerous classifications with varying conceptual underpinnings are possible at any point internationally. There are also varying classifications within any country at one time/time-point, although one tends to dominate, usually the one related to the census. Even government surveys might use different classifications and this is almost to be expected in surveys by researchers. Mostly, within a country there are relatively minor variants over time, with an evolutionary process. Nonetheless, sometimes major conceptual shifts occur, and some of these will now be pointed out.

These big shifts usually respond to major social, population, and political changes, especially political power. In the first US census people of African origin were mainly slaves, and they were

Table 2.2 Summary of some census labels for selected populations in seven countries on five continents

Country	Census year	Names for White populations	Names for Black populations	Name for mixed populations	Names for Asian populations	Names for indigenous populations	Other
United States	1850	White	Black	Mulatto	None	None	None
	1900	No options	No options	No options	No options	No options	No options
	2000	White	Black, African American, Negro	None	Japanese, Chinese, Filipino, Korean, Vietnamese, Asian Indian, Guamanian or Chamorro, Samoan	American Indian or Alaskan Native (print tribe), Native Hawaiian, other Asian, other Pacific Islander	Some other race
South Africa	2001	White	Black African	None	Indian or Asian	None	Coloured other (specify)
England	2001	White (British, Irish, any other White background)	Black, Black British, Black Caribbean, Black African	Mixed (White and Black Caribbean) (White and Black African) (White and Asian) (any other mixed background)	Asian or Asian British (Indian) (Pakistani) (Bangladeshi) (any other Asian background), Chinese	None	Any other ethnic group
Canada	1901	White	Black	(Mixed children were to be assigned to the appropriate non-White race)	Yellow	Red	None
	1951	English, Scottish, Ukrainian, Jewish, Norwegian	Negro	(Traced through the father except for mixed Indians living on reserves)		Native Indian, North American Indian	
	2001	White	Black		Chinese, South Asian, Filipino, Latin American, Southeast Asian, Arab, West Asian, Japanese, Korean	None	Other (specify)

New Zealand	1916	European	Negro	Half-caste	Chinese, Hindu, Javanese, Polynesian	Maori	Etc. as the case may be
	1951	European	Negro	Used fractions to denote percentage of racial mix	Syrian, Lebanese, Indian, Chinese	Maori	Etc. as the case may be
	2001	European			Indian, Chinese	Maori, Samoan, Cook Island Maori, Tongan, Niuean	Other (please state)
Ceylon (now Sri Lanka)	1901	Not available					
	1946	English, Scotch, Irish				Low country Sinhalese, Kandyan, Sinhalese, Ceylon, Tamil, Ceylon Moor, Indian Moor, Malay	
Ghana	1901	Whites	Blacks	Mulattos			
	1948	No options					

counted as three-fifths of a person, while Native Americans who did not pay tax were not counted at all. As Table 2.2 shows, there was no label for the indigenous Native American population in 1850 or 1900. This was a political issue, but there were also no labels for Asian or other populations (although there were in 1870). This was most likely a result of small population sizes. Censuses tend to either ignore or lump together small populations, or other populations that people don't want to know about, e.g. mixed populations. Mixed race was only introduced in the United States in 2000 (and 2001 in the UK as mixed ethnic group).

Over time, and particularly from the 1960s onwards, we saw the emergence of the label 'Black' as a political statement and a matter of pride. Currently, African American is the label that is favoured in the United States although Black is fully acceptable. Self-assignment of race or ethnic group also responds to the increasing rights and power of all individuals, but especially minorities, in relation to those in authority, particularly on matters such as identity. The disappearance, or rarity of terms such as Negro, Negroid, and mulatto also reflects these social changes. Census classifications, rightly, respond to such important matters. The racial and ethnic classifications in censuses tend to be designed for, and therefore suitable for, social and planning purposes rather than for scientific ones, and this is usually declared by those developing them. As a general rule, classifications, and the specification of groups to be captured under specific labels, have become more complex over time with recognition of the importance of within- and between-group diversity. We also see the move away from colour labels—white, black, yellow, red in Canada in 1901— to terms relating to country of ancestral origin. The main exception to this is White. (Census question tests in the UK in the 1970s and 1980s showed that adding European–White European caused confusion while White alone worked well.) Categories present at one time may disappear only to return at other times, perhaps somewhat changed and not always for the better, e.g. Chinese was present in the US census of 1870, only to reappear much later as the less specific Asian. These issues are now discussed in relation to three countries on three continents, with extra information on other countries in the Appendix.

2.4.1 The United States of America

The US constitution required a census, and this started in 1790. It collected data on race. In 1850 information on free and slave inhabitants was collected separately. The enumerators, i.e. the persons collecting the information, assigned race based on their own perceptions (White, Black, or mulatto). In 1870 additional groups were added—Chinese and Indian—that were not colour based and foreign parentage was noted. In 1890 the word colour was dropped but the list was extended, with further graduations of racial mixture beyond mulatto (quadroon, offspring of White and mulatto, ; octoroon, one-eighth Black descent, etc.). Language was also assessed. The 1900 census asked of 'colour or race' but categories were removed. Of 28 questions in total, eight attempted to describe aspects of race, ethnicity, and migration status, reflecting the perceived importance of the issue. In 1950 the word race was used and colour dropped, with categories including Negro. Completion of the form by the householder, as opposed to the enumerator, came in 1960. The householder was to report on the race (though this term was not specifically used) of the person using an extended list, including Negro.

The 1970 census saw the return of the words colour and race with a request, for the first time, for the tribe of American Indians, and a question ascertaining whether the person was of Mexican, Puerto Rican, Cuban, Central or South American, or other Spanish origin or descent (or none of these). This was the beginning of a question on Hispanic/Latino ethnicity. From 1977 the federal government sought to standardize data on race and ethnicity among all of its agencies through the Office of Management and Budget's (OMB) Statistical Policy Directive Number 15, *Race and*

Ethnic Standards for Federal Statistics and Administrative Reporting (1997). In these standards, developed with the needs of the education sector (especially) in mind, four broad racial categories were established: American Indian or Alaskan Native, Asian or Pacific Islander, Black, and White. In addition, an 'ethnicity' category was created identifying individuals as of 'Hispanic origin' or 'not of Hispanic origin'.

In 1980 the words 'colour or race' were again left out and the householder was asked to pick a race category on the basis of which one the person being classified 'most closely identifies' with. This was the first explicit link in the United States between race and self-identity. The centrality of ethnicity in its broadest sense was exemplified in this US census.

The 1990 census explicitly used the word race. It encouraged greater specificity in Asian or Pacific Islanders and American Indian but not in the White, or Black/Negro categories. In preparation for the 2000 census, the OMB revised these racial and ethnic categories, introducing new standards. In 2000, the Spanish/Hispanic/Latino question immediately preceded the race question. The race question introduced, for the first time and in the midst of great controversy, the opportunity to pick more than one category, hence indicating mixed race. The word African was introduced in the Black/Negro category. The 2010 census followed the same ideas. In the Hispanic ethnicity question three categories and a write-in section were offered. For race, only one White category was available, the word Negro was one of the options for the single Black and African American category but six categories were available for Asian groups plus a write-in space. For Pacific Islanders, three categories and a write-in group were available. For people not able to identify with these categories a write-in space was available for some other race.

In Chapter 10 I will discuss the criticism that one danger of classifications is to create a sense of reality and permanence where this is not so (reification). In the US census classification, over time, we see substantial change, indicating this kind of criticism is not really justified. Census makers seem sensitive to social context and need as important influences on the classification. The option of ticking more than one race (also provided in New Zealand) is a good illustration of sensitivity to the complexity and fluidity of race and ethnicity classifications.

Readers interested in how the United States' neighbour, Canada, has handled race and ethnicity will find a short account in the Appendix.

2.4.2 **The United Kingdom**

In every census since 1841 a question has been asked about a person's place and/or country of birth, and most censuses in the UK have also included a question about nationality. However, neither are reliable guides to determining a person's ethnic origin. In the 1991 census a question on ethnic origin was asked for the first time, although the authority for this was given in the Census Order of 1920. This authority was not acted upon for a number of reasons, including the view that country of birth was sufficient. Detailed plans to include a question on ethnicity in the 1981 census were cancelled, despite extensive work that developed an acceptable question, because of public opposition. The opposition was almost certainly because race relations were poor in the 1970s, partly because of the influence of the late politician Enoch Powell. Lawrence (1982) has written that (and I paraphrase) according to Powell, 'rivers of blood' will flow not because the immigrants are black; not because British society is racist; but because however tolerant the British might be, they can only digest so much alien-ness. This cannibalistic metaphor fits in well with the assumptions of assimilation. If blacks could be digested then they would disappear into the mainstream of British society.

While the opposition to the 1981 question may have been motivated by concerns about controversies around immigration, the question was needed because non-White ethnic groups were known to suffer discrimination and disadvantage, which could not be quantified without this key variable. The 1991 census question on ethnicity with its emphasis on non-White groups was achieved by arguments emphasizing the need for tackling inequity, inequality, and racial discrimination. These arguments overcame opposition. The ethnic group question of 1991 was developed after lengthy consultations and debate, including with ethnic minority organizations. A broader set of ethnic categories was designed for use in the 2001 census, including a specific 'mixed' ethnic group category, and this was further expanded in 2011.

The 1991, and 2001 censuses are compared in Table 2.3 and Figure 2.1 provides the actual question for the 2011 version.

Table 2.3 A comparison of the 1991 and the 2001 ethnic groupings in the UK census (English version)

1991 census—ethnic group		2001 census—ethnic category	
0	White	White	
1	Black Caribbean	A	British
2	Black African	B	Irish
3	Black Other	C	Any other White background
4	Indian	Mixed	
5	Pakistani	D	White and Black Caribbean
6	Bangladeshi	E	White and Black African
7	Chinese	F	White and Asian
8	Any other ethnic group	G	Any other mixed background
9	Not known/not given	Asian	
		H	Indian
		I	Pakistani
		J	Bangladeshi
		K	Any other Asian background
		Black or Black British	
		M	Caribbean
		N	African
		P	Any other Black background
		Other ethnic groups	
		R	Chinese
		S	Any other ethnic group
		Z	Not stated

Adapted from 1991 Census England, available from http://www.ons.gov.uk/ons/guide-method/census/2011/census-history/the-modern-census/1991-census-questionnaire-for-england.pdf and Count me in Census 2001: England Household Form, available from http://www.ons.gov.uk/ons/guide-method/census/2011/census-history/the-modern-census/2001-census-questionnaire-for-england.pdf. From the Office for National Statistics licensed under the Open Government Licence v.1.0.

16   What is your ethnic group?

Choose **one** section from A to E then tick **one** box
to best describe you ethnic group or background

A   **White**

☐   English/Welsh/Scottish/Northern Irish/British

☐   Irish

☐   Gypsy or Irish Traveller

☐   Any other White background, write in

▢▢▢▢▢▢▢▢▢▢▢▢▢▢▢▢▢▢▢

B   **Mixed/multiple ethnic groups**

☐   White and Black Caribbean

☐   White and Black African

☐   White and Asian

☐   Any other Mixed/multiple ethnic background, write in

▢▢▢▢▢▢▢▢▢▢▢▢▢▢▢▢▢▢▢

C   **Asian/Asian British**

☐   Indian

☐   Pakistani

☐   Bangladeshi

☐   Chinese

☐   Any other Asian background, write in

▢▢▢▢▢▢▢▢▢▢▢▢▢▢▢▢▢▢▢

D   Black/African/Caribbean/Black British

☐   African

☐   Caribbean

☐   Any other Black/African/Caribbean background, write in

▢▢▢▢▢▢▢▢▢▢▢▢▢▢▢▢▢▢▢

E   **Other ethnic group**

☐   Arab

☐   Any other ethnic group, write in

▢▢▢▢▢▢▢▢▢▢▢▢▢▢▢▢▢▢▢

Fig. 2.1 The 2011 census question on 'ethnic group in England'.

Reproduced from 2011 Census questionnaire, available from http://www.ons.gov.uk/ons/guide-method/
census/2011/census-data/2011-census-prospectus/new-developments-for-2011-census-results/key-changes-to-the-
2011-census-outputs-policy/differences-between-2001-and-2011-questionnaires/QEngland.pdf Source: Office for
National Statistics licensed under the Open Government Licence v.1.0.

The UK's census question on ethnic group is a pragmatic one which has proven acceptable despite
conceptual limitations. For example, the classification uses race and colour concepts (white/black)
together with national origins that are reflective of ethnic identity (Chinese, Indian, Pakistani, etc.).
In 1991 the White group combined people with distinct cultural, geographical, and religious heritage, e.g. those of Irish, Greek, or Turkish origin. The 2001 question was, with the exception of

including mixed groups and slight disaggregation of the White group, a variant of the 1991 question. The ethnic question in the 1991 census did not meet the requirements of users, who argued that extra information was needed such as languages spoken and religion, to properly describe the ethnicity of the groups. They also emphasized the need for an opportunity for people to describe mixed ethnic origins. In 2001, a question on religion was included, and although it was not legally required most people answered it. Language was included in the 2011 census. The 2011 census asked about country of birth, date of arrival in the UK, intentions to stay, national identity, main language, competence in spoken English, religion, passports held, and ethnicity. There are only 31 questions—the importance of issues related to the topic of this book to the nation as reflected in the census is apparent. The main change from 2001 is the addition of extra categories (Gypsy or Irish Traveller and Arab). Notably, in every major category there is a write-in line recognizing that respondents need flexibility in answering this question. Each of the four component countries of the UK made small variations in the nature of this question. The UK's is a story of lengthy deliberation and debate, followed by successful implementation that provided the experience for both evolution (mixed groups and much detail within categories) and new developments (religion and language).

2.4.3 New Zealand

The 1906 census stated that a separate Maori census would be done. There was no other information on ethnicity, but country of birth and religion were recorded. From 1916 race and/or ethnicity have been recorded and have been prominent components of the census. In 1916 there was a European race, examples of others and reference to admixture (half-caste). In 1926 there was a Maori census, with the Maori language written in English script that also took note of admixture. There was little change until 1976 when ethnic origin replaced race (or in some forms there was either no term or descent). In 1981 we saw the first more structured, tick box, form of question, placing much emphasis on mixed ethnic origin, with graduations of up to one-eighth, e.g. seven-eighths European. The 1986 census saw the progression of this approach to a range of questions, but the questions on mixture were left out, although more than one ethnic group could be chosen. In 1991 there was a special emphasis on Maori ancestry and tribe. The 2001 questionnaire was in bilingual format—English and Maori. Maori background was specified as ancestry. The 2006 census asked about country of birth, arrival in New Zealand if born abroad, language proficiency, ethnic group, and Maori descent and tribe separately. Again, multiple choices of ethnic group were permitted. The category New Zealand European has created controversy (as did White European in the UK when it was tested, leading to the dropping of European). In preparation for the 2011 census (postponed until 2013), there is considerable controversy about the continuing use of words such as European, with a clamour for a New Zealand identity.

2.5 Census categories are not necessarily a good match for identity

The questions in censuses and other surveys now usually allow respondents to choose their racial and/or ethnic identity from a menu, but does the menu offer a good choice? There is a case for far more subtlety and more use of open responses:

> Given the important implications for determining the ethnic origin of the increasing numbers of people who choose not to fit into one of the standard predefined categories, write in answers should be reintroduced while there is still time for local implementation to do so.

Aspinall (1995, pp. 1006–9)

What sort of terms might people use? Open questions are being seriously explored, given the development of computer software able to handle the responses. Data from a cross-sectional survey in the UK (the South Tyneside Heart Study) compared respondents' identification of their ethnicity using the census question, a description in an open question, country of birth, and country of family origin. Respondents ($n = 334$) first chose one of the categories from the 1991 UK census question, then provided a description of their ethnicity. Respondents were also asked where they and their mother and father were born. The most striking observation was the rarity of the term 'Asian' and the absence of the term 'South Asian', both of which are commonly used in the UK to describe people originating from the Indian subcontinent. These labels do not capture ethnic self-identity in this context. From the ethnic group categories in the census, 130 (39%) of respondents chose Indian. Only 81 (62%) of those who were Indian on the census question described themselves as Indian when given the open choice. Only 52/93 (56%) of respondents born in India described themselves as Indian. Using census categories for ethnic groups is insufficient to capture self-identification fully. Some sample results for Indians, Pakistanis, and Bangladeshis are shown in Table 2.4.

Table 2.4 Respondents' descriptions of their ethnic origin by 1991 English census category

Self-description	Ethnicity according to the 1991 census categories†		
	Indian, no. (%)	Pakistani, no. (%)	Bangladeshi, no. (%)
Indian	81 (62)	2 (5)	—
British/English/Anglo Indian	12 (9)	—	—
Indian Christian	1 (1)	—	—
Kashmiri Indian	1 (1)	—	—
Born in India but lived in Pakistan	1 (1)	—	—
Pakistani	—	29 (67)	1 (1)
Sikh	12 (9)	—	—
British Sikh	2 (2)	—	—
Indian Sikh	2 (2)	—	—
Bangladeshi	—	1 (2)	118 (94)
Bengali	—	—	5 (4)
British Bengali	—	—	—
Muslim	1 (1)	2 (5)	1 (1)
Kashmiri Muslim	2 (2)	—	—
British Muslim	—	1 (2)	—
British	6 (5)	5 (12)	1 (1)
British/English Asian	4 (3)	3 (7)	—
Asian	4 (3)	—	—
Black or Asian	1 (1)	—	—
Total	130	43	126

†Fifteen missing values.

The categories offered in the UK census are too few to reflect the true heterogeneity of ethnic groups. Similar issues certainly also apply to other labels, e.g. 'Black', 'White', Chinese, etc.

The obvious problem with these descriptions is their variety. How would we handle them in producing statistics? Firstly, without aggregation, numbers in many categories would become trivially small and hence not analysable, e.g. Sikhs, British Sikhs and Indian Sikhs are very likely to be similar. We may end up grouping people, thereby creating similar categories to those in the census. Region of origin within a country, religion, and Britishness are clearly important to the self-identity of these respondents. I am sure this area of inquiry will be advancing rapidly in the next 10 years.

2.6 **Towards a common international terminology**

Table 2.1 provides a commentary on some terms in the Glossary that serve as an example of what we might need to do to create an internationally workable terminology. This would need development in terms of improving geographical specificity, expansion to capture truly international scope, and greater precision. The terms and definitions in Table 2.2 are based on an amalgam of the concepts of both race and ethnicity. The terminology also needs to encapsulate the needs of migration studies. This Glossary is used in this book in full understanding that it is a work that will forever be in progress. Clearly, using the principles evident in the Glossary and Table 2.1, e.g. giving primacy to self-identity while acknowledging others' perceptions, the role of ancestry, and the link to countries, regions, and continents of origin, additional terms can be added. However, it is a controversial matter as to whether a deeper and longer glossary with truly international applications is either required or feasible. The task is enormously difficult but, in my view, if the subject of migration status, ethnicity, and race studies is to mature and become internationally valid it needs to be tackled. In the first edition of this book I wrote that in the field of health there is a case for leadership from a partnership including the WHO, the International Epidemiological Association, and an organization such as the World Association of Medical Editors. Research-funding organizations including the National Institutes of Health (United States), the Medical Research Council (UK), and equivalent organizations internationally also have a major role, working with national health-care agencies. Unfortunately, we see little sign of systematic progress even though the World Health Assembly and WHO have brought the topic to prominence. However, cross-national work has increased, bringing these issues to wider attention.

2.7 **Conclusions**

Some 200 years of effort in creating racial and ethnic classifications has led to numerous insights, particularly that the process is, perhaps inevitably, somewhat arbitrary, subjective, context-specific, purpose-driven, and imprecise. The process is atheoretical in that there is no coherent, valid genetic or social theory that underpins classifications. The view that the prime value of such classifications is in social, rather than biological, contexts and in service applications is clearly correct. It is surprising, therefore, that these imperfect classifications provide such powerful tools for analysis of difference and similarity that have so much importance in population health disciplines.

As societies are becoming more racially and ethnically diverse such classifications—despite their limitations—are in increasing demand and use. The challenge is to create a suite of classifications that meet the purpose better and that have greater theoretical underpinnings than hitherto (see Chapter 10). Editors and writers are jointly responsible for ensuring scientific rigour and high-quality writing, yet few journals or books have appropriate policies that are implemented vigorously. The *British Medical Journal* (1996) was one of the first journals to make progress on this. Their guidelines are given in Box 2.1.

Box 2.1 Ethnicity, race, and culture: guidelines for research, audit, and publication

Authors should describe in their methods section the logic behind their 'ethnic' groupings. Terms used should be as descriptive as possible and reflect how the groups were demarcated. For example, 'black' as a group description is less accurate than 'self-assigned as black Caribbean (Office of Population Censuses and Surveys [OPCS] category)' and 'Asian' less accurate than 'UK born individuals of Indian ancestry' or 'French born individuals of Vietnamese ancestry'.

If it is unknown which of ethnicity, race, or culture is the most important influence then an attempt should be made to measure all of them.

A range of information is best collected:

+ Genetic differences (using relevant genetically determined polymorphism)
+ Self-assigned ethnicity (using nationally agreed guidelines enabling comparability with census data)
+ Observer assigned ethnicity (using nationally agreed guidelines enabling comparability with census data)
+ Observer assigned ethnicity (using OPCS or other national census categorization or the researchers' own logically argued categories)
+ Country or area of birth (the subject's own, or parents' and grandparents' if applicable)
+ Years in country of residence
+ Religion

Reproduced from McKenzie K, Crowcroft NS, Describing race, ethnicity, and culture in medical research, *British Medical Journal*, Volume 312, Number 7038, p.1054, Copyright © 1996, with permission from BMJ Publishing Group Ltd.

Research by Ellison and Rosato (2002) has shown that these guidelines have not been followed by authors. Similar efforts by the *Journal of the American Medical Association* have been partially successful in authors' reports of the ethnic labels, although they seldom explain the theoretical underpinnings of the use of the concepts of race and ethnicity. Several systematic examinations of the way ethnicity and race (and related variables such as country of birth) are handled in important journals show that much more rigour is still needed.

Accurate use of concepts and words is an essential first step to good research, and ultimately improving the health of ethnic minorities and narrowing inequities. Helping to achieve conceptual and terminological accuracy remains a major and challenging goal for authors and editors alike. The search for accurate terminology will remain controversial, however, for both scientific and social reasons, not least because of the tension between the differing needs of science, services, and the public. There are other debatable issues, e.g. whether international understanding and agreement on these concepts and terms is achievable, if the comparative health of population subgroups within the populations is best defined by current categories or needs new ones, empirical demonstration that the benefits of reporting data by ethnicity and race exceed the costs, and in particular that they help improve the health status of the study populations. These are subjects amenable to research but have not been given the required priority.

Accurate terminology in minority health research requires a consideration of concepts and terms beyond those referring to race and ethnicity. For example, in comparative work terms such as reference, control, or comparison population have advantages compared with those such as White or European. They raise fewer expectations and prior assumptions and require the writer to provide detail on the populations studied, including their heterogeneity and origins.

International collaboration for exchange of ideas and expertise, as well as technical information on definitions, is a necessary part of this endeavour. We will be returning to these issues, particularly in Chapter 9. In Chapter 3 I shall consider the practical challenges of data collection by migration status, race, or ethnic group. Some readers might prefer to read Chapter 4 first, which gives some historical and international background.

2.8 **Summary**

Concepts need to be defined and in this process we aim to simplify and clarify them for widespread agreement. In simplification, and especially in implementation, the original meaning and intent of the concepts may be unwittingly altered. To use migration status and the concepts of race and ethnicity as variables in population health we create population groupings. This process is pragmatic and, in the absence of firm theoretical underpinnings, it is subjective and malleable and designed to meet perceived needs in particular populations, places, and times. The grouping process will utilize only one or a few of the many facets of complex concepts. The choice of which facets to emphasize will determine the grouping. The groups arising, collectively, comprise a classification. Each group needs to have a label. The label should be both meaningful and acceptable, both to those creating and using the classification and to those who are so classified. At present most classifications are designed for self-report of race or ethnicity, whereas in the past this was assigned by an observer.

The value of the classification achieved, as opposed to the many alternatives, should be judged by whether it serves the stated purpose. In quantitative health sciences the purpose is to establish and explain differences in the health status of populations; in public health it is to improve health through prevention and control of disease; and in clinical medicine it is to make diagnosis and treatment easier.

Classifications vary across times and places, reflecting both the pragmatic nature of the process of creation and the varying purpose for which they were designed. Many complex classifications of race have been proposed. Only those relating to broad continental groupings continue to hold influence. At any one place and time, though numerous classifications are possible, one tends to dominate, with minor variants. Usually, this is the classification used in the census or equivalent population registries.

Current racial and ethnic classifications, mostly based on the census questions, tend to be more suitable for social and planning purposes than for scientific ones. One of the biggest obstacles to scientific work is the heterogeneity within the populations described by current categories.

The terminology supporting both concepts and classifications is problematic, and despite the difficulties of the task, progress towards an internationally agreed vocabulary is a prerequisite for progress. These challenges of classification, terminology, and agreement on concepts are similar to those for other complex variables such as social class and educational status—migration status, race, and ethnicity are not uniquely problematic. Despite their difficulties, most classifications do work in the sense that they add to our capacity for analysis of similarities and differences in the health of populations and to take actions to improve health.

References

Aspinall PJ (1995) Department of Health's requirement for mandatory collection of data on ethnic group of inpatients. *British Medical Journal* **311**: 1006–9.

British Medical Journal (1996) Ethnicity, race and culture: guidelines for research, audit and publication. *British Medical Journal* **312**: 1094.

CampbellC, McLean C (2002) Representations of ethnicity in people's accounts of local community participation in a multi-ethnic community in England. *Journal of Community and Applied Social Psychology* **12**: 13–29.

Ellison GTH, Rosato M (2002) The impact of editorial guidelines on the classification of race/ethnicity in the *British Medical Journal*. *Journal of Epidemiology and Community Health* **56**: 45A.

Gimenez ME (1989) Latino/Hispanic—who needs a name? The case against a standardized terminology. *International Journal of Health Services* **19**: 557–71.

Lawrence E (1982) Just plain commonsense: the 'ropes' of racism. In *The Empire Strikes Back: race and racism in 70s Britain*. London: Hutchinson and Co. Ltd.

Montagu A (1998) *Man's Most Dangerous Myth—the fallacy of race*. Lanham, MD: AltaMira Press.

Office of Management and Budget (1997) *Revisions to the Standards for the Classification of Federal Data on Race and Ethnicity*. Washington, DC: OMB.

Shaunak S, Lakhani SR, Abraham R, Maxwell JD (1986) Differences among Asian patients [Letter]. *British Medical Journal* **293**: 1169.

Other sources and further reading

Agyemang C, Bhopal RS, Bruijnzeels M (2005) Negro, Black, Black African, African Caribbean, African American or what? Labelling African origin populations in the health arena in the 21st century. *Journal of Epidemiology and Community Health* **59**: 1014–18.

Aspinall PJ (2002) Collective terminology to describe the minority ethnic population: the persistence of confusion and ambiguity in usage. *Sociology* **36**: 803–16.

Bhopal RS and Donaldson LJ (1998) White, European, Western, Caucasian or what? Inappropriate labelling in research on race, ethnicity and health. *American Journal of Public Health* **88**: 1303–7.

Bhopal RS, Phillimore P, Kohli HS (1991) Inappropriate use of the term 'Asian': an obstacle to ethnicity and health research. *Journal of Public Health Medicine* **13**: 44–6.

Freedman BJ (1994) Caucasian. *British Medical Journal* **288**: 696–8.

McKenzie K and Crowcroft NS (1996) Describing race, ethnicity and culture in medical research. *British Medical Journal* **312**: 1054.

Rankin J and Bhopal RS (1996) Current census categories are not a good match for identity. *British Medical Journal* **318**: 1696.

Sangowawa O and Bhopal, R (2000) Can we implement ethnic monitoring in primary health care and use the data? A feasibility study and staff attitudes in north east England. *Public Health Medicine* **2**: 106–8.

Schwartz RS (2001) Racial profiling in medical research. *New England Journal of Medicine* **344**: 1392–3.

Stillitoe K (1978) Ethnic origin: the search for a question. *Population Trends* **13**: 25–30.

Williams HC (2002) Have you ever seen an Asian/Pacific Islander? *Archives of Dermatology* **138**: 673–4.

Chapter 3

Challenges of collecting and interpreting data using the concepts of migration, ethnicity, and race

Objectives

After reading this chapter you should be able to:

- Understand why migration status and the concepts of ethnicity or race that are underlying your data collecting system are crucial to the method of data collection and data interpretation.
- Accept that useful data collection by migration status, ethnicity, or race requires that individuals provide, and data systems record, the relevant data items.
- Understand that the interpretation of data rests upon the validity of the data.
- Be able to apply a framework of analysis to list the most important explanations for differences in health status by migration status, ethnicity, and race.
- Be able to offer appropriate policy, health planning, or clinical care responses to observations on the patterns of health by migration status, or racial or ethnic group.

3.1 Introduction

It is not absolutely self-evident or agreed that data by migration status, ethnicity, or race are necessary or helpful. Nonetheless, the quantity of data is increasingly rapidly, and given policy spurs (see Chapter 8) this is likely to accelerate. Arguably, the only current, ethical justification for collecting such data within health information systems, and for holding such data on clinical records, is the aim of improving health and health care for the groups being recorded. Improvement might come directly through better service delivery to individuals or through research and clinical audit leading to better policy (see Chapters 8, 9, and 10). This justification is, in my view, a sufficient reason for collecting such data—but see Box 3.1 for some more specific reasons. Box 3.2 gives some context for such information.

Box 3.1 Purposes

Health and health-care improvement needs migrant status, race, and/or ethnicity data to:

- establish the extent of health inequalities and inequity in health service provision
- monitor the impact of efforts to reduce these inequalities
- tackle racism and discrimination
- make good decisions on health needs and interventions based on evidence
- grasp scientific opportunities

Box 3.2 Contexts

- Political
- Health policy
- Health-care planning
- Clinical care
- Surveillance and monitoring
- Health services research
- Causal research

An explicit statement agreeing such an understanding of the reasons, contexts, and purposes ought to be in place before data are collected. Before reading on try Exercise 3.1, which encourages you to reflect on the reasons why migration status, race, and/or ethnicity data are necessary for health and health-care improvement and what would be lost if such data were not available.

Exercise 3.1 Data on smoking

- Examine the data in Table 3.1, making the assumption that the findings are correct.
- What potential benefits are there in having such data, particularly from the point of view of both the communities under study and those providing health care and public health services?

The data in the exercise come from a study carried out in Newcastle upon Tyne in England in the 1990s. This study was one of the earliest to put an emphasis on the differences within the South Asian population, i.e. Indians, Pakistanis, and Bangladeshis. Here, a relatively simple classification of ethnic groups based on that of the 1991 census in England shows massive differences in the prevalence of smoking. The variations are far greater than are usually demonstrated by other commonly used epidemiological variables, e.g. sex, social class, etc. Usually, when using standard epidemiological variables we are impressed by two-fold differences. Differences of the kind in Table 3.1 cannot be quantified except by using the concepts of ethnicity or a closely related variable such as country of birth, race, or religion. In this instance, dividing the Indian population by religion, e.g. Hindu, Muslim, and Sikh, would have produced even sharper variations because

Table 3.1 The Newcastle Heart Project. Current self-reported smoking prevalence in Indians, Pakistani, Bangladeshi, and European populations (%)

	Indian	Pakistani	Bangladeshi	South Asian groups combined	European White
Men	14	32	57	33	33
Women	1	5	2	3	31

Source: Data from Bhopal et al, Heterogeneity of coronary heart disease risk factors in Indian, Pakistani, Bangladeshi and European origin populations: cross-sectional study, *British Medical Journal*, Volume 319, pp. 215–20, Copyright © 1999.

Box 3.3 Lessons from the Newcastle Heart Project data

◆ Such data can show differences that are important in public health programmes

◆ Such differences can only be quantified using the concepts of race or ethnicity and can be refined by knowing migration status

◆ Ethnic groups can be extremely heterogeneous—combining them into broad populations may lose important data

◆ For self-reported data we need to maximize cross-group validity

there are firm and effective taboos against smoking in the Sikh community. However, as most Pakistanis and Bangladeshis are Muslim, analysing by religion alone would lead to a loss of the demonstrated difference between Pakistanis and Bangladeshis. Adding an indicator of migration, such as country of birth, would make the differences even greater as, mostly, there is convergence in health behaviours in ethnic groups born in the same place. These are self-reported data and we would want to check that the questions asked were valid, i.e. accurate, across all the groups.

Such differences are important to public health programmes. Clearly, the health promotion message for the three groups of South Asian women will need to be very different from that for men, and, indeed, that for European (White) UK women. The data also reinforce the point that minority ethnic groups may be extremely heterogeneous, because—as shown in Table 3.1—combining the three South Asian subgroups into one overall South Asian group loses the ethnic variation in men (the combined prevalence was 32%, i.e. more or less the same as for European (White) men). The data emphasize that using broadly defined ethnic groups may result in the loss of useful information. The usual, and cruder, classification of these populations as South Asians would have missed important variation. The lessons from examining Table 3.1 are summarized in Box 3.3.

There are many reasons why we need to examine such data critically, including problems of cross-group validity of self-reported data on the indicators of migration status, race, or ethnicity, and on exposure, confounding outcome variables. We will return to these matters later, particularly in Chapter 9.

3.2 **Data as an agent for health improvement—making better choices**

A vision of how data will be used is vital to their collection and interpretation. Before reading further, do Exercise 3.2.

Exercise 3.2 Reflection on an image of the circumstances of migrants

Look at the image in Figures 3.1 and 3.2 and answer the following questions:

◆ The image in Figure 3.1 is from the cover of the 1986 WHO book *Migration and Health*. What does it portray?

◆ Why is this an apt picture for a book on migration and health in Europe?

◆ What feelings does it evoke in you?

◆ The image inFigure 3.2 is from the cover of the proceedings of the Faculty of Public Health's 1988 annual scientific meeting. What does it portray?

◆ Why is this an apt picture for modern-day, urban societies?

◆ What feelings does it evoke in you?

Figure 3.1 is a little sad, though it is not portraying hopelessness. The family is in the shadows looking out (perhaps with hope and longing) into the brightness of the street. The family is waiting for its chance to participate. This is an apt picture as it describes the true experience of the average migrant, where a mixture of language and/or cultural barriers, socio-economic disadvantage, lack of networks in general society, and mistrust and perhaps prejudice interfere with full participation and place the immigrant on the margins. So powerful is this kind of image that, by complete coincidence, the 2010 WHO global consultation on the health of migrants also had a front cover of people crossing a bridge—and these people were also in silhouette. Clearly, the metaphor of living in the shadows does not apply to all immigrants—and probably not at all to celebrities, the rich, and the highly sought after qualified professionals. But it is particularly apt for the undocumented migrants, i.e. those who remain in a country without valid paperwork and official sanction. Figure 3.2 is a happy, celebratory image, where the figures openly face the observer and portray, without inhibition, their well-being.

Moving from the position as symbolized in Figure 3.1 to that in Figure 3.2 will not be easy, and amongst other factors it needs data. As considered in depth in Chapter 6, migration status, race, and ethnic inequalities in health, if not health care, are inevitable. Our objective in this book, set within the wider aim of improving the health of all populations, is to move from a society where minority populations are living on the margins of society (as symbolized in Figure 3.1) to a vibrant, multicultural society with equitable health and health care (as symbolized in Figure 3.2).

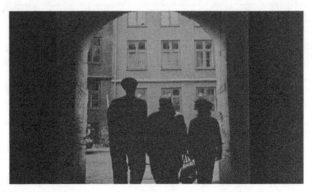

Fig. 3.1 Migrants in the archway

Source of image unknown. Previously published in Colledge, M., Van Geuns, H. A., Svensson, and Per Gunnar, *Migration and Health Towards an Understanding of the Health Care Needs of Ethnic Minorities*, The Hague, Netherlands, Copyright © 1986.

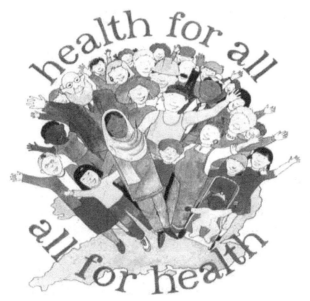

Fig. 3.2 Cartoon of a healthy society

Reproduced from the front cover of the Proceedings of the 1988 meeting of the Faculty of Public Health with permission from the Faculty of Public Health.

Laws, policies, strategies, plans, and concrete actions, thoughtfully managed and appropriately resourced, are the key to this move. Those are topics for Chapters 6 and 8. In this chapter, we focus on the collection of data, because information and research, put together as evidence, are the driving forces for change in the modern world.

Before reading on do Exercise 3.3.

Exercise 3.3 Information and research data

◆ What is the value of research data in multi-ethnic, multiracial societies?
◆ What purposes do data serve?
◆ What debates do data contribute to?

Health and health-care data that can be analysed by migrant status, race, and ethnicity are essential to establish the extent of health inequalities in death, illness, and well-being, to define inequity in health service provision, to monitor the impact of interventions to reduce these inequalities and inequities, to tackle racism in health-care systems and in wider society, to make good decisions based on evidence, and to grasp scientific opportunities for gaining insights into the causes of such inequalities and inequities and through this to develop ideas on disease causation (points summarized in Box 3.1). Unfortunately, collecting such data is not easy in routine practice, both because of a lack of appropriate coding and a lack of valid measurement instruments (the latter topic is discussed in Chapter 9).

3.3 **Collecting data on migration status, race, and ethnicity by routine monitoring: difficulties, choices, and concepts**

Examples of policies that underpin routine monitoring are discussed in Chapter 8. Here, we look at the difficulties of implementation. The move from policy to success in action is long. In 1990, the Department of Health in England proposed that data on patients' ethnicity should be collected in general practice (known elsewhere as primary care or family practice) and forwarded in hospital referral letters. The same could, of course, be done for other indicators, and is done, e.g., for age and sex. This seems a simple and efficient way of achieving comprehensive coverage of the required indicators in health databases. This is the preferred approach of most people whether the lay public, professionals, policy-makers, or politicians who have examined the issue. In England, Iqbal et al. (2012) asked 36 South Asian volunteers in five focus groups about ethnic monitoring. They favoured the idea as a means of improving health care and they recommended that general practitioners (GPs) collect the data once. They wanted more data to be collected, e.g. on language support needs. As in most countries that have tried this approach, it did not succeed in England—with a few exceptions and some very recent signs of success (about 80% completeness in England but much less in Scotland). It is worth reflecting on why this was, and continues to be so. In most countries primary health care is a highly devolved function, with a multiplicity of largely independent service providers who have their own priorities, distinctive populations, and locally developed information systems, including computer software and hardware. Primary care providers may not be subject to national policies or even laws, as they are often set up as independent businesses (as in the UK). There may be no overarching binding management system and no effective means of enforcement. Finally, when we aim to collect data from primary care we are, effectively, requesting information from the entire population. Even if only those who consult primary care services are included, that means about 70% of the entire population in a single year alone. Data collection via primary care works well in small scale, ad hoc projects but implementation on a population scale—whether regional or national—has proven both problematic and expensive. Achieving routine monitoring via primary care can be largely achieved through contractual methods based on payments. The 1990 Department of Health proposal was quickly abandoned, but later I will discuss its reintroduction.

As primary care-based approaches were not working, in the early 1990s recording of the ethnicity of patients admitted to hospitals in the National Health Service (NHS) in England was made mandatory in April 1995. This was not satisfactorily achieved, with only patchy progress until about 2010. In 2000 (implemented in 2002) the UK Race Relations Amendment Act imposed a duty on public bodies to promote racial equality and through the publication of biennial reports to show that this was achieved. The NHS responded by improving ethnic coding, but the quality and completeness of the data remained questionable. It was as late as 2009 before we saw such data being used in publications (on cancer). In Scotland, where policy was even more clear cut than in England, ethnic coding lagged far behind, so much so that an innovative record-linked retrospective cohort study was developed to solve the problem (the Scottish Ethnicity and Health Linkage Study).

In the UK the circumstances were, and remain, highly favourable for the collection of these kinds of data—there is a strong legal basis, supportive national policy, political support, and a national health service that is generally good at data collection. It is not surprising, therefore, that the somewhat disappointing example of the UK applies to virtually all other countries; indeed, progress in the UK is better than most. We need to understand why this is so and whether there is something unique about migration/ethnicity/race or whether the barriers are generic to all data collection.

Health-care systems across the world only routinely collect a few personal data items—usually name, age, date of birth, sex, and address. These act as identifiers for administrative purposes. A unique number may be added, again as an identifier. An address gives a postcode that can yield information about the kind of place a person lives in, and hence can be an indirect neighbourhood indicator of socio-economic status, the actual data being collected outside the health service, e.g. at the census. In this context we see that requesting additional routine items relating to migration, race, and ethnicity is a substantial addition. In recent years the movement towards proactive management of chronic disease and population health has led to either specific registers (e.g. a diabetes register, breast cancer screening register, etc.) or the addition of disease codes or summaries into routine information systems. The burden of data collection has increased significantly, adding to the workload of administrative and clinical staff, and challenging the capacity of the software and hardware of information systems. Additionally, we have seen significant tightening of data protection rules and laws, especially on personal data. In virtually all countries migration status indicators and race and ethnicity are sensitive personal data. In some countries, including Germany, France, and Belgium, for historical and current ideological reasons ethnic group and race are near taboo subjects. Laws in all countries place strong safeguards on the collection and publication of such data, but these laws are interpreted differently—in some countries they are interpreted so as to effectively block routine data collection using race or ethnicity categories and in others the opposite.

To some extent there is a resistance to collecting such data, including a view that their value has not been demonstrated. The data on smoking prevalence by sex and ethnic group, shown in Table 3.1 and discussed in Section 3.1, are a simple but powerful reminder that such data are vital for rational policies and plans. However, it is true that there are few practical, easily available examples of how such data from routine health care (rather than research) have demonstrably improved the patient experience or health services. There are questions of cost-effectiveness that are difficult to answer.

The need for data by ethnic group is contested, but usually because of the dangers of abuse, or almost as bad, non-use. Sometimes, professionals say the public or patients don't like to give data, but practice and research show that in health-care contexts this is generally untrue, especially when the reasons for collecting them are explained.

Given an appropriate context (see Chapters 8 and 10) and agreement on collecting ethnicity data in health databases and research studies, investigators must make choices about the concept that meets their purposes (i.e. race or ethnicity or both), and which aspects of migration status, race, or ethnicity are to be emphasized and hence captured in the information system. These choices must be governed by the reasons for which the data are being collected and the historical and social context. Without this essential first step the data are unlikely to meet the need. For example, if the purpose is to study migrants/non-migrants, country of birth is an excellent choice and is often a reasonable, indirect indicator of ethnicity. The country of birth of a person and his/her parents is the preferred indicator in The Netherlands. Every indicator has limitations, as does this one. For example, those born in Suriname comprise two major populations who differentiate themselves, and are differentiated by others, as Hindus and Creoles. Suriname was a Dutch colony and much of the population migrated to The Netherlands following its independence. Some White/European Dutch were born in Suriname. The health patterns of Hindus and Creoles are substantially different. The concept of ethnicity might be needed to differentiate them, as country of birth will not. Experience has shown that in the modern-day Netherlands, with its historical legacy of the colonization of Suriname, the purposes of the health system are best met by collecting information on the fact of birth in Suriname and also on whether the person is Hindu or Creole. The former data could probably be obtained from administrative records as country of birth is commonly recorded, e.g. on the Dutch Population Register, birth records, visa applications, etc., and the latter probably by self-report. Once such basic but vital decisions have been made, the method of data collection on race or ethnicity—whether self-report or some other indicator such as name—and the classification can then be chosen. The potential, interpretation, and utilization of the data are dependent on these initial choices. The data system needs to be designed to collect, record, retrieve, and analyse data to meet the specified purposes (see Box 3.2) and should include information on the underlying concepts used and the methods applied to collect data for the benefit of future users of the data.

3.4 **Context, purpose, and measures of migration status, ethnicity, and race**

As Box 3.2 shows, there are many contexts and purposes for data collection on migration status, ethnicity, and race. Before reading on, try Exercise 3.4 which asks you to reflect on collecting such data in various contexts and purposes.

Exercise 3.4 Choosing concepts and approaches to data collection in different contexts

Which of migration status, ethnicity or race, might prove the more useful in the following contexts:

+ political decisions
+ health policy
+ health-care planning
+ clinical care
+ surveillance and monitoring
+ health services research, and
+ understanding disease causation?

In answering these questions, consider the purposes for which the data might be used. My own answers are summarized in Table 3.2 and in the text below.

3.4.1 **Political decisions**

As in the present, so in the past, politics has been greatly concerned with immigration, and hence a question about place of birth is seen in virtually all censuses and other major national information systems, e.g. death certificates and birth certificates (including country of birth of parents). Public and political interest in immigration, and the sources of immigration, is understandable at two levels. Firstly, there is an important issue of size of the immigrant population, and within a country also its distribution. Country of birth is a good marker of immigration status that meets many needs in this political context. There is, however, a second, deeper issue, and that is about the composition of the population from a cultural perspective. In this latter respect, country of birth has limited value and the concept of ethnicity—with its emphasis not only on ancestry but religion, language, etc., becomes important to politics, especially in settled multi-ethnic societies.

Table 3.2 Context, purpose and some potential measures of migration status, race and ethnicity

Context and comment	Purpose of measures of race and ethnicity	Potential measures of race and ethnicity
Political: Markers sufficient. Migration status, race (especially colour has been of key importance) Ethnicity becomes important in settled multi-ethnic societies	Discrimination, for or against, has been the perennial purpose Implement and monitor policy	Colour, and physical features Observer's assessment Ancestry Birthplace of self or parents
Health policy: Monitoring policy needs stable marker so race and country of birth may work Both ethnicity and race needed for developing policy	Quarantine, segregation and port health Alleviation of inequalities in health and health care (fairness)	Nationality Country of birth or origin Migration history Colour and physical features as marker of discrimination Self-perception of ethnicity or race Detail needed for causal understanding
Health-care planning: Race concept and country of birth may suffice for access issues Ethnicity concept needed for assessment of need to adapt service	Restrict or target a service Add a new dimension to an existing service Evaluate a service Ensure quality	Migration status/nationality Observer's classification Colour Country of birth or origin Name Language Religion Dietary preferences Self-assigned ethnicity Cultural health beliefs
Clinical care (nursing and medical): Race and country of birth sometimes valuable Detailed data needed with several facets underlying ethnicity	Make diagnosis easier Communicate better Treat better	Colour Region/country of origin Travel history Language Health beliefs and behaviours Religion Dietary preferences Genetic indicators of disease risk and response to therapy
Surveillance and monitoring: Country of birth, race and ethnicity are low-cost markers	Routine, low-cost data on previously agreed priorities to permit assessment of change and particularly whether problems exist	Migration status/nationality Observer's classification Colour Country of birth or origin Name Self-report of race or ethnicity

(Continued)

Table 3.2 (Continued)

Context and comment	Purpose of measures of race and ethnicity	Potential measures of race and ethnicity
Health services research and non-causal epidemiology: Country of birth, race and ethnicity as markers will often suffice for surveillance and other descriptive type research Details of underlying basis of ethnic differences needed when causal understanding needed	Raise attention to an issue Measure inequality in health or health care Develop a new service to meet needs Evaluate quality of care	Country of birth or origin Migration status Observer's assessment Colour Name Language Religion Dietary preferences Self-assigned ethnicity or race Health beliefs and behaviour
Disease causation: Country of birth, race and ethnicity merely as markers are little value Detailed understanding of the interaction of biology and the environment requires direct measure of underlying facets of both ethnicity and race and information on migration history as appropriate.	Test causal hypothesis Measure association between country of birth, race and ethnicity and disease Distinguish relative contribution of environmental and genetic factors	Colour, and physical features Ancestry Birthplace and migration history Family tree/racial admixing Genetic indicators of disease risk and risk factors Valid and reliable measure of ethnicity and race (avoid misclassification bias) Measure of factors which relate both to ethnicity/race and to disease (such as poverty, diet, exercise)

Historically, the most deeply rooted purpose for the collection of data on migration status and race is political. Race-based data are used to identify individuals and groups so that policies can be applied differently (in modern times mostly to the benefits of the minority groups, pre-1950 mostly to their detriment) usually on political grounds. The history of the use of race in politics is mostly an unhappy one, so caution is necessary (see Chapter 6). The modern-day argument—and it is strong—for the retention of the race concept is that it is necessary to guide actions to reverse the effect of past injustices that were based on race. As the goal and purpose is social and political, the racial classification ought to be a socially and politically generated one. For political purposes the crude division of society into White and non-White, and other simple measures, may serve this purpose because most injustices in the past used this dichotomy. The most common division in the United States is White/Black, and the groups assigned such labels are thought of as races, with the traditional biological construct of race increasingly giving way to the social one.

The concept of race as an indicator of physical differences between population groups, the physical features themselves having been in the past the foundation for racism, works, albeit imperfectly, as a basis for a classification to be used for such purposes, i.e. reversal of injustices. The problems with race, even here, should not be glossed over—physical features do not always reliably identify population groups, they merge imperceptibly across geographical areas and are not predictable, especially in people of mixed race parentage. Nonetheless, the approach has some arguments in its favour and it is easier to operationalize than the more complex idea of ethnicity. As is discussed in Chapters 6 and 8, the concept of race underpins much of law and policy, and is essential to combat racism.

3.4.2 **Health policy**

A policy is a declaration of the direction that a governing body or organization intends to take. Policies generally are written down, though they can also be informal, or simply verbal. Policies must be within the law. In the fields of migration, race, and ethnicity perhaps the most important laws that have directed policy are international rulings on human rights, and within that the right to equality, including in health and health care. The laws apply to all member states of the UN. These laws are supplemented and/or implemented variably by country or coalitions of countries as in the European Union (EU). We will consider this again in Chapter 8. The key point is that in modern times amongst the highest priorities for health policy across the world is delivery on the seemingly impossible task of reducing inequality (differences between groups) and inequity or disparity (unjust differences between groups). While the attention of public health is often directed at socio-economic inequality, it is noteworthy that this is rarely the concern of the law and, by inference, is not seen as injustice in legal terms. Rather, the law is concerned with preventing damaging discrimination on the basis of other characteristics such as gender, race, sexual orientation, etc. The topics of migration status, race, and ethnicity are, therefore, of importance across the world.

This example illustrates the importance of integrated thinking around migration, race, and ethnicity. The law in most countries does not provide protection around migration status. Migrants who are facing discrimination will need to assert their rights mostly through race-related protection. Race, under the law, is generally interpreted broadly, including colour, ethnicity, and even religion (though there are sometimes separate laws for that). An indigenous minority—say Gypsy Travellers or Roma—can assert their rights as can migrants from China as racial or ethnic groups. What about White Polish people living in another European country? On traditional race classifications they are White, or European, or Caucasian. Nonetheless, they have the right to seek protection under race relations and anti-discrimination legislation. The one major group that will find difficulty is undocumented migrants.

Some health policies can apply the concepts of ethnicity or race as considered above for politics. For example, in monitoring to assess whether applicants for jobs in the health service from minority groups are being considered, interviewed, and employed, with the goal of equal opportunities policies in mind, race rather than ethnicity may be the better concept. This is because physical features, primarily colour, led to the historical and present injustices that these policies seek to reverse. Labels of race and ethnicity in these circumstances are markers of groups of people for whom the policy is particularly relevant.

In policies and resulting interventions designed to reduce inequalities in health status, more than a race or ethnic group label will be needed. Health inequality is a result of social factors including poverty, diet, type of employment, and cultural factors such as religion, smoking habits, dietary preferences, etc. Such underlying factors, chosen carefully on the basis of the policy or research questions to be answered, need to be directly measured and studied in relation to outcomes to make rational policy. The concepts of race and ethnicity and population groupings by country of birth are a means of identifying the relevant populations and generating preliminary hypotheses for understanding why the inequality in the disease or other health problem under investigation occurs.

3.4.3 **Health-care planning**

Health-care planners use migration status, race, and ethnicity as a guide to better assessing and meeting the health needs of the populations they serve. Usually, but not always, the populations are geographically constituted. Planners require markers to identify groups they wish to consult with, or modify services for, in accordance with health needs. In these cases ethnic or racial labels, colour labels, nationality, and migration status alone are usually not enough, though there are exceptions. Country of parental or grandparental birth or the racial or ethnic label alone do occasionally help, e.g. in the targeted delivery of BCG immunization for children of Indian subcontinent origin as one step in the prevention and control of tuberculosis. Here, the classification Indian, Pakistani, Bangladeshi, or even South Asian as an overall term either for the child or for the parents will do. Usually, however, more detail will be needed on characteristics which directly affect the need for, or utilization of, a service. Sometimes needs will be the same across a number of racial or ethnic subgroups. If this is the case, an umbrella term such as 'Asian' or 'Hispanic' may be applicable. Usually, there will be heterogeneity, in terms of language, religion, etc., making the provision of specifically targeted and appropriate services a huge challenge. (The smoking data in Table 3.1 have demonstrated the importance of population heterogeneity in planning health promotion services.) Usually, the concept of ethnicity, rather than race or migration characteristics, will be more valuable, particularly because it can easily accommodate the complexity of factors that impinge on health care, e.g. language, religion, and other aspects of culture.

To take a practical and common example, health planners need to work out what kind of interpreting and translation service will be needed over a 5-year period for their population of say, a million, people. Migration status, race, and ethnic group are, obviously, indirect and inaccurate indicators of need, but the information does indicate the range of languages that may be priorities. Also the information points to the populations who need to be asked about their needs. Of course, there is no substitute for gauging the language capacity directly, but this is very difficult, especially for those who do not speak or read the main language of the country. Health-care administrative information systems would benefit from being able to support the language needs of the population. How would we do this? One practical way would be to flag patients who were born outside the country or who identify as being from a minority racial or ethnic group, and acquire information on language needs at first registration with the health service or at referral to specialist services. As language is a changeable variable this information would need updating.

3.4.4 **Clinical care**

Racial and ethnic labels are sometimes used routinely to introduce the clinical history, as in 'this is a 45-year-old Indian/White/Caucasian/Black/African/Chinese woman', etc. This practice is open to criticism, although there are counter-arguments in favour of its continuation. The practice is summarized in the American context in the following quotation from Caldwell and Popenhoe (1995):

> *In regions of the United States such as ours, where the population is predominantly of European-American or African-American descent, the description of race is often distilled down to 'black' or 'white'. Thus, in our institution and in those with similar demographics, the fourth spoken word of many case presentations broadly describes the patient as black or white. Exactly when and how this form of introduction became common is unclear. In the United States, the format of the opening line seems to have been established a priori in case reports in the early and mid-20th century.*

Caldwell and Popenhoe (1995, p. 614)

Understanding individuals and their personal and social histories is important for good clinical care. Indeed, it could be argued that more such information would be useful, including migration history, e.g. 'Mrs B. is a 32 year old African-origin woman born in Nigeria and living in The Netherlands for the last 15 years, having arrived as an asylum seeker. She is a Muslim. She speaks Hausa and English fluently, and Dutch moderately well'. This account is richer than an ethnic or racial label, and is potentially useful in many ways. The criticisms, therefore, are more about superficiality, the danger of stereotyping, and thoughtless and possibly insensitive use of labels, rather than about the information itself.

There are, however, some circumstances in which a racial or ethnic label on its own may be helpful in diagnosis or case management. For instance, in a person of African origin with abdominal and joint pain the diagnosis of sickle cell crisis ought to be considered much more readily than in a person of European origin (even though sickle cell disease does occur in people of European origin, especially in the Mediterranean area). Even then, we must remember the huge heterogeneity in Africans. Sickle cell trait is particularly common in equatorial regions of Africa and not particularly common in people of North African or South African origin, where malaria is uncommon. Nonetheless, in such circumstances the racial label might be valuable in triggering an association between the symptoms and the diagnosis. Another example would be cough and weight loss over a month: in an Indian person this ought to trigger an association with tuberculosis, whereas the same symptoms in a White Scottish person might be associated with lung cancer. The clinician is simply using probabilities. Potential problems such as stereotyping, and hence misdiagnosis, need full acknowledgement.

Clinicians should promote thoughtful use of race and ethnicity labels and data on migration status. A rounded understanding of the social and cultural circumstances of the patient is essential for good care. The concept of ethnicity can provide the level of complexity and flexibility required. For example, a physician treating diabetes in people originating from the countries of the Indian subcontinent will need to give advice on what to do during fasting. It is not uncommon among Hindus, particularly women, to fast for one day a week. By contrast, fasting during daylight hours is fastidiously observed by many Muslims in the month of Ramadan (even though the religion does exempt the sick, it is still common for patients to fast). Race is not helpful here, and often country of birth will not help enough either. Information on ethnic grouping provides a reminder that the patient may need to be counselled on fasting. Religion is even better, since Indians, in particular, are heterogeneous in religion and culture. Even so, the physician could be seriously misled by an assumption that all Muslims fast in Ramadan or that the sick have exempted themselves from the religious requirement. A detailed cultural history from each individual is needed to ensure that errors are not made. For clinical work ethnicity is a key concept, but delving deeper than the ethnic label is almost always necessary. The purpose is to deepen understanding of the culture and circumstances of the individual.

3.4.5 **Research**

In Chapter 9 I discuss research challenges in detail. Different forms of research may apply different concepts of race and ethnicity and differing aspects of migration status. The racial, ethnic, and migrant group classifications are likely to vary according to the type of research. Finally, the type of research will determine the depth of inquiry into the specific underlying characteristics. Here, I consider causal research seeking to understand why something happens. For text relevant to the entries in Table 3.2 on surveillance, health services research, and non-causal epidemiology see Chapter 9; further details can be found in Bhopal (2000).

The concepts of ethnicity and race, and migration status, may help identify problems which merit causal investigation as well as providing ways of solving more general causal questions. They also provide a means of identifying relevant populations and interesting hypotheses, but they are not a direct source of causal knowledge. Typically, using an 'off-the-shelf' classification of race, ethnic group, or country of birth, an investigator finds large differences in death rates, let us say, for liver cancer. Since all disease arises from the interaction of the genome and the wider environment, here both the race (biology) and ethnicity (ancestry, culture) concepts are potentially of interest. In the example of liver cancer, where the main causes are infections, alcohol, and toxins, birthplace and family origins are also important.

Historically, the role of biology has been invoked (too readily) as the prime explanation for racial differences. Unfortunately, modern research also gives prominence to genetic explanations and downplays environmental (and especially economic) ones. The high rates of hypertension in populations of African origin are often attributed to genetic factors with comparatively little effort to test other explanations, including stress, diet, poverty, and racism. Cooper et al. (1997) have contested this kind of thinking, and have examined hypertension in African populations across the world; they concluded that there is so much variation that genetic factors are outweighed by environmental ones.

To develop an understanding of variations and causal paths requires direct measurement of the concepts reflected by country of birth, race, and ethnicity categories. This task will often need to include genetic studies. For example, the rate of breast cancer in South Asian women is lower than in White women in England and Wales, as recently shown by Wild et al. (2006). Since genetic factors are a demonstrated cause of breast cancer, it is important to ask whether the differences are attributable to genetic differences. It is imperative that the question is answered by direct measurements of the presence or absence of the relevant gene variants. There is no need now to use poor proxy indicators of gene distributions such as birthplace, race, or ethnicity. Equally, the differences in breast cancer might arise from social factors which vary across groups, e.g. diet, economic circumstances, contraception, or age at first pregnancy. Information on such social factors needs to be collected directly. It must not be assumed that differences between groups are genetic, or cultural. The validity of explanations must be demonstrated.

3.5 Collecting migration status, race, and ethnicity data in health contexts

Only when the purposes and contexts of the proposed work have been defined, can practical issues in relation to data collection be tackled.

Migration status, race, and ethnicity are not easily assessed, as for any complex variable. In addition, we have the problem that in some societies people are uneasy about questions on these topics. People are fearful of causing offence, or worse of being, or perceived to be, racist. Fortunately, in a health-care context the reasons for collecting data are clear and the purposes are accepted, i.e. health-care improvement. Before reading on try Exercise 3.5.

Exercise 3.5 Assessing migration status, race and ethnicity

◆ Reflect on methods of assessing a person's migration status, race, or ethnicity. Consider methods that would allow self-assessment and assessment by others.

◆ What method have you used, or would use?

◆ What method would you prefer in the assessment of your own race or ethnicity (and migrant status if you are a migrant)?

Box 3.4 Main methods of assigning migration status, race, and ethnicity

- Skin colour/physical feature
- Country of birth of self or parents/grandparents
- Name analysis
- Family origin, and ancestry or pedigree analysis
- Self-assessed ethnic or racial group
- Self-reported migration status details—length of residence, country of birth or origin, whether asylum seeker, refugee or undocumented

Three broad approaches to collecting these data are used: self-assessment, assessment by an observer on the basis of relevant data (whether self-reported or otherwise), and assignment by an observer on the basis of visual inspection. The last is becoming unacceptable now, though it was normal practice in the past and is still in use, particularly when staff feel embarrassed to ask the questions required. Box 3.4 summarizes the main approaches to assigning migration status, ethnicity, and Table 3.3 lists the markers that would help assignment—sorting them by whether they are most relevant to migration status, race, or ethnicity or all three.

I propose that most people would prefer to provide such information themselves than to have it either extracted from other records secretly or assigned by guesswork by observers.

3.5.1 Self-assessment of group identity

Historically, race was assigned by an official, whether on inspection or on the basis of parentage, ancestry, or migration history. Over the last few decades both race and ethnicity have been seen as primarily matters of self-perception of group identity, as influenced by factors such as ancestry, physical features, culture, religion, language, and country of birth and family origin. Others' perceptions of our race or ethnic group is also factored into our self-perception, as the vignettes in Chapter 1 illustrate and as is acknowledged in the definitions given in the Glossary. Voluntary self-classification of race or ethnicity, albeit selecting from a limited range of options, is rapidly becoming the most acceptable and most widely adopted method of collecting such data. Typically, the options include a write-in section of 'other group' for people who are unable to select from

Table 3.3 Potential markers of migration status, race or ethnicity for self- or observer assignment

Relating mainly to concepts of race	Relating to concepts of both race and ethnicity	Relating mainly to concepts of ethnicity	Relating mainly to migration status
Skin colour, and other physical features, such as hair texture and facial features	Skin colour, and other physical features, such as hair texture and facial features	Sense of group identity	Country of birth
Ancestral origin	Ancestral origin	Name	Country of parental/grandparental birth
	Family origin	Language	Duration of residence
	Migration history	Religion	Nature of migration status
		Dietary preferences and taboos	
		Family origin	
		Migration history	

the limited options. As shown in Chapter 2, this principle has guided the classifications currently used in international censuses. The principle of self-assignment has been widely endorsed by the populations' representative bodies.

As discussed in Chapter 1, ethnicity is a highly complex matter, and race is only a little simpler. The freely chosen responses generated by people describing their perceived race or ethnicity, such as those in the vignettes in Chapter 1, are not suitable for statistical purposes, for which easy aggregation of responses is essential. Indeed, this task of aggregation may be done by automated computer programs (which, in future, may be able to handle free text responses). The increasingly adopted compromise in public health, epidemiological, and statistical work is to invite self-assessment of race and/or ethnicity using a limited set of categories. The development of these categories requires considerable qualitative and quantitative research to ensure that they are acceptable, workable, lead to high response rates, and produce useful outputs. The ways that categories change over time and some of their strengths and limitations were discussed in Chapter 2. This approach requires continual research and updating so categories remain meaningful.

From a scientific standpoint, the problem is that self-assessed race and ethnicity are changeable over even very short time periods and are not subject to the control of the investigator. These factors are counter to the principles of repeatable and accurate measurement in science, including epidemiology. Often, however, principles are set aside, particularly when a pragmatic approach is both feasible and delivers good results. This is the case for most data that underpin social policy and public health. For example, virtually all surveys of cigarette smoking accept self-report, even though it is known there is under-reporting. Some surveys will include some form of data validation, e.g. an objective measure of tobacco use such as carbon monoxide in the breath or a tobacco metabolite such as cotinine as measured in saliva. These objective measures are by no means perfect, but they provide additional evidence to help interpret the main, self-reported data. So it is with race or ethnicity. Respondents are free to either mock the exercise by giving nonsensical data (e.g. Jedi warrior) or giving a response that is not in line with expectations, e.g. a Chinese person foregoing the Chinese (or Asian) option and choosing White. Sometimes there are simple errors, as answering the question is not always either familiar or easy. Having said this, it is remarkable that quantitative research shows there is great stability in self-report of ethnic group amongst White, Indian, Pakistani, Bangladeshi, Chinese, and many other populations. The greatest instability in self-report has been seen in populations of Black/African, Hispanic, and Native American origin. There is also good testimonial evidence that some populations such as the Roma and indigenous populations in urban areas may hide their minority status for fear of discrimination. The following quotation from Gomez et al. (2005) is fairly typical of a number of studies examining this issue, although the finding on the Black population is both encouraging and surprising:

> In our comparison of self-reported ethnicity with ethnicity recorded in the Northern California Kaiser administrative records, we found that the sensitivities and positive predictive values were excellent among blacks and whites; slightly lower, yet still high, among Asians; fair among Hispanics; and poor among American Indians. These patterns are consistent with previous studies of ethnic misclassification in administrative databases.

> Gomez et al. (2005, pp. 76, 78), reproduced with permission from Elsevier.

The implication is that more research is required with these populations to find terms that are more consistent over time, and that probably means finding terms that fit better with self-perceptions. Terminology must help maximize the self-respect and dignity of the population. Also, terminology needs to find the right balance between being highly specific yet maintaining a set of options that are workable in routine practice. An option list of 80 categories would be highly specific but would make completion of the question difficult, whereas five options would be quick and easy but sometimes too crude to be useful.

The question of how to categorize people of mixed origins is an extremely difficult one. Self-report methods allow respondents to resolve the matter, and the capacity to either describe their own race or ethnicity in free text or to choose more than one category. Self-report may be the only solution. This is certainly far superior to the now largely historical terminology of mixed race (mulatto, quadroon, octoroon, etc.) and the application of the 'one drop of blood rule' whereby any non-White ancestry meant that the person was treated as non-White.

Overall, extensive experience of self-report shows it to be acceptable, particularly to minorities who can quickly grasp the reasons for it, and produce sufficiently accurate and useful data at low cost in routine practice. The public is not as sensitive about answering such questions as professionals tend to think. For example, the health authority NHS Lothian that serves 650 000 people in the east of Scotland requested ethnic group information from patients attending hospital. Fewer than 1 in 1000 patients refused and the exercise went well, especially given staff reticence. Furthermore, staff in accident and emergency were exempted from the NHS Lothian target of 90% completion given the nature of the patients they served but they achieved 99% anyway.

3.5.2 Country of birth of self, parents, and grandparents (family origins)

These variables are obviously related to migration status. Migration status can be important in itself, independently of race or ethnicity. For example, what is the health status of Japanese people born and living in Japan compared with those born in Japan and living in the United States? Studies of this kind are classical and important to the scientific elements of epidemiology. This is not, however, the common way that these variables are being used in modern times. Rather, this information is used as an indirect, or proxy, indicator of racial or ethnic group, usually because the latter data are not available. Sometimes, country of birth is used as a way of cross-checking racial or ethnic group, e.g. if a person says he is Chinese, we confirm Chinese ethnicity by birthplace data. In the context of this book, migration status is considered in the context of race and ethnicity, and not primarily as a means of doing migration studies. Data on country of birth are especially valuable because they are widely available in many administrative systems. Why this should be is unclear, but race and ethnicity studies have benefitted enormously. Reported country of birth is commonly collected in birth and death certificates, censuses, and in population registries. A question on country of birth is in most censuses internationally, and usually over long periods of time, e.g. in the UK it has been included in each census since 1841. Country of birth is a relatively objective but crude method of ethnic group classification for recent migrants.

It is objective in the sense that it is factual information that most people know and that is recorded in documents they have, e.g. their passport. A person born abroad is, by definition, an immigrant. Such a person is commonly referred to as a first-generation immigrant. Most people also know their parents' place of birth, but may be hazy about grandparents and beyond that. Imagine a Greek family immigrates to the United States. Greek background is important to health for a number of reasons including the relatively high prevalence of blood disorders known as haemoglobinopathies (e.g. thalassaemia). The offspring of two Greek parents will carry this raised risk. Maintaining some record of their ancestral roots is potentially important for many generations. Such offspring are not strictly speaking, second-generation immigrants—they did not immigrate. This kind of label is commonplace. In some contexts it is important because it maintains the immigrant (alien) identity across generations when it might be detrimental to full settlement status. Notwithstanding the reservation about terminology, the fact of Greek (or Turkish, or Japanese, or Polynesian) origin remains potentially important.

The value of country of birth as an indirect indicator of ethnic group is reduced when a person's parents are from different places. When two parents of a child, let us say in Germany, are Turkish born the child may be reasonably described as Turkish (or Turkish German or German Turkish), or at least treated this way in statistical analyses or in health-care delivery. What do we do when one parent is a White European German born in Germany and the other parent is born in Turkey and of Turkish ancestry? There is no logical single label. At different times and contexts countries have used either the mother (as currently in The Netherlands) or the father to denote the proxy racial or ethnic group.

The country of birth may not, however, relate to self- or other-perceived ethnic group at all. For example, a large number of elderly people living in European colonial countries were born in the colonies governed by their countries. In Scotland, for instance, at the 2001 census more than 50% of those aged 65 years or more who were born in India classified their ethnic group as White.

People may be born abroad when their parents are travelling on vacation or on work assignments, e.g. in the diplomatic service. (Such a circumstance of birth gives rights of residence and nationality in some countries, e.g. the UK and United States.) This method of assigning ethnicity does not take account of the diversity of the country of origin of the individual. India is culturally diverse, with innumerable distinct ethnic groups, a complex caste system, at least eight major religions, and many official languages. Yet Indians are grouped as one by this method, a classification comparable in its heterogeneity to European. It is possible in ad hoc research to ask for the region, state, and city/village of birth, but such data are not in administrative data systems.

The ethnic group of children of immigrants is not directly identifiable using this method. Country of birth as a proxy for ethnicity, therefore, becomes more inaccurate with time. One answer is to ask for the country of birth of parents and/or grandparents, and so on. The further back one goes the greater the difficulty of obtaining accurate data, and the greater the chances of parental/grandparental birthplace being in more than one country, creating difficulties in assigning a single ethnic group.

The St James survey in Trinidad and the Newcastle Heart Project used parental and grandparental national origin and birthplace, respectively, to help assign more accurately the ethnicity of those being examined. Whilst it can help to more accurately assess individual origins and ethnicity by complementing other data sets, the method using country of birth requires more information, adds rigidity to assignment, may override self-perception, and yields a potentially large 'mixed' group (e.g. people with fewer than three grandparents from the same country).

Self-reported family origin has been used. This approach is also based upon ancestry and birthplace, usually of parents or grandparents. It is relatively straightforward except when the origins are diverse. Both self-perception and family origin are closely related. The difficulty with this approach occurs, as with many methods of assigning ethnicity, when an individual responds as having mixed family origins. In recent decades we have seen large-scale movements of people whose forebears were born in one country, themselves in another, yet are residing in a third one. For example, the long-established Indian settlements in Kenya and Uganda moved in large numbers to the UK in the 1960s and 1970s, and in smaller numbers to Canada, Australia, and the United States following political unrest. The same happened to Surinamese Indians (Hindus) moving to The Netherlands. What are their family origins? Are the origins India or Kenya/Uganda/Suriname. Curiously, the immigrants may see themselves as Kenyan/Ugandan/Surinamese but their children may see themselves as Indian/Asian etc.—a reversion to historical identities. While it is usually possible to extract country of birth from records, perhaps by computer linkage (except in the case of anonymized data sets), it seems good practice to seek informed consent first—or ask the person directly.

3.5.3 **Assessment using name analysis**

Methods of classifying racial and ethnic group that do not rely on direct contact with individuals are highly sought-after, particularly in societies and situations where people are uncomfortable about asking questions directly or even giving out a self-completion form.

One popular method is assignment of ethnicity using the name of an individual. Classification of group ethnic status by inspecting names has been used to identify a range of populations including South Asian, Chinese, Hispanic, Polish, and Irish. Experience of this method in the UK and Canada is fairly substantial where, in particular, it has been used to identify people with origins in the Indian subcontinent and China. South Asian names are distinctive and often relate to religion, region of India, occupation, and caste. Marriage with other Indians is the norm even for Indians throughout the world. For South Asians the method is reasonably sensitive and specific, i.e. it successfully identifies most South Asians from a list of names from a mix of ethnic groups (sensitive), and when a name is said to be non-South Asian that judgment is usually correct (specific). The method is imperfect: some South Asian names are not distinctive (e.g. Gill); South Asians may deliberately Europeanize their names or adopt nicknames; South Asian Christians often adopt European names (e.g. Rodrigues); South Asia Muslims have similar names to Muslims elsewhere; and marriage outside the South Asian community does occur and is increasing, meaning that South Asian women, in particular, may be difficult to identify by name, and women of other ethnic groups might be wrongly identified as South Asian.

Computerized name search algorithms are available, e.g. to allocate Polish, Irish, Chinese, and South Asian ethnic group status. The performance of some computer packages has been studied in detail. The Nam Pehchan program developed in Bradford, England where there is a large South Asian population performed well in that city and in other places in England. It was found to identify names of Pakistani ethnic origin better than those of Indian ethnic origin. The proportion of those judged by the computer program to be South Asian who actually turn out to be so (known as the predictive power of a positive test) depends on the percentage of the population that is actually South Asian. The predictive power of this program was found to be low in Scotland, because only 1% of the population there was South Asian. In places where the population is proportionately small it is essential that the ethnic group assignments of the program are checked by name-expert observers. This is probably good practice everywhere.

The concept of name searching is, however, simple enough, and the methods could be adopted for other populations. The problem is that for some populations the name is not distinctive, e.g. many people of African origin, and particularly those coming from the Caribbean, may have traditional European names, or names associated with religions they have adopted. Of course, this might help if one were searching for people with a particular religion. Muslims share a naming system that transcends countries of origin and ethnic groups. Such names are poor at identifying country of origin, or self-assessed ethnic group, but are excellent for identifying Muslims. The method's validity needs to be demonstrated in other ethnic groups, as experience is more limited.

It is not uncommon for researchers to do a name search on their lists of people with a disease or health problem (the numerator of the rate) but take information on the population at risk (denominator) from the census. This creates a mismatch between numerator and denominator and is a serious potential bias. In a study in Canada examining mortality by ethnic group, Sheth et al. (1997) took the unusual step of validating name search against country of birth, as indicated in the following quotation:

> Our approach to this problem is unique in that we combined last names and country of birth criteria in classifying South Asian and Chinese ethnicity. This study is also unique in that we have selected

self-reported ethnicity as the denominator for mortality rate calculation and validated its comparability to last name as a measure of ethnic status. We found that last names correspond to self-reported ethnicity among South Asians with high sensitivity and specificity. These results would suggest that last names and self-reported ethnicity are indeed comparable measures of ethnic status.

Sheth et al. (1997, p. 293), with permission from Taylor & Francis Ltd.

Even if such methods can be developed further, they fail to address the needs of all ethnic groups in an equitable manner and may, therefore, be unable to meet the requirements of race relations legislation requiring people to be treated equally (here it favours those with distinctive names). Self-evidently, name searching also ignores the increasingly common recommendation that ethnic group should be self-assigned, and usually there is no consent for the use of names in this way. An ethical committee should, therefore, be consulted before using names analysis for research. Where there are no other viable options name search methods provide a starting point—perhaps a springboard for better methods—and so should be part of the repertoire.

3.5.4 **Assessment on the basis of visual inspection**

A classification based on physical traits (phenotype, or physiognomy) seems an obvious and logical way to assign race, if not ethnicity. The physical features most closely associated with race are the skin colour, facial contours, and colour and type of hair. These features are largely, but not wholly, genetically determined, and are clearly central to the concept of race. Visual cues have been, currently are, and probably always will be of great importance to humans. Observers have classified people using such features, indeed this was the standard method until very recently, and is still in use, even when staff are instructed not to use it.

This approach is now generally judged as distasteful, subjective, imprecise, and unreliable. Some of the criticisms, however, may derive from the political misuse of the concept of race in numerous societies throughout history (see Chapters 6 and 9). Clearly, some people would be difficult to differentiate and classify, even in broad groupings such as Black and White, on looks alone. This approach is currently out of favour, but it continues to be used.

Perhaps observer-assigned methods should not be discarded, but seen as a component of a more sophisticated approach. In a recent Australian study of myopia, as part of a package of information to assign ethnicity a photograph of the subjects was placed in the records. In practice, the photograph was not used, but the idea is a reasonable one. The greatest limitation of this approach from a research point of view is that it is crude, and is unlikely to differentiate at any more than the continental or subcontinental level, which is similar to modern-day genetic methods. It is not credible that the method can differentiate accurately between subgroups of Indians (e.g. Muslim Punjabi or Hindu Punjabi), Chinese (e.g. Mandarin or Cantonese speakers), Africans from a variety of countries and tribes, and Europeans (e.g. Italian or French).

Nonetheless, observations can help to assign ethnicity. In addition to physical features, the observer can look for other clues, e.g. the type of dress, the type of food eaten, or the language spoken. Some types of dress are highly distinctive, e.g. the wearing of a kilt is closely associated with Scottish identity, the hijab with Islam, the sari with being Indian, etc. Even taking into account physical features and these additional cultural clues, an observer could not accurately distinguish, by observation alone, between Muslim and Hindu Punjabis, who are in several important respects culturally distinct, though in others similar, or between people from Norway and Ireland. Given an opportunity to define their own ethnicity in health studies these people would probably not place themselves in the same ethnic group. However, they are likely to be in the same racial group (though it is unclear which of the currently available racial groupings the South Asians above are in). Observation can be seen as a potential adjunct to other methods, but probably no more. It is evident that visual inspection provides no data on migration status, except from the angle of ethnicity and race.

3.5.5 Combining self-reported data and observation

An observer might use a range of data to assign race or ethnicity including self-assigned race or ethnicity, reported country of birth of self and parents, and family origins and observations of physique and dress. As ethnicity is a multifaceted concept it makes some sense to assign it using several variables. Hazuda et al. (1988) identified Mexican-American Hispanics using father's surname, mother's maiden name, birthplace, self-assessed ethnic identity, and stated ethnicity of grandparents. The method was valid in reflecting both common origin and current identification, but such approaches require many data. Investigators would need to be sure that this adds value to simpler approaches before going down this path. To this data set we may want to add years lived in the country and other indicators of migration status. Even with detailed information of this kind the assignment might be wrong.

3.6 Practicalities of assigning migration status, race, and ethnicity in health settings

It is very difficult to put these ideas, even the simplest, into practice. Collecting data on birthplace, race, and ethnicity in the context of censuses is demonstrably achievable, presumably because of the combination of a national integrated effort, earmarked funding, a long-standing research base, and legislative force (Chapter 2). Even here, the issues have been, and remain, controversial. The controversies are general and concern the right of the state to collect personal data and the potential harms of disclosure and misuse of these data. Data on the issues of migration, race, ethnicity, and religion are among those seen as highly sensitive. The key learning point from censuses is that collecting such data is not only feasible but acceptable, and, in a multiplicity of ways, extremely valuable. Censuses were considered in Chapter 2 so we will now focus on health service records. The bigger challenge is in following the same (census) path in health-care settings, but on a smaller scale and especially in places where the minority population is small (where the need for data may be particularly acute). There are substantial gaps in the information available on the health status of, and the utilization of health services by, migrant, racial, and ethnic groups in most countries, and the main exception internationally is the substantial work by broad race and ethnicity categories in the United States, especially on the Black/White population dichotomy. Monitoring the race and/or ethnic group of users of services is advocated to fill such gaps and to encourage a focus on the health needs of local minority populations. The main clinical records in places for such monitoring are in primary (family medicine, general practice) and secondary (hospital care, non-clinical administrative records), and through linkage. The policies underpinning such monitoring are discussed in Chapter 8. The following account draws on the UK where ethnicity is the core concept in use, although the difficulties illustrated are international.

3.6.1 Primary care (incorporating family medicine and general practice)

Primary care is defined by the WHO as essential health care, but it is used here in the narrower sense of care by non-specialist staff who are normally the first point of contact for a patient (accidents and emergencies excepted). In some countries, especially in private practice, a great deal of primary care is delivered by specialists working in general roles. In some countries access to a specialist is by referral by a generalist. As we have already discussed, in principle, and logically, the background details of the patient—including migration status, race, and/or ethnic group etc.—could be collected at registration with a primary care team and the information could then be shared widely across the health-care system, given the patient's consent. This has the potential to work well where patients do register and use a defined service, and do not visit different primary care teams for different problems. Where patients are entitled to visit any carer, whether in primary or secondary care, the idea of collecting migration, race, and ethnicity data once is less likely to succeed. As we discussed in Section 3.3, even in the ideal situation ethnic monitoring in primary care has proven difficult.

We have reviewed how in 1990, the Department of Health in England proposed that patients' ethnicity should be collected at a patient's first point of contact with the NHS and made available on referral via GPs' letters. (Instead, recording of the ethnicity of hospitalized patients was introduced nationally from April 1995. This was not wholly successful, and acknowledging that the original proposal was probably better new efforts were made in primary care in the 21st century.)

Collecting ethnicity data in primary care settings makes sense, because virtually everyone in many countries, including the UK, is either registered with or regularly consults one GP (family practitioner) or group of doctors. Even if this is not the case most people have regular contact with the local primary care services. This gives an opportunity for capturing ethnicity data on a large proportion of the population. The primary care team could use the data for clinical care to treat diseases better, for targeting health promotion and preventative services referrals to secondary care, and helping in health planning and policy development for the population. The problem is one of putting an apparently good idea into daily practice. Several studies have shown that the idea is generally accepted and can be implemented.

Sangowawa and Bhopal (2000), amongst others, demonstrated the feasibility and acceptability of ethnic monitoring in primary care even in an area where only a small proportion of the population was from ethnic minority groups, i.e. north-east England. Eight GPs and eight practice managers who were interviewed from eight general practices all supported ethnic monitoring in primary care, and thought that it may lead to improvement in provision of health-care services and potential benefits for both patients and service providers (Table 3.4).

Table 3.4 Summary of responses to interview questions

Question	Number of 'yes' responses ($n = 16$) (%)
Are you aware of ethnic monitoring in primary care?	5 (31)
Do you think that GPs may benefit from ethnic monitoring?	16 (100)
Do you think that patients may benefit from ethnic monitoring?	16 (100)
Do you feel that provision of health-care services may improve with ethnic monitoring?	16 (100)
Do you support the implementation of ethnic monitoring in primary care across all Cleveland?	16 (100)

They thought it would be more beneficial to implement monitoring across the whole of their area rather than in selected practices. Other issues raised include the need for incentives to encourage compliance, for training staff, and education of the patient population.

A system for ethnic monitoring of patients attending two practices (called A and B here) and inclusion of ethnic group data in GP referral letters was put in place for 6 months (August 1995 to January 1996). Effectively, the practice receptionists collected ethnicity data on attending patients, entering it on the computer system. In practice A ethnicity was entered onto referral letters manually and in B it was done automatically. In general practice A none of 2559 patients refused to indicate their ethnicity but more than one-third of patients were missed. In practice B, only 5 of 4096 patients refused to indicate their ethnicity and about one-fifth of patients were missed. Overall, of the 181 referral letters sent 160 (88.4%) had a note on the patient's ethnic group—100% in practice B where it was automated. This and several other projects have demonstrated that data on ethnic group can be collected and used to inform hospitals. The very high compliance achieved when a field was created in the referral letter template demonstrated the power of automation using computer technology. The special learning experience from this project was that even in a place where the minority population was small, and where ethnicity had not previously been an issue of prominence, staff and patients supported data collection and quickly made it a success. (No payments were made to practices but Sangowara and Bhopal provided support and expertise.) The secret was to start by coding the ethnic group of patients attending for health care.

Despite a number of successful demonstration projects, ethnic monitoring in the UK did not become routine on any large scale, despite general support from regulatory and professional bodies. In the early 2000s pressure to collect more and better data came from law (the Race Relations Amendment Act 2000), health policy, and the need to better target resources for chronic disease management. Many projects aimed to spur ethnic coding in primary care, mostly by practice-level education, advocacy, administrative support, and funding. One initiative has had particular, though not universal, success and has provided lessons that can be generalized internationally. This was done via a national negotiation of terms and conditions of service between 2006 and April 2011. A small financial incentive was provided for general practices to collect the ethnic code of 100% of newly registered patients through the Quality and Outcomes Framework.

Local health authorities also have the opportunity to supplement this with locally negotiated schemes. Despite the trivial level of payment, ethnic coding reached around 80% in England, with data of sufficient quality to permit publishable research. Given this achievement the payment was withdrawn on the agreement that ethnic coding should continue as part of good processional practice and that funding was not of further importance. Interestingly, Scotland did not match England's achievement. Even with a locally funded supplement, e.g. as in the NHS Lothian area, estimates of ethnic coding lie at around 40%. We await new statistics to show what will happen to ethnic coding in England after the withdrawal of funding. The generalizable insights from the UK experience seem to be that there is widespread support for diversity coding but achieving it comprehensively is difficult. Ad hoc projects work, but at a national scale contractual approaches can help even with modest funding where there is a perceived clinical need (England) but not where there is not (Scotland). It may be that incorporation of migration, race, and ethnicity data will be easier as part of a larger package of information on diversity or additional needs incorporated into an electronic medical record. This remains to be seen. What is clear is that for any country the challenges of collecting data in primary care settings are formidable. Given the utmost importance of these services for minorities, however, the challenges need to be overcome so equity can be demonstrably achieved and quality improved. Data from England are already showing us how to do this, especially in relation to diabetes and chronic disease management.

3.6.2 **Secondary care (specialist and hospital services)**

Secondary care is, in many health-care systems, accessed by referral from primary care. It is true that in some countries, especially where health care is paid for privately, there are few or no barriers to self-referral. Even then, hospital admission will likely be through a private specialist or through an emergency department.

For reasons that are not fully understood, migrant and ethnic minorities attend accident and emergency departments more than would be expected. Otherwise, the picture tends to be unclear. Many studies from the United States have shown that minorities—African Americans in particular—have lower use of high technology services and poorer health outcomes. In other countries the picture is either unknown or less clear cut.

It is widely accepted that, in a number of countries, a mixture of institutional, language, and cultural barriers affect both the utilization and quality of hospital care of migrant and ethnic minority groups (see Chapter 8). Whether this is true or false is an important matter that needs to be evaluated using quantitative and qualitative research. A fundamental requirement for evaluation is ethnic monitoring of patients using the service. As already discussed, this would be easy if patients' migrant status, race, or ethnicity details were sent on referral, but this is generally not happening sufficiently often so hospitals and specialist services need to develop their own systems. As with primary care, this has proven difficult in secondary care, though far more progress has been made. Again, I will concentrate on the UK experience and generalize from that.

Two national pilot studies took place in 1992. Ethnic monitoring was then, as stated above, introduced as a matter of Department of Health policy in hospitals in England in 1995. The codes were based upon census categories, though recognizing that they might be insufficient to meet the needs of the local population. The guidelines indicated that categories should be adapted for the particular service and the data system might include other relevant items such as religion, language, or dietary requirements (but no mention of migration status). However, ethnic group was the only mandatory field for inpatients and day-case patients (outpatients was optional). Accident and emergency services were also exempted from a mandatory requirement. The guidance was extremely detailed, running to more than a hundred pages. Despite this enormous effort the policy failed for many years, only being revived by the stringent requirements of the Race Relations Amendment Act of 2000. It was as late as 2009 before we saw published, and clearly valuable, data (on cancer). Scotland followed the path of England; the field was not mandatory but recommended. By about 2008 around 10% of inpatient records in Scotland had an ethnic code. These failures have required a great deal of advocacy, prompting by regulators, and ad hoc projects to rectify. Many general lessons can be learned.

Collecting valid data on race or ethnic group of people using hospital services has proven difficult, even when such monitoring is national policy and mandatory, and generally the information remains incomplete and of variable quality, making it useless or at best difficult to interpret. This incompleteness reflects variable managerial, administrative, and clinical commitment to collecting data; lack of awareness, or relevant training, about its importance; lack of custom-designed information systems; and lack of use of data in research, clinical audit, service planning, and delivery because when data are used their limitations are quickly apparent. Alternatively, there may have been an underestimation of the difficulties, sometimes interpersonal ones, of collecting ethnic group data in the context of busy hospitals dealing with large numbers of sick people needing urgent attention. The difficulties include the possibility that staff do not like to ask questions about ethnicity because of the possibility that they might seem to be 'racist'. Ultimately, the failure of a policy is a failure of management, management accountability, and monitoring of performance. Table 8.3 outlines some of the perceived obstacles and solutions, in the context of the implementation of the new Scottish ethnic monitoring programme.

Optional completion of data does not work. Between 1996 and 2004 a code for ethnic group was optional in the Scottish hospital admissions and discharges record. The guidance stated 'Although not mandatory, it is strongly recommended that these items be completed whenever the information is available'. Ethnicity was missing in around 94% of records at the end of this period. Furthermore, it was not clear whether ethnicity was based on assessment of appearance by administrative staff or whether patients (or relatives) were asked to state their ethnic group. Ethnic group was recorded in only 18% of Scottish cancer registrations.

An ethnic monitoring toolkit has been developed in Scotland, and is currently being implemented. Ethnic monitoring is seen as vital and is promoted by the Race Relations Amendment Act 2000, the Scottish Fair for All policy, and the Scottish Ethnicity and Health Research Strategy. It is also a central component of policies in other countries, including the United States.

High-level ethnic monitoring in secondary care is certainly feasible at a population level, as recently demonstrated in the NHS Lothian Board (health authority) area. In 2008 it was apparent that the local ethnic coding rate of about 6% was unacceptable. A task force set a target of 90% coding by the end of March 2012, 3 years later. This was perceived as an idealistic but nigh impossible goal. Accident and emergency services were excluded from the target. Through a programme of hospital visits, listening exercises, and discussions with managers, clinicians, administrative staff, and information system managers an agreed plan was implemented. Managers agreed to move from an optional to mandatory system. The 90% target was achieved and the best performing service was the one excluded from the goal, i.e. accident and emergency. The challenge now is to show that the availability of such data can improve the health care of ethnic minority patients and is good value.

Interpretation of data in ethnicity and health is often difficult, as illustrated in relation to mortality in Chapter 5.

3.6.3 **Linking data using exact and probability computer linkage methods**

Data on migration status, race, and ethnicity are sometimes available but not within one database or even the databases of one organization, whether a statistics office or a health service. Linkage of records is proving immensely powerful in helping to fill information gaps. While it is possible to manually link records, and this may occasionally be required even now, it is the increasing storage of data electronically that has made linkage practical, ethical, quick, and inexpensive. There are exact and probability linkage methods and both are useful. In some countries such as Norway, Sweden, and The Netherlands population registers have a unique identifying code that is a personal number that can be used to link individuals across data sets. The populations registers of The Netherlands have country of birth but no other indicators of race or ethnic group. The personal number is also found on many data sets, whether relating to health care, death certificates, or social security or education records. Given that the linkage of data is approved, researchers can generally request the linkage they need and analyse the data. Typically the unique registration number is issued to all residents. The important exception to this is undocumented migrants.

If the registration number were included in research studies, the participants in such studies could be followed up to assess health and other outcomes over very long periods, even to death. In many countries personal identification numbers are not issued, are issued but not to the whole population, or are not used sufficiently consistently to permit exact data linkage. The UK is a good example. There are several numbers that identify people—passport number, driver's licence number, and NHS number but the proposal to have a unique number for each citizen has been politically controversial and tends to be blocked, most recently on cost grounds. This is one of many examples of the important role that political context plays in our field of work. In the UK self-reported ethnicity and religion data are fine but a national identity number is not, while in several countries in continental Europe, e.g. The Netherlands, the opposite applies. In the absence of a single identifying number other data can be used for linkage, e.g. name, date of birth, sex, address, and other such variables. Linkage is then said to be based on probability methods. These methods are very useful.

One major source of data on demographics, economics, migration status, race, and ethnicity is the population census (the UK example is discussed here). Strictly speaking the UK census captures the ethnicity assigned either by the person who fills in the census form, usually the head of the household, or if this task is delegated by the head of household, the individual. There is an understandable concern about linking health data to census data, particularly as the uses of the latter are often tightly controlled by law. In a recent project in Scotland, the Scottish Health and Ethnicity Linkage Study (SHELS) such a linkage approach was considered acceptable only if the information on individuals remained strictly confidential except to those with previous authorized access. A strict protocol using computerized methods that prevents disclosure of personal information has been developed and tested. This study succeeded in its goals of linking census data to a wide variety of health data, achieving the pre-set standards for linkage by ethnic group of 80% or more in every group.

These methods provided an innovative, cost-effective, and ethical way to analyse information by ethnic group in health databases. Figure 3.3 illustrates the core idea of linkage methods. On the assumption that probability linkage accurately links individuals in the census to individual health outcomes as in health records, on a one-to-one basis, the result is a retrospective cohort study, with the census providing baseline data. The numerators of the incidence rate in SHELS were the morbidity and mortality counts based on the hospital discharge and deaths databases. As such we get an estimate of the incidence of disease based on new cases. Sample analysis is shown in Table 3.5.

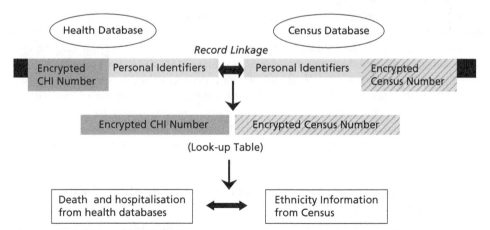

Fig. 3.3 Anonymized linkage of health databases to census databases: conceptualizing the procedure (CHI, Community Health Index).

Table 3.5 Directly standardized hospital admission rates for first chest pain per 100 000 (incidence) using a matched population of 30 years and older from the Scottish census population 2001 as reference

Sex/ethnicity	Population size	Adjusted rate/100 000	95% confidence interval
White Scottish	1 212 686	590.5	585.4–595.5
Pakistani	5354	1276.8	1137.1–1416.4

From Bhopal et al, Ethnic variations in chest pain and angina in men and women: Scottish Ethnicity and Health Linkage Study of 4.65 million people, *European Journal of Preventive Cardiology*, Volume 19, Number 6, pp. 1250–7, Copyright © 2012 by European Society of Cardiology. Reprinted with permission of SAGE.

Linkage methods are transforming epidemiological and health services research in numerous ways, and hold promise of relatively rapidly transforming the baseline of knowledge in the migration, race, ethnicity, and health field internationally. This has already been demonstrated in The Netherlands, New Zealand, and Scotland, among other countries—all countries where large-scale (unlinked) prospective, multi-ethnic cohort studies are unlikely to be cost-effective or practical.

What can we do, however, if there are no data and linkage is not feasible?

3.6.4 Modelling data

To prevent and control diseases it is necessary to know about the frequency and distribution of disease patterns and risk factors. However, there may be no such data, particularly in small areas. A potential way out of this dilemma is to extrapolate from data sources in other populations with a similar population structure, e.g. apply data on risk factors for chronic disease from England to the ethnic groups in the Scottish population or from Oslo in Norway to Bergen. The assumption behind this approach is that the distribution of risk factors for chronic disease is about the same in the ethnic groups in both populations (England/Scotland and Oslo/Bergen) except that demographic and social structures differ.

In England, risk factor data by ethnic group are available in relative abundance compared with Scotland and most other European countries, e.g. from the 1999 and 2004 Health Surveys of England and many local surveys.

The Scottish retrospective ethnic coding project (mentioned in Section 3.6.5), aimed to use these data, together with population data on ethnic minorities in Scotland, to model the burden of some risk factors. The data source for this approach was the Health Survey for England 1999 with a boost sample for ethnic minority groups (see Erens et al. 2001). The project was able to demonstrate that it is possible to impute estimates for prevalence of health-related risks that have apparent validity. Also, it was possible to estimate the distribution of continuous variables and present these as averages (means) in a distinct ethnic group and give confidence limits.

While this approach might work conceptually, it is unlikely on its own to satisfy the public, policy-makers, and researchers. The approach, of course, uses fictitious estimates and is not likely to meet legal and policy obligations.

3.6.5 An overview of retrospective addition of migration status, race, or ethnic codes

Routinely available health and health-care surveillance data generally provide incomplete, and very often no, information about migration status, race, or ethnicity. In 1983 a WHO (European Region) consultation on migration and health placed heavy emphasis on the importance of improving information systems in this area. In the 2010 WHO Global Consultation on migration and health this emphasis needed repeating as very little progress had been made, even though the WHO World Health Assembly of 2008 had adopted a resolution on migration and health that also prioritized better information systems. Given the need, the difficulty in making progress, and the cost and delays in acquiring prospective data, each nation needs to ask whether, in some way, existing data can be 'mined' to shed light quickly and at low cost on migration, race, and ethnicity. In about 2000 Scotland was a typical such nation. Scotland's generally favourable stance on equity, and equality in health, and its high-quality information systems had not been accompanied by data shedding light on whether equity goals for migrant and ethnic minorities were being achieved. The need to 'mine' existing data sets retrospectively was recognized.

The Scottish retrospective ethnic coding project was the result of a collaboration between several Scottish agencies between 2002 and 2005. Its objective was to see whether we could use existing health-related databases to create analyses by ethnic group, particularly by adding ethnic codes retrospectively. It demonstrated that the data can be obtained at relatively low cost, and reasonable timescales, given cooperation between agencies and appropriate skills within the research team. Our conclusions and recommendations from this project included the following:

1. Name search methods offer value but need considerable extra refinement if they are to be used in automatic computer mode, i.e. without visual inspection by experts. While technically valuable, these techniques do not achieve equity as they cannot be applied to some minority groups.

2. Country of birth is a reasonable proxy for ethnicity for recent ethnic minority migrant populations in the middle years of life and is of interest in itself. Such analyses are practical in many countries and are a good alternative, and sometimes, as in Scotland, produce surprising and important results.

3. Modelling as a means of extrapolating from data available elsewhere has some value as a stopgap measure. However, as the resulting numbers are fictitious there is an inherent suspicion and dissatisfaction with the outcome.

4. Linking ethnic codes in the census to mortality and morbidity databases is an approach that has great potential. The probability linkage method is likely to be exportable internationally wherever there is a database recording ethnic codes and an electronic health database with administrative details.

The project recommended that record linkage be emphasized, a recommendation that has been supported by the Scottish Ethnicity and Health Research Strategy and by research funding agencies.

3.7 **Interpreting data**

The above discussion of approaches to collecting data on migration status, race, and ethnicity, and the examples of the strengths and weaknesses of the resultant outputs, should make it self-evident that data systems need to be designed to record, retrieve, and analyse data to meet specified purposes, and should include information on the underlying concepts and methods for the benefits of data users. The users need to interpret the data and come to valid explanations for population group differences and similarities, or at least valid questions that guide interpretation.

Systems for data interpretation are fundamentally important and the real/artefact framework is particularly important. This is explained in textbooks, including in my book *Concepts of Epidemiology* (Bhopal 2008). In brief, variations in disease across population groups are often illusory, and arise from data errors and artefacts. A systematic approach to the analysis of variation in disease begins by separating artefactual from real differences. Differences can arise from: data and system error; random error; bias in data collection; socio-economic and lifestyle differences; other cultural factors and genetic factors. Misinterpretation, particularly reaching hasty conclusions that differences between population groups arise from genetic factors, needs to be avoided. Real differences occur because there are differences in populations' susceptibility, in external agents' capacity to cause disease, and in the influence of the environment. In these circumstances, the challenge is to pinpoint the causal factors.

Most quantitative research on migration, race, ethnicity, and health is epidemiological, or uses closely related survey methods from the social sciences. Epidemiological and similar studies are prone to error, because they study human populations in natural settings and this is a complex matter especially when faced by time and cost constraints. The potential problems will be discussed in more detail in Chapter 9. In brief, three major broad challenges confront epidemiologists: unbiased selection of populations, high and equal quality of information across populations, and confounding. Confounding causes an error in the assessment of the difference in the association between a disease and a postulated causal factor in the compared populations. It results from comparing groups which differ in characteristics other than the postulated causal factor under study. Vander Stoep and Link (1998) gave a great example of failing to account for confounding. Essentially, in the 19th century an investigator in Massachusetts, USA (Edward Jarvis) jumped to the conclusion from a study he conducted that the Irish population had a high rate of insanity. However, once social class differences were taken into account—so that like was being compared with like—their rate of insanity was lower than in the comparison population. We will discuss other examples in Chapter 9.

Some principles which apply to all studies and help minimize these kinds of errors include: constructing research questions and hypotheses carefully, so as to benefit all the subgroups of populations; studying representative populations; measuring accurately and with equal care across groups; comparing like with like, and when this is not possible adjusting statistically so comparisons are valid; and checking before assuming that inferences and generalizations apply across groups.

The importance of interpreting health data on migrant, racial, and minority ethnic groups with care cannot be overemphasized, especially when these show a higher degree of disability or disease than the population as a whole. It is normal practice to compare health data in minority groups with those of the ethnic majority, usually the White/European origin population. A comparative approach has many strengths. However, this is potentially an ethnocentric approach that can be misleading by concentrating on differences and diverting attention from the more common causes of morbidity and mortality. For example, while there may be some differences between groups in health patterns, generally the big picture will follow that of the whole population, e.g. in most of Europe and North America cardiovascular, neoplastic (cancers), and respiratory diseases are the major fatal diseases for all ethnic groups. In a recent analysis of mortality in England and Wales by Gill et al. (2007), the top five causes of mortality by the chapter headings of the International Classification of Diseases (ICD) in all ethnic groups were:

- diseases of the circulatory system (ICD 390–459)
- neoplasms (ICD 140–239)
- injury and poisoning (ICD 800–999)
- diseases of the respiratory system (ICD 460–519)
- endocrine, nutritional and metabolic diseases, and immunity disorders (ICD 240–279).

To minimize misinterpretation, and to avoid an overemphasis on differences, actual (or absolute) and relative disease patterns are both examined because they give a very different picture. This issue is discussed in some detail in Chapter 7 on priority setting.

3.8 **Making use of data**

Collecting data has a cost. This is, obviously, partly financial, but there are less tangible costs, e.g. public perceptions. To justify the cost it is imperative that the data are analysed and used well. In health-care, public health, and epidemiological contexts, there is an ethical and professional obligation to use data to do good (see Chapters 8, 9, and 10 for further discussion). Turning data into useful recommendations that can be used to alter law, policy, strategy, or plans, in turn to improve services or health status, is no easy matter. Usually, the benefits are intangible, long-term, and diffuse. This will be a recurrent theme throughout this book, but will be tackled specifically in Chapters 5 and 8. At this point, however, it is worth noting that data are sometimes never analysed, and even if they are they are not used. Sometimes, the incompleteness or poor quality of data on migration status, race, or ethnicity makes it difficult to use them. The completeness and quality of data improves if they are used—a virtuous circle. The number of people interested in using such data, with the exception of in the United States, is generally small, certainly in comparison to the members involved in the analysis of more general inequality variables, e.g. socio-economic inequalities.

3.9 **Conclusion**

Collecting data by migration status, race, or ethnicity is sometimes difficult, and requires agreement on concepts and terminology, excellent information systems, excellent communications, and understanding between data providers and data holders. The choice of population group classification should be driven by the uses to which the data are to be put, though pragmatism will be essential. In practice, classifications will follow, at least in part, those used in the national census. There should be a widespread understanding of the concepts underlying the classification to permit valid interpretation and utilization of data. It is, in fact, unlikely that exact explanations for differences between population subgroup will be achieved, and more likely that the findings will raise questions that focus attention on priorities. In Chapter 4, as a foundation for moving from theory to practice, we trace an evolutionary pattern in the development of interest in migration, race, ethnicity, and health, before turning to the use of data in health needs assessment.

3.10 **Summary**

The only ethical justification for collecting data by ethnicity and health is health improvement, either directly through law, policy, or practice or through better understanding achieved through research. People setting up health databases and research studies need to make choices about which aspects of migration status, race, and ethnicity are to be captured. These choices ought to be governed by the purposes for which the data are being collected. The method for collecting data on migration status, race, or ethnicity—whether self-report or some other indicator such as name—and the classification can then be chosen. The interpretation and use of the data are dependent on these choices. Purpose and context will influence the concepts to be adopted, the methods to be applied, and how data are interpreted and used.

There are three main approaches to assigning migration status, ethnicity, and race: self-assessment, assessment by another on the basis of relevant data, and assessment by another on the basis of observation. The last is not recommended in modern societies, though is still in use and was normal practice in the past. Major sources of data include censuses, population registers, death and birth certificates, health-care records, and disease registries. Data linkage holds great promise.

The data system needs to be designed to record, retrieve, and analyse data to meet the specified purposes, and should include information on the underlying concepts and methods for the benefits of data users. Users need to interpret the data and come to valid explanations for differences and similarities, or at least valid questions that guide interpretation. A conceptual framework for interpretation of differences includes data and system error; random error; bias in data collection; and differences in socio-economic, lifestyle, other cultural factors, and genetic factors. Misinterpretation, particularly unsubstantiated conclusions that differences arise from genetic factors, needs to be avoided.

References

Bhopal RS (2001) Race and ethnicity as epidemiological variables. In Macbeth H (ed.) *Ethnicity and Health*, pp. 21–40. London: Taylor and Francis.

Bhopal RS (2008) *Concepts of Epidemiology*. Oxford: Oxford University Press.

Caldwell SH and Popenhoe R (1995) Perception and misperceptions of skin colour. *Annals of Internal Medicine* 122: 614–17.

Cooper R, Rotimi C, Ataman S, McGee D, Osotimehin B, Kadiri S, et al. (1997) The prevalence of hypertension in seven populations of West African origin. *American Journal of Public Health* 87: 160–8.

Erens B, Primatesta P, Prior G (eds) (1999) *The Department of Health. Health Survey for England 1999: the health of minority ethnic groups*, Vols 1 and 2. London: The Stationary Office.

Gill PS, Kai J, Bhopal RS, Wild S (2007) Black and minority ethnic groups. In Raftery J (ed.) *Health Care Needs Assessment. The Epidemiologically Based Needs Assessment Reviews*, pp. 227–389. Abingdon: Radcliffe Medical Press Ltd. Available at: http://www.birmingham.ac.uk/research/activity/mds/projects/HaPS/PHEB/HCNA/chapters/index.aspx

Gomez S, Kelsey JL, Glaser SL, Lee MM, Sidney S (2005) Inconsistencies between self-reported ethnicity and ethnicity recorded in a health maintenance organisation. *Annals of Epidemiology* 15: 71–9.

Hazuda HP, Haffner SM, Stern MP, Eifler CW (1988) Effects of acculturation and socioeconomic status on obesity and diabetes in Mexican Americans: the San Antonio heart study. *American Journal of Epidemiology* 128: 1289–301.

Iqbal G, Johnson MR, Szczepura A, Wilson S, Gumber A, Dunn JA (2012) UK ethnicity data collection for healthcare statistics: the South Asian perspective. *BMC Public Health* 12: 243.

Sangowawa O and Bhopal R (2000) Can we implement ethnic monitoring in primary health care and use the data? A feasibility study and staff attitudes in north east England. *Public Health Medicine* 22: 124–5.

Sheth T, Nargundkar M, Chagani K, Anand S, Nair S, Yusuf S (1997) Classifying ethnicity utilizing the Canadian Mortality Data Base. *Ethnicity and Health* 2: 287–95.

Vander Stoep A and Link B (1998) Social class, ethnicity, and mental illness: the importance of being more than earnest. *American Journal of Public Health* 88: 1396–402.

Wild SH, Fischbacher CM, Brock A, Griffiths C, Bhopal R (2006) Mortality from all cancers and lung, colorectal, breast and prostate cancer by country of birth in England and Wales, 2001–2003. *British Journal of Cancer* 94: 1079–85.

Other sources and further reading

Alshamsan R, Lee JT, Majeed A, Netuveli G, Millett C (2012) Effect of a UK pay-for-performance program on ethnic disparities in diabetes outcomes: interrupted time series analysis. *Annals of Family Medicine* 10(3): 228–34.

Aspinall PJ (1995) Department of Health's requirement for mandatory collection of data on ethnic group of inpatients. *British Medical Journal* **311**: 1006–9.

Bhopal R (2006) Race and ethnicity: responsible use from epidemiological and public health perspectives. *Journal of Law, Medicine and Ethics* **34**: 500–7.

Bhopal RS, Unwin N, White M, Yallop J, Walker L, Alberti KG, et al. (1999) Heterogeneity of coronary heart disease risk factors in Indian, Pakistani, Bangladeshi and European origin populations: cross-sectional study. *British Medical Journal* **319**: 215–20.

Bhopal R, Fischbacher CM, Steiner M, Chalmers J, Povey C, Jamieson J, Knowles D (2005) *Ethnicity and Health in Scotland: can we fill the information gap? A Demonstration Project Focusing on Coronary Heart Disease and Linkage of Census and Health Records.* Edinburgh: University of Edinburgh.

Bhopal R, Fischbacher C, Povey C, Chalmers J, Mueller G, Steiner M,et al. (2011) Cohort profile: Scottish Health and Ethnicity Linkage Study of 4.65 million people exploring ethnic variations in disease in Scotland. *International Journal of Epidemiology* **40**(5): 1168–75.

Bhopal R, Bansal N, Steiner M, Brewster DH, on behalf of the Scottish Health and Ethnicity Linkage Study (2012) Does the 'Scottish effect' apply to all ethnic groups? All cancer, lung, colorectal, breast and prostate cancer in the Scottish Health and Ethnicity Linkage Cohort Study. *BMJ Open* **2**:e001957.

Blakely T and Salamond C (2002) Probabilistic record linkage and a method to calculate the positive predictive value. *International Journal of Epidemiology* **31**: 1246–52.

Bos V (2005) *Ethnic Inequalities in Mortality in the Netherlands: the role of socioeconomic status.* Rotterdam: University Medical Center.

Bos V, Kunst AE, Deerenberg IMK, Garseen J, Mackenbach JP (2004) Ethnic inequalities in age- and cause-specific mortality in the Netherlands. *International Journal of Epidemiology* **33**: 1112–19.

Cabinet Office (2000) *Minority Ethnic Issues in Social Exclusion and Neighbourhood Renewal.* London: Cabinet Office.

Coldman A, Braun T, Gallagher R (1988) The classification of ethnic status using name information. *Journal of Epidemiology and Community Health* **42**: 390–5.

Coupland VH, Lagergren J, Konfortion J, Allum W, Mendall MA, Hardwick RH,et al. (2012) Ethnicity in relation to incidence of oesophageal and gastric cancer in England. *British Journal of Cancer* **107**: 1908–14.

Cummins C, Winter H, Cheng KK, Maric R, Silcocks P, Varghese C (1999) An assessment of the Nam Pehchan computer program for the identification of names of South Asian ethnic origin. *Journal of Public Health Medicine* **21**: 401–6.

Ecob R, Williams R (1991) Sampling Asian minorities to assess health and welfare. *Journal of Epidemiology and Community Health* **45**: 93–101.

Faculty of Community Medicine and the WHO (1988) *Equity: a prerequisite for health. Intersectoral Challenges for Health for All 2000.* Proceedings of the 1987 Summer Scientific Conference of the Faculty of Community Medicine of the Royal Colleges of Physicians of the United Kingdom in collaboration with the World Health Organization, 1987.

Harland J, Unwin N, Bhopal RS, White M, Watson B, Laker M, Alberti KGMM (1997) Low levels of cardiovascular risk factors and coronary heart disease in a UK Chinese population. *Journal of Epidemiology and Community Health* **51**: 636–42.

Heath I (1991) The role of ethnic monitoring in general practice. *British Journal of General Practice* **41**: 310–11.

Home Office (2001) *Race Relations (Amendment) Act 2000. New Laws for a Successful Multi-racial Britain.* London: Home Office Communication Directorate.

Miller GJ, Beckles GL, Maude GH, Carson DC, Alexis SD, Price SG, et al. (1989) Ethnicity and other characteristics predictive of coronary heart disease in a developing community: principal results of the St James Survey, Trinidad. *International Journal of Epidemiology* **18**: 808–17.

Miller GJ, Maude GH, Beckles GL (1996) Incidence of hypertension and non-insulin dependent diabetes mellitus and associated risk factors in a rapidly developing Caribbean community: the St James survey, Trinidad. *Journal of Epidemiology and Community Health* **50**: 497–504.

Nanchahal K, Mangtani P, Alston M, dos Santos Silva I (2001) Development and validation of a computerized South Asian names and group recognition algorithm (SANGRA) for use in British health-related studies. *Journal of Public Health Medicine* **23**: 278–85.

Newcombe H (1988) *Handbook of Record Linkage: methods for health and statistical studies, administration and business.* Oxford: Oxford University Press.

Nicoll A, Bassett K, Ulijaszek S (1986) What's in a name? Accuracy of using surnames and forenames in ascribing Asian ethnic identity in English populations. *Journal of Epidemiology and Community Health* **40**: 364–8.

Office for National Statistics (2005) *Ethnicity, Identity, Language and Religion Census Topic Group; Working Paper no. 1.* Unpublished draft.

Patel KV, Eschbach K, Ray LA, Markides KS (2004) Evaluation of mortality data for older Mexican Americans: implications for the Hispanic paradox. *American Journal of Epidemiology* **159**: 707–15.

Patel VV, Rajpathak S, Karasz A (2012) Bangladeshi immigrants in New York City: a community based health needs assessment of a hard to reach population. *Journal of Immigrant and Minority Health* **14**: 767–73.

Pringle M (1996) Practicality of recording patient ethnicity in general practice: descriptive intervention study and attitude survey. *British Medical Journal* **312**: 1080–1.

Razum O, Zeeb H, Akgun S (2001) How useful is a name-based algorithm in health research among Turkish migrants in Germany? *Tropical Medicine and International Health* **6**: 654–61.

Senior P and Bhopal RS (1994) Ethnicity as a variable in epidemiological research. *British Medical Journal* **309**: 327–9.

Shaw J (1994) *Collection of Ethnic Group Data for Admitted Patients (EL(94)77).* Leeds: NHS Executive.

Sheth T, Nair C, Nargundkar M, Anand S, Yusuf S (1999) Cardiovascular and cancer mortality among Canadians of European, south Asian and Chinese origin from 1979 to 1993: an analysis of 1.2 million deaths. *Canadian Medical Association Journal* **161**: 132–8.

Unwin N, Harland J, White M, Bhopal R, Winocour P, Stephenson P, Watson W, Turner C, Alberti KGMM (1997) Body mass index, waist circumference, waist–hip ratio, and glucose intolerance in Chinese and Europid adults in Newcastle, UK. *Journal of Epidemiology and Community Health* **51**: 160–6.

Wild S and McKeigue P (1997) Cross sectional analysis of mortality by country of birth in England and Wales, 1970–92. *British Medical Journal* **314**: 705–10.

Chapter 4

Historical development of health and health-care services for migrant, racial, and ethnic minorities

Objectives

After reading this chapter you should be able to:

♦ Trace the development, using international case studies, of the social and institutional response to migrant and minority racial and ethnic group health and health-care challenges.

♦ Based on this, see and discuss a pattern of response and action.

♦ Understand the crucial role that both research data and case studies play in instigating and directing social and institutional responses.

♦ Understand that without data on migration status, ethnic group, and race a directed and rational response is not possible: hence the need to make progress on the complex task of conceptualizing migration status, race, and ethnicity and devising locally relevant terminology and classifications.

4.1 Introduction: migration, race, and ethnicity

As we considered in Chapter 1, migration is the driving force that creates multiracial, multi-ethnic societies. Migration and exploration are fundamental human behaviours, possibly relating to the evolution of humans as hunters and gatherers, moving from place to place both as a way of life and as a way of meeting the need for food and other resources. This migratory drive has permitted modern humans (who all originated in Africa) to inhabit virtually the entire globe and adapt to local environments as diverse as the tropics, mountains, deserts, and the Arctic. There are many reasons for migration in the modern world, including the need for work, education, aspirations for a better life, trade, reunion, political refuge, and curiosity. All are worthy and important motivations.

Migration, race and ethnicity are closely linked. The *Oxford Dictionary of Current English* defines an immigrant as 'one who immigrates; descendant of recent (especially coloured) immigrants' and to immigrate as 'come into a foreign country as a settler'. The emphasis here upon coloured immigrants is an important acknowledgement of a reality, illogical though it may seem. Race, the concept so closely related to 'colour', is important in relation to migration. The immigration experience of a White person migrating to the UK, North America, or Australasia from northern Europe even though unschooled in English, may be more favourable than for an African, Chinese, or Indian person even one educated in English. Whether consciously or subconsciously, the field of immigrant health is usually focused on non-White people—especially the more recently settled and also the poorest ones—the field recognizes the interrelationship of socio-economic status, migration, race, and ethnicity. This is unfortunate for disadvantaged White migrant minorities, for their needs may be overlooked. Immigrant and minority health cannot be disentangled easily, if at all, although the issues change over time and generations (so-called 'second generation, third generation' and so on).

Even in the absence of statistical data, ethnically diverse societies are generally conscious that the health status and health-care needs of their subpopulations vary. When the direction of variation is not known there tends to be a perception that the health of the minority is disadvantaged compared with the majority. Such perceptions of disadvantage may not exist in relation to immigration of businessmen, academics, and senior professionals. (In fact, as we will see later, most migrants, even poor ones, tend to be healthier than the host population—the healthy migrant effect.)

Historically, most if not all societies have been suspicious of immigrants as outsiders, and as potential carriers of disease, particularly contagious diseases. There are many historical examples of the dangers of such suspicions, but the slaughter of Jewish people to control infectious diseases is particularly gruesome. The contagion theory was once one of two dominant theories in explaining the occurrence of plague (the other being based on miasmata). Jews, a minority population in Europe that was discriminated against in many ways, were incriminated in a poorly defined causal pathway of contagion and thousands were executed in organized efforts in various places and times to control plague, particularly in the 14th century. Tesh (1988) says 16 000 Jews were killed in Strasbourg, while Porter (1997) estimates 2000 Jews were slaughtered in Strasbourg and 12 000 in Mainz. Suspicions, prejudices, and stereotypes can be very dangerous to minority populations.

Societies do have reason to be suspicious of migration, of both humans and animals, because infectious diseases can be transmitted quickly over large areas before immunity can develop. Influenza and measles can be particularly dangerous in populations previously unexposed to them and therefore lacking in immunity. Over the last few hundred years isolated groups have been rapidly exposed to populations of strangers, with devastating consequences for their health. The Tasmanian Aborigines were made extinct largely by the diseases developed following their interaction with European settlers, and North American Indians were decimated by the new patterns of disease arising from their interaction with Europeans. In 1857, the British colonized the Andaman Islands (east of India, west of Thailand) where 5000 people comprised the Great Andamanese tribe. In 1988, 28 were left. Measles and influenza took a major toll. The record shows that when populations mix the smaller, rural, isolated groups fare worse than migratory urban populations—at least from infectious diseases.

Migration and population mixing have a profound effect on the disease patterns of society, even for non-infectious conditions. As a generalization, over some generations, the migrant population takes on, or at least converges towards, the pattern of disease prevailing in the country to which migration takes place. The pattern of cancers is an excellent example of this. The process of change is usually slow, but it can be very fast. An example of a slow change is the way that taboos against women smoking and drinking alcohol tend to hold in migrant South Asians. Sometimes the incoming people can overshoot the rate of disease seen in the host population, and two of the best examples of this are the high prevalence of hypertension in populations of West African origin moving outside Africa, particularly those living in the United States, and the high rate of heart disease in South Asians in numerous countries outside the Indian subcontinent. In both instances a low rate in the country of origin is converted to a very high one by migration. The explanations are highly complex and provide high-level research challenges (in Chapter 8 I deal with this topic to show the influence of research on policy).

Populations that are physically different, whether in terms of biology (e.g. facial features) or culture (e.g. wearing a burqa), are destined to be seen as immigrants and minorities. This is reflected in the persistence of illogical terminology such as second-, third-generation (etc.) immigrant—offspring of immigrants born in the receiving country are obviously not immigrants. Immigrant health is, nonetheless, usually focused on immigrants and their descendants, i.e. racial and ethnic minorities, and in the case of Europe, Australasia, and North America this primarily means non-White people even though some White migrant populations are themselves disadvantaged, e.g. the highest all-cause mortality rates in England and Wales are in Scottish and Irish immigrants, as demonstrated by Wild and McKeigue (1997).

Most non-White immigrants, in general and in comparison with White populations including White immigrants, tend to live on the margins of society, occupying the poorly paid jobs, the lower-quality housing, and a lower social status. This is particularly true in the early years of migration but it may persist over long periods. Arguably, many African Americans are still shrugging off the disadvantages of the legacy of their immigration into the United States in the era of slavery and after that a long period of state-sanctioned racism.

The key potential contribution of work on migration, race, and ethnicity in epidemiology and public health is to point to actions that can directly help minority populations, and also contribute indirectly to the well-being of the whole population. An awareness of the harm done by misuse of the concept of race, including scientific racism, in the past is necessary. As discussed in Chapter 1, race has been used to justify slavery and colonialism, to abet eugenics, to contribute to the unfortunate and damaging debate on the IQ of human subgroups, to underpin harmful medical research, and to promote genocide as in Nazi Germany, to give just some examples: Figure 4.1 lampoons the IQ and race debate. This historical burden now lies heavily on the shoulders of those who advocate the active use of migration status, race, or ethnicity to promote the well-being of populations, and the creation of harmonious, dynamic, multi-ethnic societies. In Section 4.2 I consider how six countries have responded to the issues of race and ethnicity. I focus on the UK and the United States, the countries I know best, with some other illustrative and complementary observations on the other four countries.

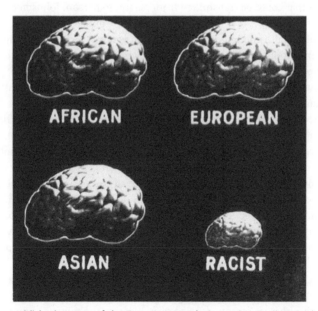

Fig. 4.1 A cartoon published as part of the European Youth Campaign Against Racism, supported by the Commission for Racial Equality.

Reproduced with permission from the Equality and Human Rights Commission (EHRC), originally published by Commission for Racial Equality which has been replaced by the EHRC.

Before reading on try Exercise 4.1

Exercise 4.1 Potential responses of societies to migration, and subsequent racial and ethnic variations in health status or health care

- ◆ What range of responses can you foresee–in general terms?
- ◆ Can you outline the likely chronological order for these responses (a) in practice and (b) ideally?

4.2 Characterizing society's response to the health aspects of migration

In an ideal world, where migrants are welcomed and perceived as new and necessary contributors to the receiving community, one might anticipate that there would be a rapid assessment of their needs followed by the delivery of the services needed to prepare the newcomers for their roles. In a health setting, newcomers might be introduced to the health threats facing them in their adopted (usually industrialized and wealthy) country, e.g. pressures to drink alcohol, smoke cigarettes, and eat a high-fat, high-energy diet. Newcomers would be helped to use the health services they needed. In due course, these newcomers might be invited to take part in health research and to participate in the health services as volunteers or as employed, trained staff. The reality tends to be different.

Mark Johnson (1984) has identified four broad phases in the development of interest in the health of migrant, minority ethnic groups in the UK, and these may be internationally generalizable. There was early interest in the unusual diseases of minority ethnic groups, particularly unusual infections that could be transmitted from person to person. Johnson called this the port health or exotic disease phase. In many respects, this phase builds upon general interest in tropical and international health and imported infections. It is not surprising that migration was, until recently, focused in seaports, particularly in the days when merchandise was often transported by sea, and shipping was the main means of international travel. Now, migration of people is mainly through air and land travel, and health units tend to be established in these locations.

The second phase, according to Johnson, was around the study of biological differences, with a focus on genetically inheritable diseases, such as the haemoglobinopathies. There was also an interest in the relationship between genetics and cultures, as in cousin marriage, which is associated with a relatively high incidence of genetically caused birth defects. This interest was easily linked to mother and child health, especially as migrants tend to have relatively larger families.

Third there came a focus on the population patterns of disease, including attention to mental health, with a strong emphasis on group comparisons. In trying to explain variations, it became necessary to examine the impact of immigrants' culture, and social and economic standing, on their health. Comparisons of the patterns of diseases were usually, if not invariably, with the majority White population. These variations drew the attention of researchers, professionals, and policy-makers.

Once noted, such variations were not easily ignored. (In Chapter 3 we examined some of the strengths and limitations of this approach, and will develop the theme in Chapters 5 and 9.) The health policy and health-care response varied from blaming the minority population's culture or habits for their health problems to setting up special initiatives; then a general policy of equity followed—equal service for equal need. The response depended largely on the social context and political and public views on race and ethnicity.

Johnson notes that following this there was an interest in the issue of adapting health-care policy, research, and services to meet the needs of ethnic minority groups, and arguably this fourth phase was surprisingly late. Even then the aim was to adapt policy and services to meet specific needs, rather than to try to ensure that the health-care system as a whole was primed to meet the challenges of multicultural health care. This latter more ambitious goal was set very late (in the late 1990s), and remains a current challenge.

In Johnson's view two issues were under-emphasized in this evolution: racism, and acknowledgement of the delivery of substantial amounts of health service by ethnic minority staff.

While Johnson's framework does not necessarily work as a rigid chronological account, it makes sense, assuming an ongoing interaction between the four phases. The framework predicts that society's response follows a pattern: an awareness of problems and especially of a risk of infectious disease harming society as a whole; formal study of health status and health care by ethnic or racial group; articulation of policy and plans, sometimes backed by legislation; a move from policies of indifference towards minorities to the promotion of the welfare of minorities; specific actions to redress inequities; and, finally, an attempt to adapt general service to meet needs.

With this framework in mind, we will examine, briefly, the response of six countries to the issue of ethnicity and health. Before reading on you should reflect on whether this framework fits your country, and then on your knowledge of the evolution of the response to ethnicity and health in one or more of the following: Australia, the United States, South Africa, the UK, Hungary, and The Netherlands. I have chosen these countries so to permit discussion of indigenous/aboriginal minorities (Australia), long-settled minorities tracing roots to enforced migration and slavery (the United States), the use of race as a political tool (the apartheid era in South Africa), rapidly changing multi-ethnic nations (the UK and The Netherlands), and Roma Gypsys (Hungary).

4.2.1 The UK

As trading nations in command of the biggest empire in world history, the countries of the UK (England, Scotland, Wales, Northern Ireland) were hubs for international travel and migration—particularly emigration, but also immigration. Ships were the main means of transport of people and goods overseas. Ports in the UK have been home to small multi-ethnic populations for centuries. The country was also deeply involved in tropical medicine, both from the perspective of safeguarding the health of British emigrants, particularly those holding important roles in empire or serving in the armed forces, and the local people being governed. Until 1962 there was, ostensibly, a free flow of people across the Empire and Commonwealth as there was no legal or institutional block to immigration (in practice, paying for tickets and obtaining passports and visas was not always easy). In 1962 came the first of a series of immigration acts that stopped this freedom.

In the 19th and early 20th centuries Britain was home to large numbers of immigrants, mainly from Europe, in particular Ireland, but also some from further afield. This changed after the Second World War when substantial numbers of non-White people from the Commonwealth or Empire, particularly from the Caribbean and the Indian subcontinent, and smaller numbers from Hong Kong, China, and Africa, settled in the UK. The reasons for this immigration are complex, but include Britain's need for labour for post-Second World War reconstruction. Also, there was a great deal of political and social turbulence following decolonization, e.g. in the creation of Pakistan in north-west and north-east India. This either compelled or motivated tens of millions of people to migrate, and some went abroad. Relatives and friends followed the early emigrants.

The NHS was formed in 1948 and funded through taxation, with the aim of providing high-quality, comprehensive health care free at the point of delivery for all people in Britain. Although, in truth, there is no such thing as a culturally or genetically homogeneous population or nation, the NHS at that time provided a model of care for, comparatively speaking, a fairly stable culture, rooted in northern European traditions and based on the English language and the Christian religion. In its early years the NHS was not expected to adapt itself to meet the needs of ethnic minority groups. Such populations were small-scale and expectations were, compared with the present day, low. Some conference reports and papers in the UK research literature discussed the challenges of meeting the health needs of minority ethnic groups in the 1960s. Many of the issues of concern observed then remain a challenge today, for instance the need for communication between professionals and patients which bridges language and cultural barriers. Interest in the health and health care of immigrants then accelerated, at least partly in response to the rise of the minority ethnic population following immigration from the 1950s through to the 1970s.

Mark Johnson's analysis of the evolution of interest in the health of minority ethnic groups was based on his observations in the UK. Numerous documents demonstrate that there was interest, first, in the unusual diseases from which minority ethnic groups suffered (the exotic diseases phase), second, in the impact of their culture on their health, and, third, in comparing the patterns of their diseases with those of the majority White population. Interest in adapting health-care policy, research, and services to meet the needs of minority ethnic groups came late. Even then the aim was to adapt policy and services to meet specific needs, rather than to try to ensure the NHS as a whole was primed to meet the challenges of multicultural health care. This latter more ambitious goal was the prime purpose of the NHS Ethnic Health Unit which served in England for 3 years from 1994 to 1997, closing down with the task only just begun. Following the Race Relations Amendment Act 2000 this task has been renewed in all the devolved nations of the UK, as discussed in Chapter 8.

Despite the multi-ethnic and multicultural nature of the modern UK, and notwithstanding the enormous efforts of both institutions and individuals, NHS health-care provision and training are still struggling to respond to diversity. Health service provision in the UK is largely based on an understanding of what constitutes illness, disease, and health care in terms of so-called 'Western medicine' and this is firmly based on the teachings of British medical schools. Nonetheless, the regulatory body, the General Medical Council, and medical schools have both emphasized ethnic and cultural diversity.

Throughout the UK many projects on ethnic health and health care start and stop each year and their focus is usually basic, e.g. communication or health promotion services. Nationally, even basic services such as translation have not yet become integral, properly funded, effective, and accountable parts of routine NHS care. (Such services are devolved to local health authorities.) While there have been attempts to adapt services to take into account Britain's multiracial, multicultural, multifaith society, inequitable health care for minority ethnic communities continues as a consequence of linguistic difficulties and social and cultural differences between patients and staff. Often the minority ethnic groups are blamed for their failure to adapt, e.g. for not learning English faster, or for their behaviours, e.g. vitamin D deficiency due to lack of sun exposure. Such barriers to equity of access and quality of care undermine the assumption that because the NHS is free to all then it is equally available to all. This said, recent work increasingly indicates that in many respects equity is being achieved.

In the UK, as in the United States, the issue of racism in health has been comprehensively discussed, particularly in relation to employment of staff (see Chapter 6). Laurence Ward (1993) reviewed the history of racism in the employment of staff in the NHS. Nurses were specially recruited for the NHS by waiving immigration restrictions in the 1960s, but most overseas nurses went into, or were channelled into, the lower-status grades. They were concentrated in the fields of psychiatry, geriatrics, and mental handicap, which were unpopular but which arguably needed an understanding of local cultures greater than would be the case for other higher-status acute care specialities. British nursing schools trained very few local people from minority ethnic populations—the reasons for failure to recruit them are complex, and include the perception amongst some South Asian groups that nursing is an undesirable profession for women. The recruitment, promotion, and retention issues remain an acknowledged and major challenge to this day, and even now recruitment of overseas trained nurses remains essential to NHS staffing.

Doctors were recruited from India and Pakistan from accredited colleges. As many as a third of all doctors in the NHS, at various times, were from overseas, mostly from the Indian subcontinent. Again, perhaps surprisingly from a socio-cultural perspective, but not from an understanding of the competition for posts, many went into general practice, psychiatry, and geriatrics. These might have been, comparatively speaking, somewhat inappropriate specialities for immigrant doctors but they were the least popular for home-educated graduates. As problems with the quality of care were perceived, the overseas doctors were blamed. The General Medical Council's requirement for most overseas doctors to sit an examination (known as PLAB, the Professional and Linguistic Assessments Board) to gain full registration was subsequently introduced.

Studies demonstrated that race and ethnicity, sometimes distinguished by indicators as crude as a person's name, was a factor in obtaining entry to some medical schools and also employment opportunities following graduation. The distribution of both merit awards (subsequently distinction and now in England clinical excellence awards) and specialist/consultant status showed huge disparities by ethnic group, which are not easily explained. Medicine is a popular profession among UK-born South Asians. The question of whether such doctors will enjoy equality of opportunity and career progression is of interest and is being monitored. The charge of racism in health care in Britain is less vocal than in the United States, but the issues are similar enough to learn from the experience there.

In the UK the focus in the area of ethnicity and health has been on immigrants and their descendants. Each group of immigrants, whether Irish, Jewish, or Indian, has been perceived to raise the risk to wider society of infectious diseases and environmental hazards. Since the 1970s the potential value of studying ethnic variations in disease patterns has been increasingly recognized. This has been followed by a policy response to tackle health problems usually seen in excess in minority groups. Where minority groups have a lower prevalence of a problem, the issue is usually ignored—wider society thereby misses the chance to learn from the minority, e.g. on the social forces that maintain a low prevalence of smoking in women from the Middle East, South Asia, and China. A new and better approach to making comparisons is discussed in Chapters 6 and 9.

The 1990s and early 21st century saw the rise of a social justice agenda accompanied by powerful legislation to promote equality in Britain's multi-ethnic society. As predicted by Johnson some 20 years ago, the prime current interest in ethnicity and health is the challenge of delivering equitable services, and this topic is the focus of Chapter 8.

While the UK is not a paragon of virtue, it has not in the last few centuries created laws and structures that embed racial inequality, as has been the case in South Africa, Germany, or the United States, to mention a few countries. It has vigorously done the opposite. To counter the then pervasive socially generated racial discrimination that imposed barriers to employment, housing, and social exchange (e.g. 'No Coloureds' signs in bars) the Race Relations Acts of 1965 and 1976 were passed to outlaw such actions. The racist murder in London in 1993 of a British-born teenager, Stephen Lawrence, followed by an inadequate response by the police led to the Macpherson Inquiry that identified a core problem to be institutional racism, and this spurred the Race Relations (Amendment) Act 2000. This Act required a major shift in the way all public bodies approach issues of employment and service provision. Above all the Act placed a duty on public bodies to actively promote racial equality. One of the principal outputs from public bodies are race equality schemes that comprise detailed plans of the actions to be taken, and then regular reports on progress. This legislation did not mandate ethnic monitoring of employment practices and service delivery, but it is clear that without it compliance with the legislation cannot be demonstrated. In Scotland, in parallel to these legislative moves, the Scottish Executive Health Department (2002) implemented a wide ranging policy called Fair for All. This policy requires NHS staff to meet the health and health-care needs of minority ethnic communities, and is being extended to other groups that are potentially at risk of discrimination. The principles and processes established by the Fair for All policy were judged worthy of wider application, e.g. in the fields of inequalities in services for the disabled, the elderly, etc. (see Chapter 8 for details). As awareness grew of the damaging effects of prejudice and discrimination, and the importance and public acceptability of legislation and policy became clear, so did appreciation of the commonality of the principles and actions across the equality fields. The Equality Act 2010 provided a unifying antidiscriminatory framework where nine protected characteristics were identified: age, disability, gender reassignment, marriage and civil partnership, pregnancy and maternity, race, religion or belief, sex, and sexual orientation. The integration is a potential strength for each of the equality 'strands', as in the previous approach it was hard to implement and monitor effectively a wide range of disparate work. Race in the UK context includes colour, nationality, citizenship, and ethnic and national origins.

With a legislative and policy backing that promotes equality, as in the UK, epidemiological data can be both generated and applied to the good of public health, as will be discussed in Chapters 5, 6, and 9. Certainly, the risk of harm is reduced in this environment. These laws and policies have had an impact on local strategies, plans, and services, as will be discussed further in Chapter 8.

4.2.2 **The United States**

The modern history of the United States is traceable to 1492 when Columbus's landing changed the course of its history dramatically. The native population of the North American continent plummeted in just a short period from some 20 million to as few as 0.5–1 million, while the population of immigrants, especially from Europe soared. The United States rapidly became one of the most diverse nations in the world. The United States has a long and sustained tradition of race and health research, scholarship, and health-care practice with a strong focus on populations of African origin, especially in comparing them with the White population—the 'Black/White' dichotomy is deeply ingrained (see Chapters 6 and 8 for examples).

Johnson's framework applies very well here, but over a much longer timescale than in the UK. From the 16th to the 18th centuries when West Africans were imported as slaves the medical interest was in the exotic illnesses they had, and on biological differences, particularly those that made them effective slaves, e.g. endurance of long working hours, heat tolerance, and their comparative immunity to the tropical infectious diseases that were a scourge in the United States. Much of this work was, in retrospect, scientific racism as mentioned in Chapter 1, and discussed briefly below and in more detail in Chapters 9 and 10.

Medical practitioners were important contributors to racialized science, i.e. a science that saw race as a primary means of analysis (see Chapter 10). As discussed by Kiple and King (1981), and referred to earlier, the idea of a package of specific 'ethnic' diseases was of much interest to medical science and practice. The susceptibility of Africans to some diseases was sometimes explained by nonsensical hypotheses on causation that veered away from the probable and obvious ones of poverty, captivity, demotivation, lack of opportunity, overcrowding, and lack of previous exposure to some infections. Impressive Latin labels such as drapetomania—defined as an irrational and pathological desire of slaves to run away—and dysaethesia Aethiopica (rascality) were used to label and explain their normal human behaviours.

These ideas, essentially based on an ideology of biological differences, were attractive as a way of maintaining differences in social positioning in which White people were superior and Black people inferior. They were not, of course, completely unchallenged. Krieger (1992) discusses the work of Dr James McCune Smith who was the first Black US-trained physician. In 1859 he challenged the assumption that Black inferiority was innate and pointed out, amongst other things, that rickets was similar in poor Black and White children. He also argued that the division of people into White and Black categories was artificial and that race was a social category. It is no coincidence, perhaps, that it took a Black person to state something that now seems so obvious. The American Civil War was fought over slavery, and its practice was only abolished legally in 1865.

Until the latter half of the 20th century the research and health-care work on race and health in the United States was, probably, detrimental to minority groups, with negative stereotyping being the norm and open discrimination being common in limiting access to health-care facilities. Black Americans have legally been free and fully equal citizens with voting rights only since 1968, shortly after the Civil Rights Act in 1964. This is a very short period in comparison to a history of 250 years of slavery and 100 years of racial segregation following the end of slavery. As a reminder of this it is worth remembering that Rosa Parkes, the woman who was arrested when she refused to give up her seat for a White person on a bus in Alabama, thus further catalysing the Civil Rights movement, only died on 24 October 2005.

Following the Civil Rights Act in 1964 the aim of narrowing the gap between the health of African Americans and White Americans came to the fore. The major US classification for race and ethnicity, released as Directive 15 of the Office of Management and Budget, was created to help achieve this goal (see Chapter 2). Those who created it explicitly stated that it was designed for that purpose and did not have anthropological or scientific validity.

This goal of equality and equity has not, however, been achieved, and the gap even widened rather than narrowed in the 20th century, as shown by La Veist et al. (1995), probably reflecting increasing inequalities in wealth and incomes. This is not to say that the health of African Americans has not improved, just that it has not improved faster than that of the White population, which it needs to do if the gap is to be narrowed. African American people are disproportionately represented in physical environments that are likely to produce ill-health. One of the staggering statistics of the 1990s that has been widely publicized is that men in Harlem, New York, one of the most advanced cities on Earth, have less chance of reaching the age of 65 than men in Bangladesh, one of the poorest places on Earth. Cirrhosis and homicide are the third and fourth causes of death in men from Harlem:

> Boys in Harlem who reached the age of 15 had a 37 percent chance of surviving to the age of 65; for girls, the likelihood was 65 percent.
>
> Geronimus et al. (1996, p. 1552)

As a group, Native Americans are even worse off than African Americans, with the worst health of any defined population in the United States, even though they have their own Indian Health Service to help tackle the challenge. Like the Australian Aborigines (see Section 4.2.3), Native Americans are a people who were displaced by colonists, often by force of arms, with a catastrophic loss of population, and from a historical perspective, loss of perceived and actual dignity, respect, status, and resources. Fortunately, this is changing for some groups. For example, the Apache of Arizona and the Navaho have become well-organized and wealthy—but wealth is bringing its own problems, e.g. the rise of diabetes and obesity in Pima Indians.

Such persisting inequalities pose political, social, and ethical problems, and the analysis leads to many questions and potential explanations. Of the explanations, those relating to racism are the most disturbing yet least amenable to open discussion and corrective action. In Chapters 6 and 8 we will consider this matter in more detail in relation to policy. Empirical evidence is complex to interpret but much public opinion and some scholarly analysis in the United States (as in the UK) places racism at the hub of ethnic and racial inequalities in health and health care. Racism is most clear-cut, surprisingly, in health research rather than health care, and the most infamous example is the Tuskegee Syphilis Study which has done more to substantiate the charge of racism than anything else in North American medicine. As already mentioned in Chapter 1, this was a government-sponsored research study of the natural progression of untreated syphilis which took place in Alabama from 1932 to 1972. The 600 subjects of the study were deceived into cooperating with the study, thinking they were receiving free health care from the government. The study actively denied them effective treatments and hastened many deaths. Syphilis in Blacks had been a matter of long and considerable interest to the medical profession, and this work was done to test a viewpoint that the disease was less serious in Black people than in Whites; a viewpoint that was wrong, and predictably so, even then.

Gamble (1993) has painted a picture of a legacy of mistrust by African Americans of health care and health research, showing that the Tuskegee Syphilis Study was not unique as a racist experiment. Gamble recounts Thomas Hamilton's experiments on a slave called Fed, testing remedies for heat stroke, and the work of Dr J. Marion Sims on an operation for vesico-vaginal fistula. The slaves, of course, had no right to refuse as they were property. The legacy has meant, according to Gamble, that participation in research by Blacks is low, and it offers an explanation for the distrust of health-care workers in the modern United States. It is true that the number of Black people in US health research, particularly clinical trials, is disproportionately low, and that has required special efforts by National Institutes of Health. However, the problem is unlikely to be an unwillingness to participate but the inability of researchers to recruit (see Chapter 9).

The issue of racism in health care has been the underlying, if sometimes understated, focus of the extensive debate and research on the disparities in the intensity of activity in the health care received by Black compared with White Americans. This matter will be discussed in Chapter 6.

A panel on racial and ethnic disparities in medical care has reviewed the evidence, making 24 policy and 11 research recommendations (Institute of Medicine 2002). These recommendations are easily generalizable internationally. Among the observations were the following: racial and ethnic disparities are persisting and may be widening; only recently has the focus turned to health care; there is evidence of both stereotyping and bias against racial minorities in the United States; there are inequities in relation to health insurance; data collection is vital to redress the balance, including data collection for clinical records; and the legal and policy basis for redressing racial and ethnic disparities is already in place, but underused. In particular, the panel believed that narrowing these disparities is a civil right.

It appears that in the United States too attention is turning to the effective and equitable delivery of health care and health promotion. In Chapter 8 we will discuss the massive policy response there. In terms of Johnson's framework, we see once again that the collection of epidemiological data has preceded the call for action to redress inequalities. We also see that action has been minimal, even discriminatory, until the social and political circumstances became favourable, i.e. after civil rights were granted. The United States is one of the few countries that has made attempts to redress past injustices through a programme of affirmative action, whereby quotas were placed to allow inclusion of historically disadvantaged minorities in public services and posts. As in other countries that have done this, e.g. India with the disadvantaged castes, the policy has been highly controversial. The topic, though relevant to the issue of health, lies outside the scope of this book.

4.2.3 The case of aboriginal/indigenous populations: Australia's Aborigines

The terms indigenous and aborigine (see Glossary) are used here (and more generally) to refer to original peoples who have become minorities in their land, usually following colonization. The number of such people globally is estimated at about 400 million. As a generalization, within the countries in which they live in substantial numbers indigenous populations usually have the worst recorded health status. This applies to the indigenous peoples of Canada, the United States, South America, India, Australia, and New Zealand. The latter is an exception in having made great progress in improving the health and health care of the indigenous people there (Maori). In most places, notwithstanding governmental efforts, inequalities in health status remain largely unaltered and have sometimes widened. Indigenous people are not, of course, migrants but they are ethnic (or racial) minorities. This minority status is not always welcome to aboriginal indigenous people, but it has a demographic and political reality. In this regard, at least, I propose there is reason to include indigenous populations within the umbrella of migration, race, and ethnicity, rather than following the historical approach of considering indigenous minorities as a separate case, with separate services, budgets, and leadership. In this section I consider the case of Australia and its indigenous population, the Aborigines. Australia is a country fundamentally shaped by relatively recent immigration but, surprisingly, ethnicity and race have not loomed large in the health-care response. The reasons for this may include the fact that the country promoted a White Australia immigration policy through much of the 20th century; the populace regarded the country as belonging to a mostly homogeneous group of northern Europeans (though this is not so); and responsibility for health and health care is constitutionally by state, rather than central (Commonwealth) government. In the last three decades of the 20th century Australia became one of the world's most multi-ethnic nations, with migration from numerous countries, but especially the Indian subcontinent, and south-east and eastern Asian countries. Despite this, the academic and service response has been relatively muted, with only a few studies examining variations in health status and health care by ethnicity, race, or country of birth. As is so often the case following such migrations, there has been a political backlash with a rise to popularity of politicians advocating a pro-European stance in national life, culture, and immigration.

There has been a sustained focus, however, on the indigenous populations, the Aborigines and Torres Strait Islanders, who have exceptionally poor health. Aboriginal people have inhabited Australia for about 50 000 years. After the European settlement started in 1788 their population declined fast, to a large extent because of imported diseases including smallpox, tuberculosis, and measles but also because of hostilities. Although population counts are difficult, estimates suggest that the population of Aborigines was over 300 000 and up to 1 000 000 at the time of settlement and less than 100 000 at the beginning of the 20th century. At times, predictions of population extinction were made, and this indeed happened in the Australian state of Tasmania, in the sense that the last 'full blooded' Tasmanian Aborigine died in 1905. In 2005, about 2.5% (517 200) of the Australian population was estimated as aboriginal. The population has risen greatly, and this is a good sign. Population counts depend on definition. Currently, self-determination of ethnic group is given primacy, although the definition is highly controversial and has required several court rulings. The nub of the definition is that the person must self-assign as an Aborigine but also be accepted as such by the aboriginal community. This focus on the health of Aborigines and Torres Strait Islanders was boosted by a referendum giving responsibility for the welfare of these populations to central government. The poor social, political, and economic circumstances of the aboriginal people had been noted for a long time but sympathy was in short supply, especially in the settlement era. Instead political and institutional efforts were directed towards reducing the aboriginal presence and culture, either through assimilation, enforced settlement, or resettlement in reserves, and at times even force and violence. At one time there was an acceptance that the aboriginal peoples of Australia were dying out; now there is acceptance that aboriginal health and well-being need to be improved.

The late 20th century saw an awakening to the appalling health status of Aborigines and limited health services and a resolve by central government to improve matters. Unfortunately, this has not proven easy to achieve. A high proportion of Aborigines now live in urban areas, and so it may be easier to take effective action than in remote reserves. Whether seen in terms of general indicators of health (life expectancy, infant mortality), specific diseases (coronary heart disease, stroke, diabetes, infectious diseases), social problems (alcoholism, tobacco use, illegal drugs, violence), or utilization of high-quality preventative or curative services, the picture is grim. Inequalities appear to be widening. The size of the inequalities is surprisingly large—up to ten-fold or greater risks for a range of infectious diseases and two- to four-fold higher risks for a range of chronic diseases. Life expectancy of Aborigines is estimated at about 10–20 years less than the population as a whole. The cause of these health problems is widely accepted as, fundamentally, social and economic deprivation, together with inadequate or suboptimal uptake of a range of services, whether health care or education.

The critical response, and one that holds promise in the face of a seemingly intractable challenge, is a national approach through the Office for Aboriginal and Torres Strait Islander Health. The essence of the strategy will be outlined in Chapter 8.

In terms of Johnson's framework, in relation to indigenous populations, we have seen in sequence: a long period of hostility during the colonization and settlement phase; indifference including the expectation of population extinction; a curiosity around aboriginal culture and lifestyle including development of pride around the heritage; an examination of their health status bringing to international light a catalogue of woes; and finally an attempt at national level to create strategies and services to redress inequalities. While Australia is a multicultural nation that is slowly leaving its openly racist and Eurocentric era behind (despite some politicians' attempts to turn the clock back), social attitudes towards aboriginal populations remain largely negative or indifferent. The era of equality for them is in the distant future, but at least part of the solution is building their dignity and self-respect.

It would be simplistic to imply that the problems and solutions we see in the health of indigenous populations and in recent migrants and their descendants are the same, or require the same response. Nonetheless, the factors in common are many and include: inequality in health status and health care; the need for adapted and targeted services; the concomitant presence of infectious and chronic diseases; the relative socio-economic deprivation; and the need for national strategy that emphasizes involvement, empowerment, and legal protection (especially against racism).

4.2.4 South Africa (under apartheid)

Apartheid is an Afrikaans word meaning a system of racial segregation. Afrikaans is the language of the people of Dutch origin who colonized and settled in South Africa. The policy was, perhaps astonishingly, introduced by the government in 1948 and lasted until 1994. Apartheid followed the atrocities of Nazi race crimes and the subsequent Nuremberg trials which laid bare the hollowness and dangers of the biological race concept.

South Africa during the period of apartheid exemplifies, *par excellence*, how concepts of race and ethnicity can be applied over very long time periods to bolster a society's efforts to justify, institutionalize, and sustain major inequalities in access to economic opportunities and services. South Africa has exemplified a struggle between populations—whether the indigenous ones living there when the settlers arrived, the African ones migrating there after that, or between the Dutch and British colonialists. The history of South Africa disabuses us of the notion that race and ethnicity are not central to human affairs.

South Africa under apartheid exemplified the damaging effects of a policy institutionalizing, with the full force of the state, separate and unequal social development and services for different racial groups, defined in arbitrary and unscientific ways. The population was divided by officials into native (Black), White, Coloured, and Asian groups. Among the many impositions, residential areas were segregated by race and intermarriage and sexual relations across races were forbidden. South Africa's health researchers in the apartheid era expended much energy in studying racial differences in health and disease, using the statistics generated by the state-sponsored compulsory racial classification, itself designed to maintain the so-called purity of the White population.

The results of apartheid were, predictably, comparatively excellent services and economic development for the country's White population and comparatively inadequate services and relative poverty for the other groups, especially the Black African majority.

South Africa was, and still is, the richest country on the African continent, with about 5 million people classified as White who were (and still are) in command of a large share of the resources, while the 30 million plus others were politically and economically marginalized.

After the dismantling of apartheid in 1994 the situation is changing, albeit slowly. While the public health sector does most of the training of staff, and most of the research and development for the population, the private health sector focuses its attention (and 50% of the total spending on health care) on the 20% of the population that has health insurance, i.e. mainly the White population.

In some ways, Johnson's framework still applies, with the major difference being that for a long period of time the interest in race and ethnicity led to state-sponsored discrimination favouring White people. In South Africa, we see an evolution from interest in infections, tropical diseases, and exotica, to biological differences, to discriminatory practices under apartheid, and then to the study of epidemiological variations (partly generated by the apartheid policy) based on rigid, politically driven and official-assigned racial classifications. Once again, following the era of apartheid, we see the appearance of an interest in equity and equality in health and health care. The Gluckman Commission of Inquiry in the 1940s pointed to the need for a new direction, but little happened, and in the 1950s the Freedom Charter of the African National Congress offered a new vision for South Africa, but at the time did not have the political power to deliver it. It took the arrival of democracy and the demolition of apartheid to deliver change. The current health and health-care challenge is equality. As elsewhere, South Africa is finding that racial equality cannot be delivered without data and without racial classification. Ironically, the very racial classifications that suppressed ethnic minorities for so long are needing to be put back into service to rectify the same problems. There are tensions around the collection of data about ethnicity in South Africa. One major change between this second edition and the first edition of this book (see the Preface) is my greater acceptance of the value of race. I am persuaded that in South Africa, as in the United States (and elsewhere where similar circumstances applied), the same kinds of classifications that gave arise to inequalities are now needed to reverse them. However, there is little mention of race or ethnicity on the website of the National Department of Health, South Africa (http://www.doh.gov.za/; last accessed 26 July 2013).

4.2.5 **The Netherlands**

Like the UK, The Netherlands has a long and successful history as a colonizing, trading nation with its colonies stretching across the globe. The country is typical of much of the western and northern parts of Europe, and yet offers contrasts with the UK scene that provide important insights. The Nazi atrocities are relevant to understanding the wariness about the topics of race and ethnicity in mainland Europe to this day. It is sadly also true that the political far-right—associated with anti-immigrant and minority culture sentiments—is still strong in a number of countries, including The Netherlands. This creates an interesting tension, given the liberalism that permeates so many facets of Dutch society. The Netherlands became a multi-ethnic society with substantial numbers of non-White people in the latter half of the 20th century, with the entry of people from its previous colonies, particularly Indonesia and Suriname, but also from the Antilles, Turkey, and Morocco. As in other European countries, decolonization, the need for labour, especially after the Second World War, and humanitarian asylum policies promoted this immigration. As also applies to the UK, the EU's freedom of movement and settlement across borders has attracted people from other European countries, especially eastern Europe, given the excellent economic opportunities.

The Netherlands has been famous for its egalitarian and liberal politics. Examples of this include legalizing gay marriage in 2001 (the first country in the world to do so), and liberal rules on euthanasia and the private use of drugs such as cannabis.

The Netherlands' policy response in relation to the welfare of ethnic minority populations has followed this liberal tradition; however, it has been unstable in the light of political change. Initially, the response was minimal. The earliest major immigration of non-White people was from Indonesia, an ex-colony, so the settlers were familiar with Dutch culture and language. These Indonesian immigrants seem to have settled and assimilated very well, both in terms of economic development and use of services. In the 1990s there was increasing awareness that this early experience was not being replicated in other ethnic minority groups, e.g. the Turks. Policy was reviewed and research was started, with an emphasis on ethnic variations in mortality and morbidity and utilization of health care. Since then, despite some setbacks, The Netherlands has become a leader in this field. The results of recent research by Vivian Bos and colleagues (Bos et al. 2002) examining mortality data indicate substantial variations that can, in large part, be accounted for (statistically) by differences in socio-economic status. Studies of quality of care have pointed to some challenges in delivering equity in services, although in many respects these are satisfactory. Agyemang et al.'s study (2005) gives typical findings. It examined blood pressure in Black Surinamese, South Asian Surinamese, and White Dutch people in Amsterdam (as a comparison) in the period between 2001 and 2003. Blood pressure was, comparatively, higher in both minority groups. There were no differences between study populations in awareness of the problem or the utilization of treatment, but the most important issue was the level of control, which was worse in Black Surinamese, and there was a suggestion this might also be so for the South Asian Surinamese. The study is not untypical of findings for many countries, that is, utilization of services tends to be as high or higher than the population as a whole but may not result in outcomes of equal quality in minority groups.

Unfortunately, just as the major programme of work in the 1990s and early 2000s was leading to discussions on policy and strategic actions the political climate changed. At the turn of the century The Netherlands saw new and negative attitudes towards some ethnic minority groups. The assassination of a prominent right-wing politician (Pim Fortuyn) and of a film producer who portrayed Islam negatively (Theo van Gogh) created a shockwave through the country. Fortuyn argued on an anti-immigration stance, stating that The Netherlands was full and describing Islam as a backward culture. Within the first few years of the 21st century the country has moved from a liberal, perhaps even *laissez-faire*, attitude to an exploration of needs, imminent policy, and service change to a less understanding and tolerant perspective. The current view is that while special efforts may be required for the foreign-born, rapid integration and assimilation should occur such that the descendants of migrants ought to require no special services. Several policies have been imposed or proposed that restrict the freedoms of ethnic minority groups and seemingly are targeted at non-White groups, especially Muslims. For example, apart from those from the United States, Canada, Australia, the EU countries, and Japan, immigrants must take an exam on Dutch language and culture and a Dutch language course at their own expense. There are proposals to restrict the wearing of the burqa in public on the grounds of public safety. These are, at least arguably, racist policies in that they treat some groups better than others without a sound case. For example, what logic is there in exempting immigrants from some countries from the need to take the exam? Why single out the burqa rather than generalize to forms of clothing that are associated with religion, or cover the face? Fortunately, in more recent years the earlier more tolerant approach has returned. Academia has played an influential part in making progress, not just in The Netherlands but more widely. Symbolic of these academic actions was that the first ever European Conference on Migrant Health that took place in Rotterdam in 2004. Two of the most important multi-ethnic cohort studies in adults (HELIUS) and infants (Generation R) are also based in The Netherlands.

The recognition of The Netherlands as a multi-ethnic nation is apt, not least because its major cities, such as Amsterdam, rank amongst the most diverse in the world. Ironically, however, and in common with several other countries including France and Germany, it is not fully acceptable to talk of ethnicity or race. Rather, concepts relating to migration, primarily country of birth but also foreign/not foreign, are wholly acceptable, and are used widely in official statistics. A consultation on the concept of ethnicity recommended the use of country of birth of self and parents (mother's country of birth being given priority when the two parents differ) as the means of assessing ethnicity. This is partly pragmatic (country of birth is already collected) and partly attitudinal (ethnicity and race are constructs people are wary of). Unlike in the UK, official policy documents do not offer strong, national priorities, but research and health-care practice are still surprisingly strong.

4.2.6 Hungary: the case of the Roma

Hungary is a country of about 10 million people in central/eastern Europe. Its geographical situation has meant that it has been one of the world's great crossroads with vast movement of people—whether traders, conquerors, or merely travellers. Its history is one of political turmoil and a great deal of war. This history makes Hungary, inevitably, an ethnically diverse place, but also a place where there is great sensitivity around the issues of migration, race, and ethnicity. Following its independence from the Soviet Union in 1989, Hungary has developed within the EU, gaining membership in 2004. I wish to focus here on the Hungarian health-related response to its Roma population, which, without doubt, is a test case of how eastern Europe as a whole fares in the field of migration, race, and ethnicity.

The Roma (or Romani and sometimes called Gypsies) people are generally perceived to be an ethnic group, although there is of course much diversity among them. They originate from north India, having started migrating in the 10th/11th centuries AD. They arrived in eastern Europe, including Hungary, in the 14th century. Despite being greatly persecuted, including an estimated 500 000 being killed by the Nazis (up to 30 000 in Hungary), they now number 6–8 million people worldwide, many of them in eastern Europe.

Characteristically, Roma populations are considered to be close-knit communities who value and preserve their culture. They are usually among the poorest populations, with low levels of education and employment and with poor health. Both international (World Bank, UN) and European-level attention has led to policy and service development, but massive health problems remain. The Roma people illustrate how immigrants become ethnic minorities, and how, without careful nurturing of the human potential, long-term, almost intractable problems can arise. That time alone is not going to lead to equality, integration, and full participation is illustrated by the Roma. The following brief account of the Hungarian scene provides lessons that are of the utmost relevance to the public health goal of health equality across populations.

The Hungarian state has had a varying relationship with the Roma people. It appears that for several centuries they maintained their distinctive lives while contributing importantly in national affairs including wars against the Turkish enemies of Hungary (from the 15th to 17th centuries). However, in the 18th century a policy of assimilation was enacted, including prohibiting the label Gypsy (to be replaced by New Peasant or New Hungarian), the raising of Roma children by non-Roma parents (similar to Australia's approach to mixed ethnic group Aborigines), and prohibition of Roma languages. This partly succeeded, for most Roma descendants are now Hungarian speakers and are called Romingros. Under the communists, by decree in 1961, Roma were not to be treated as an ethnic minority but integrated. Under this regime virtually everyone had a job, including the Roma, but after the advent of democracy and privatization following democratic elections in 1990 the circumstances of the Roma population worsened dramatically, with heavy unemployment.

The Roma population is estimated at 450 000–1 000 000 and the count (based on self-report) of 190 000 in the 2001 census is officially accepted as an underestimate. This is attributed to the stigma in the country attached to being Roma, and a fear of declaring Roma identity. Roma in Hungary are known to be poor, to live in poor-quality housing, and often in the poorest villages and towns, to have low educational qualifications and extremely poor health: life expectancy is estimated at 10 years lower than in non-Roma. At the same time prejudice against Roma has increased. Solutions on a grand scale have been proposed and, indeed, a huge amount of action has taken place in a short time. This impressive action is spurred by the fact that while the profile of the Hungarian population as a whole is aging, with a decline in fertility, the Roma population is growing and is relatively young. So, Roma are important to the economic well-being of the country.

The government's actions include the following: equality under the constitution and the law; the setting up in 1990 of the Office for National and Ethnic Minorities; a 1993 Act on the rights of national and ethnic minorities which promoted self-government at a local level and the development of cultural institutions; a wide range of practical funded measures and projects, including health care; an Equal Treatment and the promotion of Equal Opportunities Act (2003); and increasingly work in partnership with the EU. Large numbers of educational scholarships are being provided to ensure children complete schooling and higher education.

This is affirmative action of the scale and kind seen in the United States following the Civil Rights Act of 1964. As there, the measures have provoked a right-wing backlash, undoubtedly worsened by the economic crisis in 2008. In 2010 the anti-Semitic and anti-Roma Jobbik party won an unexpected 17% of the vote in the general election. The challenges raised in this context are, on a grander timescale, much the same as in the other countries we have looked at—how do societies promote both integration and cohesion and at the same time enjoy the differing cultures and customs? How do we maximize the contributions of all population, and enhance the health of all?

4.3 **A pattern of response—derivation of principles**

From the above and other accounts (see also Chapters 6 and 8), it is clear that the study of health and health-care differences by migrant, racial, and ethnic groups will be influenced by the prevailing ethos in society. If our society is a racist one (as in South Africa under apartheid), the study of migrant status and racial/ethnic difference is likely also to be racist in effect, even if not in intent. The act of seeking differentials by migration status, race, and ethnic group is simultaneously both essential to understanding the population's needs and potentially a great danger to the people studied. The outcome is dependent on the interpretation and use of the data. While racist attitudes and behaviours persist, the danger of misuse of research for racist purposes will remain. Law and national policy is key to the response.

Over the last 200 years, biological and medical sciences have made key contributions to the eugenics movement, immigration policies, and the practice of medicine. Some of these were referred to in Chapter 1, and others will be discussed in Chapter 9. Essentially, differences in health status were attributed to biological or social inferiority and this was used to justify discriminatory policies and practices, which were sometimes explained as being in the interests of the minority group being discriminated against. The greatest of all abuses, by Nazi Germany, is discussed in a little detail in Chapter 6. One major change has undoubtedly occurred in the last few decades which distinguishes the research and scholarship of the 1990s and 2000s from that of the 1890s. The current focus is not only on the description of disease patterns for the sake of science (or pseudoscience), but also on ensuring the use of the information for the betterment of the health of minority groups. This subtle change, which reflects a change in society's attitude, is all-important. UN declarations on human rights and international human rights laws have promoted equality and equity and have been instrumental in this kind of change. The strategy in science has, however, remained unchanged, with the basic method being the comparison of the health of the minority population with that of a majority population, with the health status of the latter acting as the norm or standard for comparison. This ethnocentric view, which is potentially misleading and damaging, remains the paradigm for scientific inquiry in this century as in the last two. In Chapter 9 I will offer alternatives to this approach. The paradigm change that we now need to work in is that the study of minorities benefits the entire population, and surprisingly often the majority population.

Perhaps surprisingly a resurgence of racial prejudice is also under way in the new millennium, which is coincident with the hardening of immigration and welfare policy in both Europe and North America, and adverse media reporting about migrant and ethnic minorities. The economic crisis starting in 2007–8 has worsened the situation. The proposed denial of education and health-care rights to the children of 'illegal' immigrants (most of whom are non-White ethnic minorities) in California is one effect of such new thinking that I drew attention to in the first edition of this book. As of April 2006 these proposals were rejected, a result that almost certainly reflects the power of Hispanic and other minorities in the state. This power derives from their numbers and contributions to the economy. However, in 2012 these issues remain unresolved and politically controversial. In Chapter 1 I referred to the use of genetic testing by Hungarian politicians to establish their 'racial purity'.

In seeking to understand why societies and institutions either respond to or fail to respond to the challenge of equality and equity across migrant, racial, and ethnic groups, one is reminded of the question 'which came first—the chicken or the egg?' (Or, in our context, the awareness or the data?) Clearly, social and political awareness will generate the impetus for collecting research data and undertaking case studies, and will provide the willingness to interpret the information objectively and take appropriate actions. Equally, such information can be used to generate social and political awareness. As the same data can be interpreted in many ways, the social and political milieu is clearly vital in both promoting the collection of data and in guiding interpretation. Those aspects of migration status, race, and ethnicity—colour, language, dress, etc.—that may stimulate prejudice, discrimination, and racism may also lead to inequalities in the quality of, and access to, health care. In societies that foster justice, equity, and equality, strategies to tackle such inequalities are needed, and in turn, these need to be based on data that quantify the inequalities, set targets for improvement, and monitor progress to the agreed goals. In addition, opportunities for the advancement of understanding in the social, public health, and biological sciences should be sought and grasped. In societies that are hostile to ethnic minorities, data collection is likely to do harm rather than good. In such societies people will, and rightly so, resist the collection of identifiers of migration status, race, and ethnicity.

Earlier, and especially in Chapter 3, we considered why data are so important to national action, using the example of smoking (Table 3.1). This example also drew attention to the issue of within-population heterogeneity. Most societies are slow to appreciate, or at least to accept, the implications of heterogeneity. This also reflects both lay and media perspectives. The portrayal of populations as White/Black, immigrant/native, foreigner or alien/local is commonplace. In Chapter 2 we considered the label Asian and how it is used so broadly and also so differently, e.g. in North America (for Eastern Asians) and the UK (Indian subcontinent/South Asia). Our sketch of the response in six countries helps us to understand how lay perceptions and government goals intertwine with and influence the conduct of research and surveillance. Box 4.1 highlights the diversity in terms of birthplace, region of origin in the Indian subcontinent, religion, and language of Indians (one group of South Asians) living in the UK. In a sense everyone knows this, and yet this knowledge does not have much impact. In the United States, in most work to data Indians are amalgamated within Asian and Pacific Islanders, in the UK a breakdown at a level finer than Indian is rare, and in The Netherlands at best all Indians are grouped (Hindus) and sometimes included within the group Surinamese. In Australia and Hungary Indians do not figure large in health studies. In South Africa Indians and Chinese (and others) were placed in the category Asian. Why are countries responding in this way? Possibly the response is in accord with the primary purposes of the data collection. In the United States data are collected to redress historical disadvantage—Asian Indians are not a priority, the Black population is. Similarly, in Australia and Hungary there are other priorities, i.e. Aborigines and Roma, respectively. In the UK, Indians are doing reasonably well socio-economically, and pragmatically the category works well. In The Netherlands there are pragmatic issues around the use of country of birth as a primary indicator of ethnicity so more nuanced considerations are difficult. In South Africa, the aim of the classification was to divide people, effectively in a social hierarchy in accord with racist ideology, so a finer gradation was quite unnecessary. Box 4.1 shows the heterogeneity of the South Asian populations in the UK. It is safe to say that most immigrant populations are highly heterogeneous.

Such differences within populations are of paramount importance, and it is hard to imagine how we can develop effective public health responses without data on them. In recent years there has been increasing recognition of within-group heterogeneity—the term granularity has become popular in the United States. Returning to the example of differences in smoking prevalence in subgroups of South Asians (Table 3.1), there are other questions that need answering before we can proceed to action, e.g. on the cross-cultural validity of self-report data, on the beliefs, attitudes, and social conventions that underpin such variations, and on the effectiveness of public health programmes. The immediate need, nonetheless, is for data for discussion and consideration. We have already seen that each country tends to focus on particular populations,

Box 4.1 Religions, languages, and origins of South Asians living in the UK

Religion	Language
Sikhism	Punjabi
Islam	Urdu
Hinduism	Hindi
(Jainism)	Gujarati
(Christianity)	Bengali
Buddhism	Pashto

Region of Origin	Birthplace
Punjab	Born in the UK
Mirpur and Northwest Frontier	Born in the Republic of Ireland
Gujarat	Born in western Europe
Bengal	Born in Africa
East Africa	Born in South Asia
	Born in North America
	Born in Oceania

and the choice is dictated by historical circumstances, current purposes, and pragmatism. In The Netherlands the focus is on disadvantaged 'non-Western' groups—the inevitable consequence is the equating of immigrants and minorities as problems. In each country, some groups are ignored or effectively ignored as their data are subsumed with larger populations. Try Exercise 4.2 before reading on.

Exercise 4.2 Assessing the health needs of a minority group that has not been studied (invisible minority)

- What do you think of the phrase 'invisible minority'?
- Why are some groups not studied or noted and hence become, effectively, invisible?
- Given the challenge of reporting rapidly on the health needs of an invisible minority group, how would you feel?
- Thinking about an invisible minority in your country, e.g. Iranian, Polish, or Bosnian people, what can you do to make progress?

This exercise, asking you to report on a difficult question, ought to provoke anxiety, because the dangers of misinforming policy-makers and planners are very high. Even the phrase 'invisible minority' is a charged one, though highly descriptive. Some populations' specific needs have never been studied systematically though there is usually some awareness of their needs, e.g. few high-quality quantitative research data exist on Polish immigrants or Gypsy travellers in Scotland. The reasons include that they have little political power, they have not asserted their needs, they have few champions for their cause, and, perhaps above all, they were not captured in census or health statistics until 2011. Without data, a report is likely to be based on stereotypes and general impressions that may well be wrong. In recognition of these points the Scottish government agreed to include specific categories for these two (and other) populations in the ethnic group question in the 2011 census.

It is quite possible that the general principles derived from general population research and policy development may not apply to the specific, 'invisible' minority groups you are asked to report on. For example, there may be a social distance between the group and the service and its professionals, leading to problems of inequitable access and poor quality of care. This may be specific to a small number of issues or general. You can make progress, nonetheless.

Your population may be similar to other populations studied elsewhere, whether in other parts of your country or internationally. You may need to learn from the country of origin, e.g. what are the issues facing Poles in Poland or the Irish travellers in Ireland (who have been studied in detail)? At least some of them are likely to be pertinent to the situation in your country. A close examination of publications internationally, both in academic journals and in other sources such as government reports, might give very useful insights. The third approach would be to do a rapid needs assessment, which would be based mainly on a dialogue with health service providers and representatives of the population on which you are reporting. Direct observation might be helpful, e.g. of the living conditions of some members of the population. Given a small budget and prioritization, you would probably recommend an assessment of the size and characteristics of the populations (possibly including a more detailed analysis of existing census data, e.g. by country of birth, or failing that a new mini-census focused on this population), and acquisition of data on mortality, major causes of hospitalization and use of general practice services, and major aspects of lifestyle that are relevant to health. Even the simplest of data, despite their limitations, can be the foundation for health needs assessment (see Chapter 5). Bangladeshis are an invisible minority in the United States (though one of great research focus in the UK). Patel et al. (2012) did a rapid, community-based needs assessment through a door-to-door survey of 167 women in the Bronx, New York. As is often the case, especially in previously unstudied populations, huge unmet need was uncovered, e.g. 60% had never had a cervical smear to screen for cervical cancer and 74% were overweight or obese (using cut-offs for South Asians). This kind of work is necessary to stimulate progress, including spurring the collection of data.

4.4 **Conclusion**

Modern and enlightened multi-ethnic societies ought to face the challenges raised by immigration and racial/ethnic variations in health and health care. Historically, the response to rising ethnic diversity has usually been, initially at least, an indifferent or even negative one, with a tendency to blame the minority populations for innate or cultural 'defects' that underlie their health problems and their ignorance or apathy in accessing services. Spurred by rising global and national movements for universal human rights in the late 20th century, and a realization that immigration is vital to their economic and demographic health, many countries are changing their stance, with equity of health status and health care being a central focus. The response to migration and racial and ethnic inequalities is, clearly, closely related to political and social trends. Researchers, practitioners, and policy-makers can learn from historical and international experience.

Data on race and ethnic group have both harmed and benefited minority populations, and will continue to do so, yet without the data the need for services cannot be established. Such data can underpin both policies of exclusion and of positive action. The lesson from this brief examination of historical responses seems to be that data need to be collected within an ethical and legal framework that safeguards the human rights of minority and majority populations alike and requires the use of data to improve the welfare of populations. This does not, of course, guarantee that data will not be abused, but it does impose obstacles to that. The goals of equality and equity, and monitoring of progress towards those goals, cannot be achieved without data on migration status, race, or ethnicity. There is, therefore, little choice but to work with the concepts and the resulting classifications, but with the goal of continuous improvement in the quality of the data and their uses. The scale of the challenge is great, and none of the six countries considered here has yet demonstrably achieved the goal of narrowing in meaningful and substantial ways ethnic inequalities in health status. This is not, however, a hopeless aspiration or a case for despair. Rather, it is an indicator that we need to think and work harder. Careful health needs assessment, the topic of Chapter 5, is a prerequisite for thoughtful action.

4.5 Summary

Generally, ethnically diverse societies are conscious that the health status and health-care needs of their population vary by migration status, or racial or ethnic group. These variations draw the attention of researchers, professionals, and policy-makers. Once noted, such variations are not easily ignored. The responses range from merely studying the differences, blaming the minority population for their health problems, excluding them from services, setting up special initiatives, adapting services to meet needs, and a general policy of equality and service equity to meet need. The response depends on the social context and political and public views on migrants, race, and ethnicity. This chapter has outlined the response in six countries.

In the UK the health focus has been on immigrants and their descendants, utilizing primarily the concept of ethnicity. Each group of immigrants, whether Irish, Jewish, or Indian, has been associated, rightly or wrongly, with raising the risk to the wider society of infectious diseases and environmental hazards, and that perception is harmful to the group. Since the 1970s there has been an appreciation of the potential value of studying variations in disease patterns, which has increased attention on ethnic minority groups. This has been followed by a policy response, backed by strong legislation, to tackle health problems seen in excess in minority groups. The 1990s and early 21st century have seen the rise of a social justice agenda accompanied by powerful antidiscriminatory legislation to promote equality in Britain's multi-ethnic society. Race equality has been firmly embedded within the wider equality agenda, being one of nine legally protected characteristics.

In the United States attention in the field of has focused on populations of African and Native American origin and more recently on Hispanic populations. The concept of race dominates. Until the latter half of the 20th century the response was generally unsupportive or openly discriminatory. Following the civil rights movement and the Civil Rights Act 1964 the aim of narrowing the gap between the health of African Americans and White Americans has come to the fore. This has not been achieved, despite much rigorous policy analysis, and inequalities may even be increasing. More recently, attention has turned to a wider range of minority populations. Race and ethnicity classifications have been designed to help redress historical discrimination, and this goal remains a top priority.

Australia is a country of immigrants but, surprisingly, immigrant health, ethnicity, and race have not loomed large in the health response. Australia has maintained strict controls on immigration, and it is probable that immigrants comprise a relatively wealthy and healthy group. Rather, the focus has been on the indigenous populations, especially the Aborigines. The late 20th century brought an awareness of the appalling health and health services they have and a resolve to improve matters. Efforts to date have paid little dividend in terms of narrowing inequality. However, the rising population of Aborigines following a near catastrophic decline in the 19th century augurs well. This challenge has implications for indigenous populations worldwide.

South Africa under apartheid (1948–94) exemplified the damaging effects of a policy promoting separate development for different racial groups, the results being excellent services for the country's White population and inadequate ones for the other groups, especially the Black African majority. Vigorous efforts are being made to redress these injustices in post-apartheid South Africa, with ambivalence about the continued value of using race and ethnicity in this context.

The Netherlands became one of the world's most diverse multi-ethnic societies in the late 20th century. It institutionalized the use of country of birth as the primary measure of ethnicity. Its policy response has been unstable in the light of recent political change, though generally it has done a great deal. The current attitude is that while special efforts may be required for the foreign-born, rapid integration and assimilation should occur such that the descendents of migrants ought to require no special services. Research in The Netherlands is advanced.

Hungary is a country that had a tumultuous history, and is currently transforming itself into a modern European state. One of its great challenges is to translate the ideal of equality—enshrined in its constitution and laws—particularly in relationship to its sizeable Roma (Gypsy) population. This ethnic minority group has been settled in Hungary for centuries, some tracing their roots to the 14th or 15th century. The Roma are very poor, with low levels of education and employment, and a multiplicity of health challenges, including a life expectancy 10 years lower than non-Roma. The vision in Hungary is a grand one and the result is of the greatest significance for Europe as a multi-ethnic continent.

The variety of responses in these countries is striking. Nonetheless, some pattern is discernible: first, an awareness of health problems and especially of a risk of infectious disease harming society as a whole; second, formal study of health status and health care by migration status, ethnic, or racial group; third, articulation of policy and plans sometimes backed by legislation; fourth, a move from policies of exclusion of minorities to the promotion of the welfare of minorities; fifth, specific actions to redress inequities; and, finally, an attempt to adapt general services to meet needs. The scale of the challenge is great and none of the six countries considered here has achieved the goal of demonstrably narrowing health inequalities or achieving equity of service.

References

Agyemang C, Bindraban N, Mairuhu G, Montfrans G van, Koopmans R, Stronks K (2005) Prevalence, awareness, treatment, and control of hypertension among Black Surinamese, South Asian Surinamese and White Dutch in Amsterdam, The Netherlands: the SUNSET study. *Journal of Hypertension* **23**: 1971–7.

Bos V, Kunst AE, Keij-Deerenberg IM, Mackenbach JM (2002) Mortality amongst immigrants in the Netherlands. *European Journal of Public Health* **12**: S41.

Gamble VN (1993) A legacy of distrust: African Americans and medical research. *American Journal of Preventive Medicine* **9**: 35–8.

Geronimus AT, Bound J, Waidmann TA, Hillemeier MM, Burns PB (1996) Excess mortality among blacks and whites in the United States. *New England Journal of Medicine* **21**: 1552–8.

Institute of Medicine–Committee on Understanding and Eliminating Racial and Ethnic Disparities in Health Care (2002) *Unequal Treatment: confronting racial and ethnic disparities in health care* (ed. BD Smedley, AY Stith, AR Nelson). Washington, DC: National Academies Press.

Johnson M (1984) Ethnic minorities and health. *Journal of the Royal College of Physicians London* **18**: 228–23.

Kiple KF, King V (1981) *Another Dimension to the Black Diaspora: diet, disease, and racism.* Cambridge: Cambridge University Press.

Krieger N (1992) The making of public health data: paradigms, politics, and policy. *Journal of Public Health Policy* **65**: 412–27.

La Veist TA, Wallace JM, Howard DL (1995) The color line and the health of African Americans. *Humboldt Journal of Social Relations* **21**: 119–37.

Patel VV, Rajpathak S, Karasz A (2012) Bangladeshi immigrants in New York City: a community based health needs assessment of a hard to reach population. *Journal of Immigrant and Minority Health* **14**: 767–73.

Porter R (1997) *The Greatest Benefit to Mankind—a medical history of humanity from antiquity to the present*. London: Harper Collins.

Scottish Executive Health Department (2002) *Fair For All: working together towards culturally competent services*, NHS HDL 51. Edinburgh: Scottish Executive.

Tesh SN (1988) *Hidden Arguments*. New Brunswick, NJ: Rutgers University Press.

Ward L (1993) Race equality and employment in the National Health Service. In **Ahmad WIU** (ed.), *'Race' and Health in Contemporary Britain*, pp. 167–82. Buckingham: Open University Press.

Wild S, McKeigue P (1997) Cross-sectional analysis of mortality by country of birth in England and Wales, 1970–92. *British Medical Journal* **314**: 705–10.

Other sources and further reading

Bhopal R (1997) Is research into ethnicity and health racist, unsound, or important science? *British Medical Journal* **314**: 1751–6.

Bhopal RS (1998) The spectre of racism in health and health care: lessons from history and the USA. *British Medical Journal* **316**: 1970–3.

Clyne MB (1964) Indian patients (general practitioners' forum). *Practitioner* **193**: 195–9.

Esmail A and Everington S (1993) Racial discrimination against doctors from ethnic minorities. *British Medical Journal* **306**: 691–2.

Hausfeld RG (1977) Social, ethnic and cultural aspects of Aboriginal health. *Australian Family Physician* **6**: 1301–7.

Krieger N (2000) Counting accountability: implications of the new approaches to classifying race/ethnicity in the 2000 census. *American Journal of Public Health* **90**: 1687–9.

Krieger N, Rowley D, Herman A (1993) Racism, sexism and social class: implications for studies of health, disease and wellbeing. *American Journal of Preventive Medicine* **9**: 82–122.

Whittle J, Conigliaro J, Good CB, Lofgren RP (1993) Racial differences in the use of invasive cardiovascular procedures in the Department of Veterans Affairs medical system. *New England Journal of Medicine* **329**: 621–7.

Wild SH, Fischbacher C, Brock A, Griffiths C, Bhopal R (2007) Mortality from all causes and circulatory disease by country of birth in England and Wales 2001–2003. *Journal of Public Health* **29**: 191–8.

Chapter 5

Assessing the health and health-care needs of migrant, racial, and ethnic minorities using quantitative and qualitative data

Objectives

After reading this chapter you should be able to:

- In outline, appreciate the purpose, principles and methods of health and health-care needs assessment at the population level.

- Understand the difficulties of undertaking health needs assessment in migrant, racial, and ethnic minority groups particularly when there is a lack of data.

- Given data, be able to devise and adopt frameworks to set out and interpret information, using approaches where the minority groups are compared against a standard (or reference) population and where data are examined for each group alone, i.e. relative and absolute risk approaches.

- Be able to explain how qualitative data can help to strengthen quantitative work, so increasing the validity and value of the health needs assessment.

- In outline, know the broad and potentially generalizable outcomes of key health needs assessments undertaken in minority groups in terms of health and demographic status, services needed, and service gaps.

5.1 Health needs assessment: an overview

Health needs assessment is a structured process to work out what the health problems of a population are and offer ways to resolve them, including estimating the resources needed. Health needs assessment requires the collection and use of a wide range of information, and hence it overlaps considerably with research, the subject of Chapter 9. Unlike research, however, its purpose is practical and specific, rather than the extension of theoretical and generalizable knowledge. The boundary between research and health needs assessment in the context of public health and health care is fuzzy. This chapter places an emphasis on understanding the ideas behind health needs assessment; the special role of epidemiology; optimizing use of existing information, whether statistics, specific reports, or general principles; the acquisition and interpretation of both quantitative and qualitative data; and taking advantage of the experience of others. In this chapter we will consider how health-care provision should be sensitive to the needs of all groups in society; how data can be used to plan better health care; and how multicultural societies might adapt to their changing population for the benefit of everyone.

5.1.1 **The concepts of health and health needs**

The ideas of health and health needs are, like beauty, to a very large extent in the eye of the beholder. Before reading on, you may wish to reflect briefly on these concepts by trying Exercise 5.1.

Exercise 5.1 Health and health needs

- ◆ What definition of health do you prefer and use?
- ◆ How would you measure health?
- ◆ Do you think definitions and concepts of health might vary by ethnic group? If so, in what way?
- ◆ What do you understand by the phrase 'health needs'?

There are many definitions of health, and most of them agree that health has physical, social, and psychological components and that it is not a static but a dynamic concept. The most famous, but sometimes derided, definition of health is that of the 1946 founding constitution of the WHO, i.e. that health is not merely the absence of disease or disability but a state of complete physical, mental, and social well-being. Some people would argue that a spiritual dimension should also be added, and this might be highly relevant to those groups whose identity is closely linked to religion, as often applies to migrant and minority racial and ethnic populations. Even then, this is not a complete definition of health. The indigenous (aboriginal) populations of the world give special significance to a connection to the land. While this is seldom made explicit, land is obviously important to everyone's health. It may have special significance for immigrants' sense of well-being, whether it be the homeland left behind or the new land adopted. Social networks also seem to be vitally important to mental health. Living close to people of the same ethnic group is sometimes decried by authorities who wish for dispersal and rapid assimilation, but there is evidence that it is good for mental health (not to mention economic progress). The main purpose of a WHO-type of definition, which is self-evidently not achievable, is to broaden thinking away from what is often described as the biomedical definition of health (the absence of medically defined illness, pathology, and disease) to embrace a psychosocial model. A working definition of health might be that health requires that people are alive, free of disabilities in so far as this is possible, and, irrespective of disabilities, are able to function well enough to achieve their potential and discharge their personal and social obligations. This working definition draws on public views of what health is.

Many tools exist for measuring aspects of health, and there are detailed discussions of this difficult task, which has been particularly well described by Ann Bowling (1997). From the point of view of this book, which is based on a public health approach, measures are needed which provide a summary of health status within populations generally and their migrant, racial, and ethnic subpopulations specifically. The best perspective for this is an epidemiological one whereby the health problems of groups are assessed in terms of their actual and relative frequency, expressed either as a prevalence or incidence or of the outcome of interest, or other summary statistics derived from such data (see the Glossary for definitions).

The phrase 'health need' is difficult to define. The book by Stevens and Raftery (1994) provides a detailed discussion. One interesting classification of need is 'Bradshaw's taxonomy of social need'.

This classification is a useful starting point because it illustrates that, as with health, the perspective of the beholder is crucial. Four types of need are identified:

1. *normative need* is that defined by an expert or professional;

2. *felt need* is what people want;

3. *expressed need* is what people want put into action (within the context of providing a service this is equivalent to the demand made upon that service); and

4. *comparative need* is identified by comparing populations.

In epidemiological and public health settings comparative and normative needs tend to dominate. Superficially, in an ideal world all needs would be met. It is possible, however, that in meeting all needs the recipients of the service are actually harmed. For example, experts and lay individuals might be wrong about a need, even one which was normative, felt, expressed, and comparative. Over the last 30 years or so we have witnessed a great demand for hormone replacement therapy after the menopause, at least partly driven by a professional view that this would protect against cardiovascular disease and even cancers and the lay view that the hormone keeps women youthful. Recently, large-scale clinical trials have concluded this is not true and this therapy increases the risk of cardiovascular diseases, does not, overall, protect against cancers, and increases the risk of breast cancer. The potential to provide net benefit after harms have been accounted for is therefore a crucial component of health needs.

Within the field of health care, most people, both health-care professionals and lay, recognize a hierarchy of need. They may not, however, find it easy or comfortable to make it explicit. As resources available to provide health care are limited it is not possible to meet all needs; those that are to be met should therefore be more important than those that are not. Clearly, one's perspective on needs changes with circumstances, over time, and with experience. A healthy person may extol the virtues of preventative medicine, but the person with serious disease, say breast cancer, may extol the value of high technology and potentially very costly health care directed at diagnosing, managing, and caring for those with the disease. Concepts of health and health-care need are shaped by culture and experience, and are likely to differ by ethnic group, particularly as the patterns of disease vary. That said, there will probably be many similarities too, as we discuss below.

5.1.2 **Health needs assessment**

The purpose of health needs assessment in public health is to assist in the planning and provision of health care. The definition that is most suitable here is the one taken from Stevens and Raftery (1994): 'the assessment of a population or community's health status and health care utilization patterns in relation to its ability to benefit from health care'. The emphasis is, therefore, on health care based on preventive or treatment services that have the potential to remedy health problems, whether the health problems are diseases, disease risk factors, disabilities, or lack of well-being. This does not imply a narrow clinical focus. Benefits go beyond the person with the health problem, such as benefit to carers; and 'health care' can include health promotion, rehabilitation, and palliative care. Some of the nuances of this definition are given in Box 5.1.

Health needs assessment requires a systematic, comprehensive overview of both quantitative and qualitative data on a population or subgroup of the population. It then needs to be applied to creating or adapting policies, strategies, and services to improve population health, through better health care. Health needs assessment in relation to migrant, racial, and ethnic minority groups is often problematic because of the lack of data, particularly at local level and at the level of subgroup

Box 5.1 The need for health care: the population's ability to benefit from health

- The population's ability to benefit from health care equals the aggregate of the individual's ability to benefit.*

- The ability to benefit does not mean that every outcome is guaranteed to be favourable, but rather that need implies the potential to benefit which is on average effective.

- The benefit is not just a question of clinical status, but can include reassurance, supportive care, and the relief of carers. Many individual health problems have a social impact via multiple knock-on effects or via a burden to families and carers. Hence the list of beneficiaries of care can extend beyond the patient.

- Health care includes not just treatment, but also prevention, diagnosis, continuing care, rehabilitation, and palliative care.†

* Sometimes the population benefit exceeds the sum of individual benefits, e.g. immunization may stop an epidemic spreading even to unimmunized people (so-called herd immunity). † Health care can also include advocacy for social and environmental change e.g. research and practice to bring about a ban on smoking in public places.

Source: Data from Stevens, A., and Raftery, J., *NHS Executive publication: Health Care Needs Assessment: the epidemiologically based needs assessment reviews*, Radcliffe Medical Press, Oxford, UK, Copyright © 1994.

detail that is required. For national health needs assessments, data available from administrative databases, usually recording broad racial or ethnic categories or country of birth, may need to be used. The limitations of such data need to be understood to avoid making poor decisions, but equally their strength and value must not be overlooked. In addition to lack of data there may be lack of time, funds, expertise, political will, and means of implementing the findings. Health needs assessment of migrant, racial, and ethnic minority health is too often limited to qualitative studies, or even simply consultations with selected members of the minority communities (sometimes only leaders) or just health professionals.

Modern health-care systems have found it difficult to adapt themselves to meet the needs of minority groups, even when legislation, policy, policy analysis, and research are in place (see Chapter 8 and 9). Health needs assessment is important to the achievement of the patient-centred and equity-oriented goals of all modern health-care systems in multi-ethnic societies, and to the narrowing of inequalities in health. The task is difficult—and it needs good quality quantitative and qualitative information to underpin it.

Before reading on, try Exercise 5.2.

Exercise 5.2 Data for health needs assessment and problems envisaged

- In general terms what kind of data would help you to assess health needs?

- What problems can you foresee in relation to gaining, interpreting, and using such data?

The quantitative component of the needs assessment for minority populations should start by examining the actual health status, disease patterns, and health-care utilization within each migrant, racial, or ethnic group. This is the so-called absolute risk approach. The findings can also be compared either with other minority groups or with the majority population; this is the relative risk approach. In most instances, at least in European, North American, and Australasian countries where non-White populations are in the minority, the standard, reference population for comparison is the White population. This form of comparison is usual practice and is done for ease, habit, ethnocentrism, availability of data, or statistical power. (The statistical power argument does not actually apply in all forms of analysis.)

An alternative approach is to set the standard or reference comparison as the group with the most desirable level of the health outcome under study. If this was done in the UK, the Chinese population would be the standard for overall mortality and many specific diseases too. That would give high-level and very challenging health targets for all other ethnic groups in the UK, including White populations. In Chapter 6 I discuss how using the relative risk approach alone could even widen inequalities, and in Chapter 9 I consider this issue in the context of research.

The problem with quantitative information is that it is difficult and expensive to obtain, it requires epidemiological and statistical skills for analysis and interpretation, and it is open to abuse, as discussed in Chapters 1 and 9. Abuses include using data to show that a minority group has worse health, and then to use this to denigrate, stigmatize, discriminate, or even directly harm the group. The extreme example of this was in Nazi Germany (see Chapter 6), but it is common to see negative portrayals in the media that focus on the health disadvantages of minorities, omitting their health advantages. The step from analysis and interpretation to beneficial use of the data is a tough one and needs an appropriate political and strategic framework for success (see Chapters 9 and 10).

Qualitative data enrich, augment, and validate the health needs analysis by adding opinions, beliefs, perceptions, attitudes, and self-reported behaviour, and often provide surprisingly effective case history material. Such data are particularly valuable when collected and analysed in a rigorous way. Having said this, we need to exercise caution in regard to qualitative data based on casual opinions and perceptions, particularly if they reinforce stereotyping. Health needs assessments using quantitative information have shown that perceptions of the needs of minorities are often erroneous, e.g. on perceived levels of immunization (perceived low, but actually often high), overall life expectancy (perceived as worse, actually often better or similar), availability of health education materials in relation to disease patterns (little material for the dominant fatal and serious conditions and more for conditions perceived by professionals to be important, e.g. birth control, hygiene, etc.). Stereotyping is easy and potentially misleading, yet it is important to use constructively the information content on migration status, race, and ethnicity. We cannot assume that a person possesses a particular behaviour or health characteristic on the grounds that they are a member of a particular migrant or ethnic group. The usefulness of recording a patient's migrant or ethnic origin, using a simple label such as refugee, Aborigine, Indian, White, or Chinese, without taking account of other factors is clearly limited. Within every population subgroup there are significant variations in social class, culture, and customs. For example, whether a person needs an interpreter cannot be judged from the label Bangladeshi, but it can from knowledge of the languages spoken and preferred. Similarly, the label Indian does not inform (and may misinform) about the need for 'halal' food in hospital but the fact that an Indian person is a Muslim indicates, but no more than that, that halal food is much more likely to be needed than in the average patient. The knowledge in the label is probabilistic and applies to groups of people but needs to be checked at individual level. This does not mean that we can always dismiss generalizations, or even that all stereotypes are wrong. Some are accurate: needs do vary substantially by ethnic group; minority ethnic groups are better off in some respects and worse in others; service quality, particularly for health promotion and preventive health issues requiring knowledge, is usually worse for minority groups; the cost of care for minority populations (but not necessarily over-all) is higher; the needs of minority groups include better communication; and meeting cultural needs often requires religious and dietary preferences being met and health professionals being educated about such matters. There is, however, a fine dividing line between general principles derived from detailed observation and research, and stereotypes based on cursory observation or no observation at all.

The central question that drives health needs assessment for minority populations is this: in what ways are their health needs similar to, and different from, the (usually majority) population that the health-care system has evolved to serve?

Before reading on, you should reflect on how you would answer this question by doing Exercise 5.3.

Exercise 5.3 Similarities and differences

- Is the approach of examining differences sound?
- What, in general terms, is such an analysis going to show?
- In what way can we give appropriate emphasis to similarities?
- What are the pitfalls of emphasizing differences?

The answer to the central question is usually complex. In fact, many differences are easily dem-onstrated but the similarities may be even more overwhelming. Differences can be exaggerated, both because of the human tendency to find them interesting and the scientific approach of using them as the starting point for research, especially in epidemiology. Health needs assessments, as a result, tend to present data to highlight and accentuate differences at the expense of similari-ties. This can give a biased viewpoint on priorities. Mackintosh et al.'s (1998) *Step-by-Step Guide to Epidemiological Health Needs Assessment* (which I led and draw on extensively in this book), shows how to avoid this problem. A comprehensive needs assessment following the principles of the *Step-by-Step Guide* was published by Gill et al. (2007), who showed that the UK's major health priorities were largely applicable to the main minority ethnic groups in the UK. In particular, Gill et al. showed that the emphasis on cardiovascular diseases, cancers, mental health, and other health problems of modern societies is applicable to all ethnic groups they assessed. However, this does not imply that no change in approach, or refinement of services, is needed. A few diseases and problems not figuring in the UK's declared priorities deserve a prominent place in the context of minority ethnic health, e.g. haemoglobinopathies and tuberculosis. This must not, however, be at the expense of the main priorities, but in addition to them. It might be argued that it is unfair for minorities to get additional priorities beyond those agreed as national ones. The point is a small one but, nonetheless, it is important to respond to it as a matter of principle. In fact there are many services that are needed in the majority population much more than in minorities, but these are seldom noted. For example, minorities are usually under-represented in the common cancer services, in services for the very elderly, and for some genetic diseases including cystic fibrosis. The point is that there is no 'special pleading' in the case of minorities—just a case of equitable treatment. The importance of not being overly swayed by differences is well illustrated by the example of stroke and CHD in the African Caribbean population of the UK. Stroke mortality is relatively high in this ethnic group, while CHD mortality rates are comparatively low. Superficially, one may judge that for this ethnic group stroke services and prevention ought to take priority over CHD. CHD, however, is a much commoner cause of death in African Caribbeans than stroke is, as a count of cases shows. Neglecting CHD in favour of stroke would miss the bigger problem and run the risk of the African Caribbean community losing its relative advantage in regard to CHD over the population as a whole. (This has already happened to African Americans who were in an analogous situation in the United States.) The remainder of this chapter concerns the thinking and methods underlying health needs assessment.

5.2 The questions driving data collection in health needs assessment

Health needs assessment is an ongoing, dynamic process, and this is particularly true when it is focused on rapidly changing migrant, racial, and ethnic minority populations. This dynamism and sense of change is reflected in the questions and steps outlined in this section. The process is based on data, but the data themselves are not the health needs assessment. Needs can be assessed in absolute or actual terms and in relative terms, or both. In practice, the relative approach plays a dominant role and this is something that can be a 'Catch 22' for migrant and ethnic minority populations—in that if there are no differences or the problem is less than in the majority population this may be interpreted as there being no (special) need. So, to gain attention, assessors of the needs of minority populations draw attention to health problems in relative excess, which creates the wrong impression that minorities are in extremely poor health. This in turn can create stigma as the minority is seen as a liability, creating a strain on health-care resources. It is for this reason that a needs assessment must be balanced and relatively comprehensive. While the focus of a needs assessment may be on minority groups, what is learnt may well be used to benefit the entire population, especially, but not solely, when examining health from a relative perspective.

Eight key questions that relate well to the ten steps in Table 5.1 that drive health needs assessment are as follows:

1. What are the demographic and social characteristics of the minority groups in the area and how are these changing? (Section 5.2.1)

2. What are the cultures and lifestyles of the minority populations and how are they changing? (Section 5.2.2)

3. What illnesses and diseases affect the minority populations and in what quantity, and how are these changing? (Sections 5.2.3–5.2.7)

4. What services are available for these conditions and how are they adapting to meet the needs of the minority groups? (Section 5.2.8)

5. How well are services meeting needs, and what plans are already in place to improve them? (Section 5.3)

6. What do the public and professionals think about the services (Sections 5.3.2 and 5.4) and are they being used efficiently and effectively? (Section 5.5)

7. How can services for minority groups be evaluated and audited? (Section 5.6)

8. What changes are needed to help services meet needs better? (Chapters 5, 7, and 8.)

Rawaf and Marshall's (1999) ten steps for health needs assessment, originally applied to drug misuse, are illustrative of the process (see Table 5.1).

Table 5.1 The ten steps for needs assessment

Step 1	Profile your population. Source of data: census data, population registries, health and social population surveys, specific surveys and research studies, projections, professional and lay judgements
Step 2	Measure the extent of the problem/issue. Source of data: analysis of national and local statistics on causes of illness, disease, and death (and of linked databases)
Step 3	Calculate the expected number of cases. Apply the best possible mortality or incidence/prevalence rate data to the population or a group of the population in a given geographical area at a given time (year) to estimate the expected number of cases
Step 4	Collect and analyse routine data on service utilization (current and trends). Source of data: General and mental hospital activity statistics; inpatient, day case, and outpatient data; community service statistics; and social service and other relevant activity statistics
Step 5	Calculate the unmet needs or excessive service provision: compare your expected number of cases with the current number of cases using services and the capacity of the service to identify the size of possible unmet needs or surplus services
Step 6	Segment your population into different strata (population segmentation): once the population structure is dissected and the estimate of the disease burden by various age groups, sex, migrant status, ethnic group, etc. has been determined, it would be useful to segment the population in terms of their ability to benefit from the intervention
Step 7	Review the current evidence on the effectiveness of intervention(s): as effectiveness studies by migrant status, or racial and ethnic group are rare, a general review will almost certainly be needed
Step 8	Measure your population's perceptions and expectations: focus in particular on people's understanding of the issues, and utilization and quality of services
Step 9	Seek the opinions of professionals about solutions to the problems, best practices, and service delivery
Step 10	Project the type and size of the action programmes and services needed to deal with the identified problem in a unified written health needs assessment that incorporates all ten steps

Adapted from Rawaf, S. and Marshall, F., Drug Misuse: The Ten Steps for Needs Assessment, *Public Health Medicine*, Volume 1, pp. 21–26, Copyright © 1999, with permission from the authors.

5.2.1 What are the demographic and social characteristics of the minority groups in the area and how are these changing?

Demography is the study of the structure of and change in populations based, in particular, on the census (or population registry) and vital registration statistics on births, deaths, migrations, and marriages. Such data are most accurate around the census year (in many countries the census is decennial, i.e. it occurs every 10 years). Between census years, and also in some places even in the census year, e.g. in the inner city, information is not very accurate, especially for small areas and younger people. Despite its limitations there is no serious alternative to a census. In some countries, such as The Netherlands, there is a population register, usually held and managed at city level. Such registers have the benefit of being continuously updated, but they have very limited data on the social and economic circumstances of the registrants. Also it is difficult for the data on registers to be verified. Census data can, by contrast, be cross-checked against estimates obtained from registers. The most reliable method of obtaining information by migration status, race, and ethnic group is a census. For those wishing to assess needs of minority populations, the highest priority is for a census that includes the relevant data. The census is usually a strictly confidential data collection exercise where the personal data cannot be used for other non-statistical purposes. By contrast, population registers are designed for other official, administrative purposes. Undocumented migrants will almost certainly be absent from registers. They are supposed to be counted in a census, although in practice they may not be. In an environment of mistrust, or when the principles of self-assignment are unclear, people may not provide the required data at census; e.g. in Chapter 4 we considered the undercount of Roma people in Hungary in the 2001 census.

For a number of reasons several countries are reviewing the needs for censuses, with the aim of phasing them out. The reasons include the desire for financial savings, the ever-present worries about the intrusiveness of the state collecting personal data, and the new potential created by computerized data linkage. If this happens there are likely to be important consequences for the field of migration, race, and ethnicity. Specifically, the assessment of health needs will become more difficult.

The 1991, 2001, and 2011 censuses in the UK offer rich opportunities for studying Britain's multi-ethnic populations. For the first time health authorities have relatively comprehensive data on the demography and social circumstances of their ethnic minority populations, which can be used to assess needs and plan services. Furthermore, epidemiology, which was previously limited largely to analysis by country of birth (thereby resulting in the omission of about half of the South Asian and Black populations who are born in Britain), has been revolutionized by the availability of population denominators from the census. Now data can be analysed by ethnic group, country of birth, and religion, and be enriched by stratified analyses. In 2011 language was added to the census, opening new possibilities.

The UK censuses, in common with those of other countries, also have questions on long-term illness, occupation, housing conditions, family structure, economic circumstances, education, etc., and so a picture of the minority population can be built up from this one source of information.

Unfortunately, members of minority groups are more likely than average to be missed by the census, which is also the case for those living in inner city areas (also characteristic of minority groups) and for younger age groups (characteristic of minority groups), and so their census-derived numbers may be erroneously low. The census offices are likely to give estimates of the undercount.

The interpretation of health statistics by migrant status or ethnic group is based on the assumptions that country of birth ethnicity categories are valid and consistently defined and ascertained, that questions are understood by the populations questioned, that participation and response rates are high and similar for all populations questioned, and that people's responses are consistent over time. These assumptions cannot be taken for granted for reasons that are discussed throughout this book, but particularly in Chapters 2 and 3.

The census usually provides information on a population in relation to population structure (age, sex, marital status, etc.) and on many aspects of socio-economic circumstances (employment, housing, and so on). Local health or government authorities may have commissioned reports or even local censuses or surveys about the local population that will augment or update the census data. Usually, however, we need to examine national data and extrapolate to our locality, either qualitatively or quantitatively, from those.

Professionals may have knowledge of the make-up of their local population, and in some instances their understanding may be deeper and more up to date than that from statistical sources, particularly where there is a rapid change in the composition of the population, possibly through recent relocation or migration, e.g. of asylum seekers and refugees, or seasonal workers, where change can be very rapid. However, practitioners usually do not know the numbers of people by migrant or ethnic group, and in particular may not be able to differentiate subgroups, e.g. Punjabi Indians and Punjabi Pakistanis. Census offices usually predict changes in the size and composition of the population. Population change by migrant and ethnic minority groups is usually only available at national level or in regions where the population is very large. Lack of such information is problematic because the size and distribution of the minority population is essential for health-care planning.

It may be surprising that in assessing health and health-care needs our most important information requirement is not health status but demography and social/economic circumstances. Without the demographic data, population-based rates cannot be calculated and health status measured, and without the social/economic data health status cannot be understood, as we consider below.

5.2.2 **What are the cultures and lifestyles of the minority populations and how are they changing?**

Demographic and socio-economic data paint the background picture and help in the interpretation of information on more specific health-related lifestyles. For example, the level of physical activity, which is so important for disease prevention, in a specific population needs to be interpreted in the light of the residential area, the fabric of the homes, the occupational circumstances, and economic well-being of this population.

Culture and lifestyle are major determinants of health. All aspects of culture and lifestyle which are important for the general population are important for minorities, including smoking, alcohol, exercise, diet, and stress. There are massive differences between migrant, racial, and ethnic groups in health-related behaviours. These will be substantially affected by cultural influences such as religion; e.g. Sikkism prohibits intoxicants including tobacco and alcohol. Of course, people may not adhere to religious prohibitions, and many Sikhs (men mostly) disobey prohibitions on alcohol consumption yet follow those on tobacco. These general lifestyle risks factors must not be overlooked when undertaking health promotion with ethnic minorities. It sometimes happens that attention is diverted by some more specific issue. Other lifestyle issues worth noting in some communities, including the Sikhs, include the use of traditional substances that may contain potential toxic metals such as eye cosmetics (kohl or surma), self-treatment with herbal and other remedies, and a strong sense of modesty, especially among women, which may affect their health (e.g. vitamin D deficiency as a result of inadequate exposure to sunshine) and health care (reluctance to have physical examinations especially of reproductive areas). Many such traditional customs have been recorded and much attention has been given to them. Indeed, sometimes this kind of topic, e.g. female genital mutilation, can become the dominating discourse in relation to migrant, racial, and ethnic minorities. However, their overall importance to health is usually relatively small in comparison with lifestyle matters that are general such as alcohol, tobacco, exercise, or diet. This poses a dilemma, especially when resources are limited and choices need to be made (see Chapter 7).

Information on health-related culture and lifestyle is almost invariably based on self-report, although there are rare studies that either use an objective measure (e.g. accelerometers for physical activity) or observations. These alternative approaches are interesting but tend to corroborate self-report data. There are many difficulties in comparing ethnic groups using self-reported health and lifestyle data.

Before reading on reflect on some of the uses of self-report data, difficulties in making comparisons, and the questions to ask, by doing Exercise 5.4.

Exercise 5.4 Difficulties in comparing self-report data on lifestyles

- What difficulties do you envisage in comparing data on the health-related lifestyles of different migrant, racial, and ethnic groups. (Examples of lifestyles you might wish to consider include smoking, exercise, diet, and alcohol.)
- What uses might you make of self-report data on lifestyles in health settings? (Consider clinical care, research, and planning.)

Some uses of self-reported data are given in Box 5.2.

The most important questions to ask to help interpret self-report data on lifestyles are these:

- Are the populations comparable? It is common practice to draw samples for different minority groups using different methods, times, or locations. Differences are inevitable when this happens, and may have little or no relation to migration status, race, or ethnicity. For example, if the minority populations are inner city ones and the comparison population is a mix of urban and rural people differences may well reflect geography not ethnicity.
- Are the data collected equally well and accurately in the different groups? The concepts underpinning questions (let us say on angina) may be interpreted differently in different groups. Where questions need translating the potential pitfalls are magnified. Apparent differences in migrant, racial, and ethnic group may arise from non-comparable questions.

Hunt and Bhopal (2004) have offered guidelines on how to maximize the cross-cultural comparability of self-report data. Some of the key principles are given in Box 5.3.

Collecting valid lifestyle data by ethnic group is difficult. Even if the topics are carefully chosen, the study is designed well, and the data collection instruments are cross-culturally valid (all tough goals), finding a list or register to use as a sampling frame, recruiting people, collecting data, interpreting the results correctly, and using them to achieve better health and health care are all taxing challenges. These and other matters will be discussed in Chapter 9 in a research context. An increasing number of surveys are available, nonetheless, with data of variable quality (see chapter references and websites).

One good example of how such data can be used is the observation of the high prevalence of tobacco use and oral tobacco in UK Bangladeshi men in particular and Muslim men more

---

Box 5.2 Uses of self-report data

- As an integral part of the clinical history taken by doctors and other health professionals.
- In standardized questionnaires for the assessment of general health status, to assess degree of disability, to check for the presence and severity of symptoms, or to gather patient-assessed outcomes.
- As a part of an epidemiological study, e.g. gathering data on health-related behaviour, and in tools such as the Rose Angina Questionnaire.
- In studies of satisfaction with health care, e.g. women's views of maternity services.
- As a component of health needs assessment for planning and targeting of services.

Box 5.3 State of the art translation/adaptation procedures

- Translation of items by a team of bilingual people
- Comparison of translations
- Negotiation of 'best' items
- Consultations with people who are monolingual in the target language(s)
- Item refinement
- Field testing with monolingual people
- Refinements as needed
- Testing for face, content, construct, and criterion validity in each language
- Testing for reliability and responsiveness
- Statistical analysis of ratings of quality of translation across different countries

Reproduced from Hunt, S. and Bhopal, R. Self report in clinical and epidemiological studies with non-English speakers the challenge of language and culture, *Journal of Epidemiology and Community Health*, Volume 58, pp. 618–22, Copyright © 2004, with permission from BMJ Publishing Group Ltd.

---

generally. Until the data became available, smoking control and cessation policies and programmes paid little or no attention to the needs of ethnic minorities, and especially South Asians. The revelation that the highest prevalence of smoking in the UK is in Bangladeshi men and that smoking cessation rates in ethnic minority groups are comparatively low focused policy, service, and research attention on the issue. In England, this problem was corrected over a period of just a few years.

Surveys tend to paint a static picture, whereas the reality is one of rapid change. In particular, the children of migrants are often growing up with strikingly different cultural influences and lifestyles compared with their parents. The picture emerging from studies of the children of migrants indicates, unsurprisingly, that many of the lifestyles of the parents are carried forward, even as those of the majority host population are acquired. Whether children will acquire the best or worst of both worlds is yet to be seen. Among the fast growing group of children are those born to parents of different races or ethnic groups. These children are usually referred to as mixed race, a term that has been shown by Aspinall (2010) to be favoured by young people. Data on this group are sparse but are a priority as there are some warning signs of health problems, e.g. a high prevalence of smoking. Keeping track of rapid change poses an additional but vital challenge to health needs assessment.

5.2.3 Which illnesses and diseases affect the ethnic minority populations and to what extent?

Most illnesses and diseases that health needs assessors will be interested in are fairly rare, and fortunately this is especially so for deaths in modern, well-off countries—just over 1% of the population dies in any year. Except in some regions with very large minority ethnic populations, usually those containing major multi-ethnic cities such as London, New York, and Amsterdam, local information on causes of death will be hard to make sense of because the numbers of deaths per year will be small and disease rates will be estimated imprecisely and will fluctuate over time. The commonest disabling or potentially killing diseases (e.g. asthma, diabetes) tend to have population prevalences of 5–10%, and this prevalence may vary considerably by migrant, racial, and ethnic group. So specific health needs assessments for such disorders are not likely to be possible at local level. The result is that a comprehensive health needs assessment that examines a range of migrant and ethnic groups will require large populations, perhaps national ones. One such comprehensive assessment was achieved by Gill et al. (2007), mostly by examining data for England and Wales around the 1991 census. The population was 52 million people. Mostly, reasonably precise and interpretable data were compiled for each of the major countries of birth and/or ethnic groups enumerated at the 1991 census. By contrast, in Scotland, where the minority populations are much smaller, even with the Scottish Health and Ethnicity Linkage Study of 4.65 million people (90% of the population) and 7–9 years of outcome data, it has been impossible to provide precise estimates across the full range of ethnic groups. Many health needs assessments are done at health authority level, typically serving populations of 100 000–750 000 people. What can such work say about migrant, racial, and ethnic minorities?

Knowing the make-up of the local ethnic minority community, however, it should be possible to infer the major health problems by applying the findings from national data to the local population. For example, if breast cancer incidence rates and rates of uptake of breast cancer mammography are both low in a minority population at national level, they are also likely to be low in your locality. Even in the complete absence of data on the causes of death in the minority group of interest remember that disease patterns are likely to be similar to those of the general population, e.g. CHD and strokes are among the top-ranking fatal diseases for virtually all groups in industrialized countries. So, we can use health needs assessments for the general population. Usually, however, there are some national data.

Another set of insights applicable to minority groups comes from the disease patterns in the countries of ancestral origin. In some cases these insights are obvious, e.g. haemoglobinopathies are common in sub-Saharan equatorial regions of Africa, the Middle East and India and these genetic problems are likely to be important in populations who originate from these places wherever they live. Genetic diseases are a relatively fixed feature of a population. The knowledge gained by studying disease patterns in countries of origin may, however, be much more subtle, especially for environmentally acquired problems. An appreciation that oral cancers are common in the Indian subcontinent and nasopharyngeal cancers common in China would alert the needs assessors (and clinicians) to these problems in the overseas populations of Indian and Chinese origin, respectively. There is, however, a demand and need for real data that pertain to the population under assessment. Leaving aside psychological factors, real data are required because of the rapid change in disease patterns. While it is likely that the disease patterns of the minority groups will converge towards those in the population as a whole the pace of change is not predictable, and for some diseases (cardiovascular diseases and diabetes especially) there may be an overshoot.

Information on the pattern of non-fatal ill-health (morbidity) in groups is usually much more difficult to obtain than death data. Morbidity outcomes are much commoner than deaths, so the problems of statistical imprecision are fewer. The challenges of migration status and racial and ethnic coding are slowly being overcome, and it is likely that morbidity data are going to become much more readily available. You may, however, have to do your own local survey. Population- and clinic-level registers of people with particular conditions, e.g. people with diabetes, are increasingly common and awareness of the importance of including migrant and ethnic origins is increasing. For example, in Scotland the NHS requires every health board to maintain a register of people with diabetes. The local diabetes centre (or other specialist centre) should have a list of all people with known diabetes and it may be possible to identify people from the minority community—perhaps using a mix of data, e.g. self-report of race or ethnicity and name analysis (although this will only apply to specific groups, as discussed in Chapter 3). Linkage methods might also help acquire additional information, e.g. on country of birth and parental country of birth that are in The Netherlands' population registries, or in the censuses of most countries.

Information on diseases or other outcomes (numerators), on its own, is of limited use (although the method for calculating proportional mortality/morbidity is one solution), but used with the census for the denominators (population at risk) it will be possible to calculate disease incidence or prevalence rates by country of birth, or racial and ethnic group, or both. With improvements in monitoring of migration status, race, and ethnicity, reliable data on numbers of people with specific illnesses ought to become available from hospitals and other service providers. (Ethnic monitoring was discussed in Chapter 3, and the policies underpinning it will be discussed in Chapter 8.) Interpreting hospital records is difficult compared with mortality data and population disease registry data, because hospitals do not tend to serve a specific geographical area and the population using them is not easy to define.

GP records in the UK and equivalent primary care/family practice records in other countries are a potentially useful source of information on numbers of people with specific conditions. These kinds of records are particularly useful when the primary care service is for a defined population, usually meaning a registered population, thus providing a denominator for the calculation of rates. This is the case in the UK. Although GP records in the UK do not routinely state ethnicity, it is common for people from certain minority groups in a city to be registered with a small number of GPs, sometimes because one or more of the GPs belong to the same groups(s), who may be able to both identify people for data collection and describe their needs based on their own experience. The case for migrant and ethnic health monitoring via GP records is strong, particularly as the relevant data can be forwarded to specialists on referral (this topic was discussed in Chapter 3.) As with hospital records, a major change is under way and we can anticipate many new data on minority health from primary care. Some important work has already been published, both on disease rates and quality of care, that has demonstrated its value.

There may have been some research carried out into the health and disease patterns of minority groups locally and so reports and scientific papers may be available. In most instances, however, local estimates will need to be obtained by applying national rates to the local population, e.g. if approximately 20% of South Asians aged 35–64 nationally have diabetes, it can be estimated that 20% or one in five of your local South Asian population within this age group will probably have the disease. This simple procedure can be applied to any condition. Where there are no national studies, it is necessary to apply data from local research studies carried out in other areas. For example, data on the health of the Chinese population are comparatively rare. However, it would be possible for someone working in, say, Manchester, England to use data from the study in Newcastle, England reported on by Unwin et al. (1997) and apply it to their population. Unwin et al. attempted to recruit all Chinese people in the city aged between 25 and 64 years, and did detailed measurements including both self-report on diagnosed diabetes and the OGTT, one of the most reliable tests for diabetes. (Blood is taken for measurement of glucose after an overnight fast and again 2 h after 75 g of glucose is ingested.) This kind of research is understandably rare because it is time-consuming and costly. From the age-adjusted figures in Table 5.2 the disease rate for men from the Chinese community in Newcastle who have diabetes was found to be almost twice that of the European origin (Europid was the preferred term of the investigators) population. (Overall, glucose tolerance is similar.)

Table 5.2 The numbers, proportions (in parentheses), and age-adjusted rates (with 95% confidence intervals) for Europid and Chinese men in Newcastle upon Tyne with glucose intolerance in relation to age group

	No.		Impaired glucose tolerance		Diabetes		All glucose intolerance	
	Chinese	Europids	Chinese	Europids	Chinese	Europids	Chinese	Europids
Men								
25–34	53	42	2 (3.8)	3 (7.1)	0	0	2 (3.8)	3 (7.1)
35–44	51	77	3 (5.9)	7 (9.1)	3 (5.9)	1 (1.3)	6 (11.8)	8 (10.4)
45–54	43	81	3 (7.0)	9 (11.1)	3 (7.0)	5 (6.2)	6 (14.0)	14 (17.3)
55–64	32	104	6 (18.8)	19 (18.3)	3 (9.4)	6 (5.8)	9 (28.1)	25 (24.0)
All	179	304	14 (7.8)	38 (12.5)	9 (5.0)	12 (3.9)	23 (12.8)	50 (16.4)
Age adjusted			8.0	10.7	5.0	2.9	13.0	13.6
(95% CI)			(4.0, 12.0)	(7.2, 14.2)	(1.8, 8.2)	(1.0, 4.8)	(8.1, 17.9)	(9.7, 17.5)

Reproduced from Unwin N et al, Body mass index, waist circumference, waist-hip ratio, and glucose intolerance in Chinese and Europid adults in Newcastle, UK, *Journal of Epidemiology and Community Health*, Volume 51, pp. 160–66, Copyright © 1997, with permission from BMJ Publishing Group Ltd.

Detailed data of these kind are often only available from expensive research projects and it is important to use them, but how can we increase confidence that the findings can be generalized? First, we can check whether the Newcastle Chinese population is similar in its characteristics to that in the other places where the information is to be applied, e.g. in age and sex structure, region of family origin in China, religion, height, weight, etc. Some of this comparison (age, sex structure) can be done using census data. Second, we can see whether the local findings on a more easily obtained data item, e.g. self-reported diabetes, are comparable between the research report and other information sources, say, national data. Self-report alone may also show diabetes to be more common in Chinese than in White Europeans (though the prevalence in self-report will be lower, the relative differences may be similar). If so, confidence on generalizability is increased.

Once the quantitative data are obtained, the description and interpretation of disease patterns is based on epidemiological approaches. Accurate interpretation is vital to health needs assessment and is discussed in Section 5.2.4.

5.2.4 Epidemiological approaches to the presentation and interpretation of quantitative data

Epidemiological approaches to health needs assessment produce data showing actual and relative morbidity and mortality rates, more complex measure such as years of life lost, prevalence of diseases and risk factors, and the impact and loss of social functioning. In assessing the health needs of minority groups, the most popular approach has been to compare their health status with that of the population as a whole or the majority, i.e. very often in this field the White population of European origin. Thus a disease that is commoner in the minority than in the White population is declared a problem and a relatively higher priority than one that is less common than in the White population. This comparative perspective, which is intrinsically ethnocentric, has some merit but it can also be misleading. By concentrating on issues where the problem is in excess, attention may be given to a narrow range of issues and drawn away from ensuring that all health services are equitable and available to all. This approach may lead to some needs of minorities being sidelined in relation to their importance—this has happened with respiratory diseases and lung cancer. The principles are illustrated with mortality data, focusing on the standardized mortality/morbidity ratio (SMR). The SMR is a summary measure of the rate of disease or death in a population that takes into account differences in the age structure of populations. The standard or reference population is given a value of 100. A SMR exceeding 100 means an excess of the health problem in the study population, and a value of less than 100 means a deficit.

Historically, and possibly even currently, the most important data on the health status of populations come from mortality registers. These data are used to make important decisions on priorities for health care and research funding at every level—from global work led by WHO or the World Bank or at health authority level, say planning for a population of 500 000. In many countries a death certificate is a legal requirement that needs completion by a doctor or other authorized person prior to burial or cremation. The death certificate typically contains personal identification data and the date and cause(s) of death. If death certificates included data on migrant status, race, and ethnic group the information could be used for health surveillance internationally. To do this usefully requires corresponding data, using similar categories, on the population in which the deaths occurred. This would permit construction of death rates, i.e. the number of deaths divided by the population at risk of death, either overall or for a specific cause. This has indeed been possible in many countries for country of birth. We will consider the value of this shortly.

Self-identified race or ethnicity is obviously problematic for mortality data, as it would need to be collected before death. One potential answer to this problem is data linkage, as discussed in Section 5.2.5. Information on the deceased's race or ethnic group could also be provided by the person registering the death (the informant). The informant is usually a close member of the family or a close friend, so the quality of the data would be expected to be good. Alternatively, the person completing the death certificate might provide the information. The information could be extracted from the medical record or administrative system if it had been collected. The United States has been a leader in this regard. In the US standard certificate of death (modified at state level) birthplace, ethnic group (Hispanic with four options, or not Hispanic) and race with 15 options is completed by the funeral director using information as provided by the informant if available. Instructions on the way to complete these questions and the reasoning for doing this are provided, i.e. for identifying and rectifying health problems. Race and ethnicity are not placed on the publicly available, certified copy of the death certificate but are used for statistical purposes.

These kinds of data, especially race or ethnicity, are rarely found on death certificates in other countries. In Scotland, in 2011, a national consultation showed widespread support for adding ethnic group to the death certificate. The registrar whose role it is to register deaths, births, and marriages requests this information from the informant, having explained that the data are being collected for health research purposes. The scheme has been a success, with virtually all informants supplying data even though they are offered the option to refuse. In many places, including the UK and across much of mainland Europe, country of birth is recorded both on death certificates and in census returns or population registries. Information on mortality by country of birth is potentially common although in many countries the data have not been analysed.

An example is shown in Figure 5.1, an analysis of CHD mortality in England and Wales by country of birth. The number of deaths, from death certificates, and the population from the 1991 census was used to calculate the rates. The bars (by sex) represent broadly based populations born in particular countries or regions of the world. The x-axis shows the SMR, which the

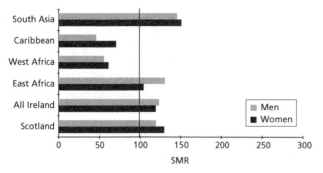

Fig. 5.1 Cross-sectional analysis of mortality in England and Wales, 1970–92, by country of birth.

Reproduced with permission of Sarah Wild. Graph presented previously on British Heart Foundation heart statistics website http://www.bhf.org.uk/research/heart-statistics/heart-statistics-publications.aspx. Source: Data from Wild S and McKeigue P, Cross-sectional analysis of mortality by country of birth in England and Wales, 1970–1992, *British Medical Journal*, Volume 314, pp. 705–10, Copyright © 1997.

measure used to take into account differences in the age distribution of the populations. Here the standard or reference population is that of people born in England and Wales. Their disease rates are represented by the line marked 100. The disease rates for other groups can be interpreted as a percentage of the rate for England and Wales. Before reading on, try Exercise 5.5.

Exercise 5.5 Analysis of heart disease mortality in England and Wales by country of birth

- In what way does this analysis shed light on the health of migrants and racial or ethnic minorities?

- What potential limitations can you see in accepting that the variations in mortality shown in Figure 5.1 are true?

- Specifically, what errors might be present in the numbers of deaths, and the numbers of the population at risk, that are required to produce the disease rates that underlie the calculation of the SMRs?

We have touched on country of birth and its value in true migration studies and its use as an indicator of race or ethnicity. Country of birth provides a fair guide to race or ethnicity for recent migrants, particularly older people. It is not good for very long-established populations, e.g. populations of African origin in Brazil, the Caribbean, and the United States, which have (largely) been settled there for hundreds of years. It is good for populations of African origin in most of Europe, Australia, and New Zealand. However, even in relatively new immigrant groups, a surprisingly large proportion of the population might be born in the host country. The reason for this is that migrants tend to be in the age group (20–40 years) when raising a family is important and they also generally have slightly larger families than host populations. Currently, 40–50% of people from non-White minority ethnic groups in the UK, e.g. Indians, Pakistanis, and Chinese, were born there (with higher proportions among younger people) so information on country of birth is becoming less useful. The country of birth of a person's parents could be used but it is not usually on the death certificate and is less likely to be available in linkable databases. Most deaths, however, occur in the older age groups, so country of birth remains of some value even when a high proportion of the minority population is young.

As discussed already, country of birth is potentially misleading for people who were born abroad but would classify themselves as of an ethnic group unrelated to the country of birth. For example, Scotland had a major role in the British Empire. While 98.9% of White Scottish people were born in Scotland or England, this still means over 1% (about 50 000 people) were born elsewhere. Some of them, especially the older ones contributing most deaths, were born in British colonies. An analysis of the 2001 census data confirmed this, with many of those people born in India who were over 65 years of age being self-classified as White. Many Scottish residents who perceive themselves as Indians, however, are born neither in Scotland nor India, but in a variety of other countries.

In the absence of valid data on ethnic group, country of birth analysis has provided insights into health and disease inequalities of the kind shown in Figure 5.1. These analyses are also of value in their own right, i.e. not merely as a proxy for ethnic group but as a marker of migration status and migration history, and in particular exposure to different countries at a particularly sensitive period in relation to health. For example, migration studies have shown that people born in northern Europe, e.g. Scotland, where there is a comparatively high risk of multiple sclerosis, but living in countries such as Australia where the risk is comparatively low, continue to have a high risk if they migrated after childhood but not if they migrated at a very young age. This is potentially important given that the cause of the disease is unknown. All this said, most such studies, including the one illustrated in Figure 5.1, are contributing to the field of race or ethnicity not migration studies per se.

The interpretation of country of birth analyses done using census denominators and death certificate data is complex, and has been discussed in some detail by Gill et al. (2007). In brief, the count of deaths (numerator) may be wrong because: (1) some people may enter a country and die there but are not normally resident, e.g. they are tourists, business visitors, or have come overseas for medical care; (b) some people who are normally resident may prefer to leave the country to die elsewhere, e.g. their country of birth (so-called salmon bias, as this fish tries to return to die at its place of birth). Even if such deaths are notified to the normally resident country, which is possible for administrative and other reasons, the cause of death may not be known. These kinds of effects are seldom studied but are probably not very important.

Cause of death may be incorrect. Diagnosing the cause of death without an autopsy is an imprecise part of the art of medicine. Whether there are variations by country of birth in the accuracy of determining the cause of death is usually not known, although on first principles one anticipates that there would be; e.g. the medical history may be less accurate in those people born overseas who do not speak the local language well, making it more difficult for the doctor to identify the cause of death. The likelihood of gaining permission for an autopsy to ascertain more accurately the cause of death will probably vary by group. There is evidence that the perceived racial or ethnic group has an influence on the stated cause of death, as has been shown in the United States.

The numerator (e.g. death) is turned into a disease rate using a population denominator, i.e. the number of people at risk. In some countries such as The Netherlands, this information is obtained from local government population registries. The death data and the population registries there can be linked exactly using a personal identification number. This leads to a relatively accurate assessment of the death rate by country of birth. In other countries, including the UK, this is often not possible, and census data are used to estimate population size and structure. In most countries, a census is held once every 10 years. Even in a census year the figures are imprecise for young mobile adults and inner city populations (though the published figures may be adjusted for undercounts). Migrants and ethnic minorities are over-represented in these populations. There are, therefore, likely to be variations in the precision of denominators by country of birth group. The data from censuses at different times can be used to estimate the between-census population sizes by simple linear extrapolation. This makes an assumption that is unlikely to be correct, that the pattern of change over time is even across groups.

Given careful interpretation the data are of potential value, especially if they are available for a long period, as country of birth data generally are. Try Exercise 5.6 before reading on.

Exercise 5.6 The value of data

- ◆ What value can you see in the data on CHD mortality by country of birth in Figure 5.1? (Another way to answer this is to ask what would be lost without such data?)
- ◆ What insights are gained by looking at these data?

International variations in CHD are well-documented. Although the rates are rising, CHD mortality is generally low in the Indian subcontinent, Africa, and the Caribbean compared with Europe and North America. On the basis of such international studies we would expect ethnic variations in CHD within a multi-ethnic country. On first principles we would expect recently migrating minority ethnic groups living in industrialized countries to have, in comparison with the population as a whole, less CHD. For example, we would expect relatively less CHD in South Asian women, particularly Indians, who tend towards vegetarianism and have low smoking prevalence.

We see from Figure 5.1 that, as anticipated, variations are indeed present, but there is an important surprise—those born in the Indian subcontinent have a considerable excess of mortality and not a deficit.

The lessons are that investigators need to be creative, because information by race and ethnicity is not always easy to obtain. In this example country of birth is a reasonable proxy for ethnic group. General principles are inaccurate in predicting mortality patterns. The differences shown have huge implications for public health, clinical practice, and epidemiological research. Country of birth can continue to be of use in the analysis of mortality data. Analysis of such data is recommended to add to our understanding of ethnicity and health for policy and service purposes, to contribute ideas for epidemiological and clinical research, and to compare and contrast findings with a large and growing international research literature. Box 5.4 summarizes these points. We need race and ethnicity, but we need to do better than hitherto, and one potentially better approach is data linkage.

Box 5.4 Lessons from studies of immigrant mortality from CHD that provide general lessons

- ◆ Coronary heart disease (CHD) is the dominant cause of death—very often the dominant causes of death are dominant in all migrant and ethnic groups.
- ◆ International variations in CHD are well documented, and in consequence we expect there to be racial/ethnic variations in CHD, including in recent migrants.
- ◆ On first principles, we would expect recently migrated minority ethnic groups to have lower rates of CHD, e.g. South Asian women, particularly Indians, tend towards vegetarianism, and have low smoking prevalence. Data often confound first principles.
- ◆ Investigators need to be creative, as information by race and ethnicity is not always easy to obtain—here country of birth is a reasonable proxy for ethnic group.
- ◆ The patterns shown have huge implications for public health, clinical practice, and epidemiological research.

Table 5.3 contains data originally presented by Marmot et al. (1984). As in this table, SMRs relative to the majority or whole population are almost invariably provided in reports on ethnicity and health (which sometimes present disease ranking by SMR as here) and are usually given emphasis in the text. Try Exercise 5.7 before reading on.

Exercise 5.7 Tables of mortality by SMRs and case numbers

- What is your reaction on being presented with a table like Table 5.3?
- What is your eye drawn to? What facts strike you as important ones?
- Which diseases would you pick out as reflecting the priority needs of this male immigrant population?Examine the data in Table 5.4. Now look at the table and confirm that the right-hand column ranks diseases by their relative frequency based on SMR and that the left-hand column shows diseases among the same men ranked by number of deaths.
- Which cause of death killed most men born in the Indian subcontinent?
- Which cause of death is greatest in men born in the Indian subcontinent relative to men born in England and Wales?
- Which is a bigger health issue for men born in the Indian subcontinent, ischaemic heart disease or homicide?)

Most people find tables like Table 5.3 daunting. It takes considerable patience to extract the key messages. The eye is drawn to summary figures. Here the summary figures are, first, the ranks (top five) and second the SMR. The raw, unsummarized data are on numbers of deaths. The diseases one would pick out depends on one's own perspectives, but most readers would be guided by the text given by the authors. In this case, as is often true, the authors emphasized the patterns shown by the comparatively high SMRs.

Table 5.4 contains a reworking by Senior and myself (Senior and Bhopal 2004) of the data originally presented by Marmot et al. in Table 1.4. The two columns give radically different perspectives on disease patterns. The priority needs would certainly include ischaemic heart disease, cerebrovascular disease, and neoplasm of the trachea, bronchus, and lung. In terms of impact on the population's health, homicide (21 deaths but ranked first in Table 5.3) is dwarfed by ischaemic heart disease (1533 deaths). Analysis and interpretation using SMRs is grounded in the classic epidemiological strategy of generating hypotheses about disease causation by focusing on differences. However, this is insufficient for assessing health needs. CHD was not ranked in the top five based on SMR in Table 5.3. The top-ranking conditions in Table 5.3 (homicide and neoplasm of the liver and intrahepatic bile duct) do not figure in the left-hand side of Table 5.4 but dominate the right-hand side.

Based on the actual number of deaths, ischaemic heart disease is the main cause, but using the SMR homicide seems to be the most important. Thus, without examination of Table 5.3 from these two perspectives, we get a misleading interpretation of major health problems in this immigrant group. The primary perspective of the right-hand side of Table 5.4 is to compare and contrast the health status of the minority groups with that of the majority population. The perspective of the left-hand side is to consider the common, dominant problems of minority groups without comparison.

Table 5.3 Deaths and SMRs among a male immigrant population (aged 20 and over) to England and Wales, by cause

Cause of death	Rank (top five)	Deaths	SMR
Ch I Infective and parasitic diseases A6–10 Tuberculosis—all forms	3	64	315
Ch II Neoplasms		722	69
Malignant neoplasm of:			
A45 Buccal cavity and pharynx	5	28	178
A46 Oesophagus		30	110
A47 Stomach		50	45
A48 Intestine		38	55
A49 Rectum		27	57
ICD 155 Liver and intrahepatic ducts	2	19	338
ICD 156 Gall bladder and bile ducts		9	139
A50 Larynx		12	127
A51 Trachea, bronchus, and lung		218	53
A53 Skin		8	73
A54 Breast		0	—
A55 Cervix uteri			
A56 Uterus (other)			
A57 Prostate		48	105
ICD 183 Ovary, fallopian tube, and broad ligament			
A59–60 Leukaemia and other neoplasms of lymphatic and haematopoietic tissue		74	96
Ch III Endocrine, nutritional, and metabolic diseases			
A64 Diabetes mellitus	4	55	188
Ch IV Diseases of blood and blood-forming organs		8	92
A73 Multiple sclerosis		2	22
Ch VII Circulatory diseases		2,377	111
A81 Chronic rheumatic heart disease		46	86
A82 Hypertensive disease		85	128
A83 Ischaemic heart disease		1,533	115
A84 Other forms of heart disease		134	96
A85 Cerebrovascular disease		438	108
A86 Diseases of arteries		101	99
A87 Venous thrombosis and embolism		37	102
Ch VIII Respiratory diseases		494	86
A90 Influenza		22	80

(Continued)

Table 5.3 (Continued)

Cause of death	Rank (top five)	Deaths	SMR
A92 Other (non-viral) pneumonia		214	100
A93 Bronchitis, emphysema and asthma		223	77
Ch IX Digestive diseases		111	106
A98 Peptic ulcer		37	105
A102 Cirrhosis of liver		25	145
Ch X Diseases of the genito-urinary system		93	151
A106 Other (non-acute) nephritis		39	160
A107 Infections of kidney		20	176
Ch XI Complications of pregnancy, childbirth, and puerperium			
Ch XVII Accidents, poisonings, and violence		333	102
AE138 Motor vehicle accidents		134	110
AE140 Accidental poisoning		15	118
AE141 Accidental falls		24	76
AE147 Suicide		69	90
AE148 Homicide	1	21	341
AE149 Injury undetermined whether accidentally or purposely inflicted		28	147
All causes		4352	98

Adapted from Marmot et al, *Immigrant mortality in England and Wales 1970–78: Causes of Death by Country of Birth (Studies on Medical and Population Subjects)*, p.132, HMSO, London, UK, Copyright © 1984, licensed under the Open Government Licence v1.0.

Generally, when the data are presented using the number of cases, or rankings based upon this, the major health problems for minority groups seem similar to those of the population as a whole. When presented using the SMR, the differences are emphasized. For example, while there are some differences between ethnic groups in the UK, circulatory diseases, cancers, and respiratory diseases are the major fatal diseases for all groups. The comparative, relative risk approach underlying SMRs, which focuses on diseases either more or less common in minority groups, refines the analysis; it should not be ignored but should be seen as supplementary.

Interpretation of data has often been misinformed by an excessive emphasis on differences rather than similarities, the uncritical use of White populations as a standard to which minority populations should aspire, and the use of data sets looking at a limited number of conditions or particular age groups. To avoid these and similar problems the following approach is recommended:

◆ Base the epidemiological component of the needs assessment on disease causes using case numbers and disease rates and rankings based on these.

◆ Refine the above understanding by looking at comparative indices such as the SMR, and rankings based on this, which will focus attention on inequalities and potential inequities.

◆ Try to explain such differences with care, and with due emphasis on social and economic deprivation as important factors.

Table 5.4 Deaths and SMRs* in male immigrants from the Indian subcontinent (aged 20 and over; total deaths = 4352)

By rank order of number of deaths				By rank order of SMR			
Cause	Number of deaths	% of total	SMR	Cause	Number of deaths	% of total	SMR
Ischaemic heart disease	1533	35.2	115	Homicide	21	0.5	341
Cerebrovascular disease	438	10.1	108	Liver and intrahepatic bile duct neoplasm	19	0.4	338
Bronchitis, emphysema, and asthma	223	5.1	77	Tuberculosis	64	1.5	315
Neoplasm of the trachea, bronchus, and lung	218	5.0	53	Diabetes mellitus	55	1.3	188
Other non-viral pneumonia	214	4.9	100	Neoplasm of buccal cavity and pharynx	28	0.6	178
Total	2626	60.3	–		187	4.3	–

*Comparing with the male population of England and Wales, which was by definition 100.

Reproduced from Senior P and Bhopal RS, Ethnicity as a variable in epidemiological research, *British Medical Journal*, Volume 309, pp. 327–330, Copyright © 2004 with permission from the BMJ Publishing Group Ltd. Source: Data from Marmot et al, *Immigrant mortality in England and Wales 1970–78: Causes of Death by Country of Birth (Studies on Medical and Population Subjects)*, HMSO, London, UK, Copyright © 1984, licensed under the Open Government Licence v1.0.

Table 5.5 The standard table for assessment of the pattern of disease, particularly for needs assessment purposes. It shows how to lay out data for a needs assessment study

Disease or condition	Number of cases	Rate	Rank position on number of cases or rate	SMR/relative risk	Rank on SMR

- Beware that inferences of biological difference between ethnic and racial groups may be particularly prone to error and misinterpretation, and may harm the standing of minority groups.

A sample 'dummy' health needs assessment data table is shown as Table 5.5.

Unfortunately, most existing reports and papers neither present analyses in this format nor provide the information to permit readers to extract it themselves. Gill et al. (2007), however, have presented data in this format in their comprehensive health needs assessment. We now consider other issues that underpin the epidemiological approach.

5.2.5 Epidemiological approaches for health needs assessment: making choices and understanding limitations

Questions which are essential to the process of epidemiological modes of health needs assessment for minority groups include:

- Which groups are to be studied?
- Are the categories used to define population subgroups acceptable, ethical, and accurate?
- What data need to be collected?

♦ Have we collected accurate, representative data?

♦ How do we derive from the data a true picture of health and health-care needs and priorities (the latter is considered in Chapter 7)?

For reasons discussed in Chapter 2, the choice of minority groups and group categories is usually influenced by the classification used in the census or population registry. For national studies reliant on census data for denominator information this is invariably the case to avoid mismatch between the outcome data (numerator) and the population at risk of the outcome data (denominator) that are used for calculating rates, but there is sometimes flexibility in local studies. For example, we may be interested in the pattern of health and disease in Punjabis compared with Gujaratis, but data are unlikely to be available, at least nationally. That said, this kind of question has been tackled using name analysis, but that makes a strong assumption that this is an accurate method, which is unlikely given that high proportions of these populations are Muslim and the names of Punjabi and Gujarati Muslims are likely to be similar. The nearest we can usually get is the appropriate category in the census, and region of origin is unlikely to be there (it is not in the UK). We could gather data on Indians and their religions. The appropriate denominators would be available from the census. Using pragmatic categories that cannot be related to the census categories can be misleading and wasteful. For example, one ethnic category that was commonly used, and sometimes still is, is 'Asian' as a label for people from India, Pakistan, Bangladesh, and Sri Lanka (and in North America for Eastern groups such as Chinese). This label may lead to an erroneous view that South Asians are ethnically homogeneous—which may have adverse consequences for health (as discussed earlier generally in Chapters 1 and 2 and in relation to the data on smoking prevalence in Table 3.1). Moreover, it may prove difficult to get an accurate denominator for the 'Asian' population, so disease rates cannot be calculated. Health needs assessors must to be aware of these kind of issues.

The limitations of census categories are discussed in Chapter 2, but as they have usually been tested in both pilot studies and in widespread community consultation they are likely to be acceptable to the populations described at the time they are devised. This generalization may not hold in societies where the power imbalance permits one group (usually the majority) to impose its will on others. Also, categories that are acceptable at one point in time may become unacceptable (as discussed in Chapter 2, we see this with words used to describe populations of African origin, e.g. Negro, and we know that Oriental to denote Far Eastern peoples is no longer acceptable). Where due consultation has taken place, and the purposes of data collection are fair, analysing data using such categories is likely to be ethical and legal (see Chapters 9 and 10 for further elaboration of this point).

Now let us return to that proposed work on Punjabi and Gujarati groups. If there are compelling reasons for a comparison of Punjabis and Gujaratis, and one could imagine that to be the case in some cities, then ethnic group categories will need to be devised and tested and local studies undertaken. Investigators should consider not only the technical issues, e.g. maintaining a match between numerators, but also those of ethics and acceptability.

The choice of data items depends on the underlying purpose. In health needs assessment the challenge is to provide both professionals, and ideally also members of minority communities, as quickly as possible with a wide range of balanced information to allow them to make informed decisions on service development. The value of mortality and morbidity data is self-evident. Reliable national statistics on hospital utilization by racial or ethnic group or country of birth are often not available, so information on the patterns of (non-fatal) ill-health is difficult to obtain. The challenge is to balance the ideal against what is available. Data on mortality and lifestyles can be reanalysed or extracted from published documents comparatively easily; it is therefore inevitable that needs assessments will use them and further reflection on their limitations is appropriate even though this was considered in Section 5.2.4 from a general perspective.

Before reading on try Exercise 5.8.

Exercise 5.8 Limitations of mortality data

- List the potential limitations of mortality data analysis by minority group status for assessing health needs

---

Death data usually include information on any person dying in a country and thereby may include deaths of visitors; these may not be germane to needs assessment, except in a specialist way. Death data may include information on residents of a country dying in other countries only if these are notified to the authorities. Again, assessing the needs of such populations is a special matter. Such reporting probably varies across different populations and thereby by migrant, racial, and ethnic group. It is evident that migrant and ethnic minority groups are both more likely to have overseas visitors and to spend time overseas. If they die overseas in their country of origin it is less likely that their remains will be repatriated—not least because of the dual nature of residency, nationality, and sense of home and belonging of recent migrants. Indeed, remains may be repatriated even when death occurs in the new country of residence.

One answer to numerator–denominator bias (see Section 5.2.4) used in previous analyses of mortality by country of birth (e.g. that by Marmot et al. 1984), is to group together countries where this is a particular issue (e.g. countries of the Indian subcontinent). This grouping approach obscures potentially important differences between people with different countries of birth, so substituting one kind of error with another.

Death certificates, and hence mortality statistics, do not provide an accurate reflection of the importance of certain conditions in the general population, e.g. diabetes mellitus which is very common but which usually ends in death from cardiovascular diseases so often is not listed as a cause of death. Variation in the accuracy of cause of death described on death certificates by country of birth or ethnic group may be especially important for deaths occurring abroad, particularly where the cause of death has not been stated by a medical doctor. Medical certification is not compulsory in many countries, and customs may dictate quick burial or cremation even before cause of death is established.

In the analysis of mortality statistics we need to align counts of cases and populations at risk (from the census). Usually the published census statistics exclude people who are not normally residents. If so, deaths of visitors should not be included in the count of cases, the numerator. Census data are invariably incomplete. The effect of this is to overestimate the calculated mortality rates. Restricting the mortality analyses to the year of, or years around (usually 3, 4, or at most 5 years), the census minimizes the effect of population change and inaccuracies in the denominator. The downside is that the numbers of deaths are reduced by this restriction so reducing statistical precision, which is a problem when the size of the minority population is small.

Country of birth provides no indication of length of stay in either the country of birth or the country of residence. Mortality by country of birth is a particularly poor measure of health needs in children, because very few minority children living were born abroad and so mortality statistics are very incomplete. In countries where even minority elders were born in that country, e.g. the United States, country of birth is of little value as a proxy for race or ethnicity.

Studies of immigrant populations show that mortality experience converges to that of the host population with time, and particularly in succeeding generations. Overall mortality of even very poor new migrants is usually either similar to or lower than the population as a whole, even when the immigrants are from countries with high mortality and even when their social and economic circumstances are worse. The 'healthy migrant effect' is the term used to describe this finding. Health needs assessors should not be misled—this is likely to be a temporary phenomenon that will not last or be transmitted across generations. Health policy must take this into account. There is also the possibility that some members of minority groups emigrate, often to their country of ancestral origin ('salmon bias') or elsewhere, as a consequence of ill-health. There is certainly a tendency to return to the place of birth or ancestral homeland in old age. Some people probably die unexpectedly during such visits. Others may go there deliberately in the knowledge they will die there. On the other hand medical facilities are likely to be poorer in the country of origin, which is a deterrent to returning. Again, needs assessments should consider those possibilities.

Notwithstanding these and other limitations, data need to be turned into information, and Section 5.2.6 summarizes what kind of information has accrued as a result of epidemiological needs assessments. The account draws heavily from an unusually thorough assessment done by Gill et al. (2007), but it also draws on similar work across the world. The principles are likely to be widely generalizable to migrant, racial, and ethnic minorities in many industrialized multi-ethnic nations.

5.2.6 **Patterns of disease in minority groups**

Armed with the cautions and principles about data interpretation outlined above it is possible to draw much of value and interest from the rapidly enlarging data sets on migration, race, ethnicity, and health internationally. The following are some of the types of conclusions that are fairly robust, and arise from a number of health needs assessments particularly, but by no means only, that by Gill and colleagues.

Minority groups are heterogeneous in their health, both in overall health (e.g. measured by the all-cause mortality or self-reported health) and specific causes (e.g. CHD or oral cancers). There is also great heterogeneity within the usual broad ethnic groupings (South Asian, Chinese, Black, White, etc.); this is still insufficiently explored territory even though it is now widely acknowledged. The reasons for research not heeding heterogeneity are lack of knowledge amongst investigators (this is becoming less common), the constraints of standard, available, and recommended categories (common), and matters of statistical precision, because small groups mean fewer cases and hence wider confidence intervals around estimates. Within the majority population—usually White Europeans—there is also much heterogeneity. It is unfortunate, therefore, that needs might be overlooked in White subpopulations for lack of data. In addition to the three reasons above, here we have another, i.e. that the interest or focus of investigators is on non-White minorities so the majority White population is merely being used for reference. This perspective needs to change. The majority population is a racial or ethnic group in its own right, and comprises many subgroups, some of whom will be recent migrants or descendants of recent migrants. Health needs assessments tend to show more heterogeneity between sexes in minority groups than in the majority. We see generational differences, and also variable rates of acculturation, not just in migrants but also their descendants. While the process of acculturation is normally understood to be the adoption of the way of life of the host majority population, this is not correct. Minorities may adopt some of the ways of life of other minorities too, and the majority may adopt some of the ways of life of the minorities. In short, the picture is both complex and changeable, so health needs assessments need to incorporate the uncertainties and also need to be updated periodically. Harnessing this heterogeneity is definitely an area for future research.

There is a common assumption, and frequently stated view, that the health of minorities is worse than expected (judged by the standard of the majority, usually White, population). This view is almost invariably expressed by those seeking resources either for research or services. This is at best simplistic, and sometimes wrong. First, such conclusions need to be cautious given the weaknesses in the underlying data. Second, even on the basis of the published statistics, overall measures such as SMRs are often around and sometimes less than 100 (i.e. the value for the reference population) in some minority populations. Recent analyses in several countries shows that many migrant and ethnic groups (especially Chinese) have all-cause SMRs well below 100. The primary explanation for this finding is the healthy migrant effect, i.e. the people who migrate are, disproportionately, the fit and healthy. They are the fit and able amongst the populations they came from. They may also be relatively well educated, and relatively free of the lifestyles that are causing the killing diseases in the host population, e.g. smoking or alcohol misuse. Both these kinds of protective factors would be expected to diminish with time and across generations, and they do.

It would be wrong to assume that the healthy migrant effect will be seen in all minority groups. First, it is likely to apply to migrants who move voluntarily, not those who are forced to migrate, e.g. trafficked people or refugees, especially those who have been persecuted and even tortured. It would not be expected in long-settled minorities e.g. Roma/Gypsy peoples. (And, of course, the opposite would be the case for long-settled majority and minority indigenous people, who find migrants in their midst. Their populations may exhibit the consequence of having lost their healthiest, most energetic members to emigration.) In evaluating whether the apparent good health of a minority is reflecting the healthy migrant effect, assessors need to exclude data artefacts, especially the incomplete ascertainment of outcomes in minorities. On a broader note, the challenge for public health is how to sustain the healthy migrant effect, and perhaps even propagate some of it to the population as a whole.

Needs assessments usually include an overview of the social and economic circumstances of minorities. While there are a few exceptions, they are generally found to be living in worse circumstances than the majority population. Given this, the finding of lower mortality rates is even more of a surprise, as adverse socio-economic circumstances are usually strongly associated with poorer health outcomes. Health needs assessments need to acknowledge that this relationship is often unclear in recently migrating minority groups. (We will consider this in more detail in Chapter 6.)

Given all this, we have the important question of how we should judge the level of expected health. Is it right to base the expected level on the majority, usually White, population which, on average, has a higher economic standing? Might it be that, taking into account social and economic factors, the health of minority ethnic groups is at about the level to be expected? Studies of mortality outcomes in recently migrated minorities show that the healthy migrant effect is even greater when such factors are taken into consideration. In studies of long-settled minorities, such as African Americans in the United States, many aspects of adverse health are greatly reduced once social and economic factors are accounted for. The implication is that social and economic advancement would eradicate or greatly reduce such differences. Sometimes the highest all-cause SMRs are not in the ethnic minority groups but in a subgroup of the White population—e.g. Irish-born and Scots-born people living in England have much higher SMRs than any other group by country of birth. Presumably, health selection effects are non-existent as migration is so easy, indeed, the not-so-healthy or wealthy may be the emigrants.

While mortality is a primary indicator used in health needs assessment (and SMR is a marker of life expectancy), self-assessed overall health status has gained attention, partly because it is a common component of health surveys and partly because in general populations it correlates well with future mortality, i.e. those who report poor health have higher mortality rates compared with those reporting good health. This applies even in the absence of specific diagnosed health problems. Surprisingly, given the observations on the healthy migrant effect above, even migrants with average or low overall mortality self-report their health as worse than reference majority populations. This paradox needs explaining before health needs assessments can take full advantage of it. (Cross-cultural comparability of the self-report method and questions is one of the issues that needs further exploration.)

One of the most important contributions of health needs assessment, unlike research which tends to focus on differences, is to emphasize similarities. In many respects the migrant, racial, and minority ethnic groups have similar patterns of disease and overall health to the majority ethnic group. This is most obvious when disease rankings are based on frequency of outcome (not relative frequency) as in Tables 5.4 (left-hand column) and Table 5.6.

Table 5.6 Commonest causes of admission (in rank order) to hospitals in Leicestershire, England

'Asians' by diagnostic category	Number	Non-Asians by diagnostic category	Number
1. Accidents/poisonings	404	1. Accidents/poisonings	7442
Fracture	93	Fracture	2204
Burns	11		
2. Digestive system	384	2. Circulatory system	6693
Appendicitis	56	Ischaemic heart disease	2155
Cirrhosis	10		
3. Respiratory system	377	3. Digestive system	6141
Obstructive airways disease	104	Appendicitis	864
4. Symptoms and signs	370	4. Symptoms and signs	5088
5. Circulatory system	352	5. Respiratory system	4606
Ischaemic heart disease	141	Chronic obstructive airways disease	749
6. Infectious disease	277	6. Neoplasms	4343
Tuberculosis	153	Lung	755
Malaria	28		
7. Nervous system	206	7. Nervous system	2887
8. Genito-urinary system	160	8. Genito-urinary system	2634
9. Perinatal	156	9. Musculoskeletal	1952
10. Congenital abnormality	126	10. Congenital abnormality	1193
11. Neoplasms	120	11. Infectious disease	872
Lung	11	Tuberculosis	128
Oesophagus	6		

For example, CHD, stroke, and cancer are among the commonest causes of death; and accidents, poisonings, digestive disorders, respiratory infections, and circulatory problems among the main reasons for admission to hospital whichever minority group you consider (illustrated in Table 5.6 by data for Leicestershire, England). Health professionals in a multicultural society caring for patients from minority groups will usually be confronted with these common problems and will see the conditions that are more specific to minorities comparatively infrequently, but these latter problems are of utmost importance too. Health professionals will usually need to make the correct diagnosis in the face of greater communication or cultural barriers than they are accustomed to. However, both health needs assessors and individual clinicians need to know of the conditions that are rare in the population as a whole and yet not rare in minority communities, e.g. typhoid fever, tuberculosis, nasopharyngeal cancer, malaria, etc. Service providers may need to modify their service priorities and practitioners their approach to diagnosis to accommodate these differences.

Some of the conditions that are much commoner in one or more recently settled minority groups (and often most) than the population as a whole include:

◆ infectious diseases including tuberculosis and malaria
◆ type 2 diabetes mellitus
◆ perinatal and infant mortality
◆ cerebrovascular disease (stroke)
◆ cancer of the oropharynx, liver, prostate, and stomach
◆ haemoglobinopathies
◆ vitamin D deficiency.

In addition, there are a very large number of health outcomes that are highly group specific, sometimes arising from particular environments (e.g. Chagas disease), ways of seeing the world (psychosocial disorders), or from specific behaviours (e.g. betel nut chewing). While these are unlikely to feature much in health needs assessment, clinicians working with specific populations may need to know about them.

Equally, there are some conditions which are less common in many recently settled minority groups relative to the population as a whole, including:

◆ many cancers, including the common ones of lung, colorectal, and breast
◆ suicide
◆ accidents
◆ peripheral vascular disease
◆ alcoholism.

The above lists are illustrative and not comprehensive. Some general explanations for such variations will be considered in Section 5.2.7.

Differences in disease patterns need careful attention, but not at the expense of ignoring potentially more important diseases that show no such differences (such as respiratory diseases). Conditions which are less common in minority ethnic groups than in the White population that tend to be ignored include lung cancer, the leading cancer in men in most ethnic groups, and among the leaders for women. It and similar conditions may be worth more attention than conditions which are actually rare, though relatively more common than in the White population, e.g. liver cancer. The consequences of not doing this are considered in relation to health inequalities in Chapter 6.

The differences are obviously complex and vary over time and between minority groups. Simplifications may easily mislead. Information is most readily available for the visible, large populations that are enumerated using specific categories in the census. Some groups in which the need may be great are often relatively invisible in health statistics, e.g. asylum seekers, refugees, Roma/Gypsies, travellers, and people from eastern Europe and the Middle East. Describing health patterns is the central issue in health needs assessment, but its value is enhanced by understanding the factors that shape the patterns.

5.2.7 **How do we explain similarities and differences?**

Description is essential but is not enough—meeting needs also requires some understanding of the causes of differences, and indeed the causes of similarities. Epidemiological strategies for understanding similarities, however, are not well developed. (Causal interpretation will be considered in some detail in Chapter 9.)

Before reading on do Exercise 5.9.

Exercise 5.9 Categorizing the explanations for migration status/ethnic/racial differences

◆ List the differences between minority groups that could explain their different patterns of disease. (You may wish to focus your thinking using the disease rickets or osteomalacia, a bone disorder caused by deficiency of vitamin D, which in the UK is more common in most minority groups than in the host population.) Vitamin D is a vitamin that is synthesized by the body and exposure to the sun is essential to this process.

◆ Can you put them into categories?

Osteomalacia in adults, and rickets which is its equivalent in childhood, are both caused by a deficiency of vitamin D. The biochemistry of vitamin D is very complex and beyond this discussion, except to note that in understanding health phenomena, health needs assessors may need to seek the advice of clinicians and laboratory scientists, and not just epidemiologists and other public health scientists. This understanding is essential to formulating an appropriate response.

The exercise informed you that most vitamin D is produced in the body, and this requires exposure of the skin to direct sunlight (and even then at certain times of the day and year so UV-B radiation from sunlight can reach the skin). However, some vitamin D is found in foods and supplements are available. The potential causes for the observation, now made in numerous countries and in many populations, that minorities have comparatively low levels of vitamin D in the blood and a higher risk of osteomalacia and rickets include the following:

1. Those minorities that have a dark skin are less likely to synthesize enough vitamin D because the UV-B radiation is absorbed by the pigment cells.

2. Some minorities are less likely to expose their skins to sunlight, either because their skin is covered up by clothing or they do not spend time in the sun. Sunbathing may be abnormal behaviour or there may be no time or opportunity.

3. Some minorities are less likely to eat the kind of foods that contain vitamin D either naturally (oily fish) or by fortification (cereals, margarines).

4. Some minorities are less likely to take vitamin supplements.

5. The constituents of the diet of some minorities interfere with the absorption of vitamin D from the gut.

These five explanations illustrate the point. Of course, all five may be correct, but they are unlikely to apply equally to all groups in all places. Health needs assessors may need to prioritize some explanations to generate local workable solutions.

This question of causality poses great difficulty because inequalities (or disparities) are very complex—they combine cultural, socio-economic, and, for a few diseases as in our example above, genetic factors as underlying causes. In understanding differences we must be wary of the idea, based on the race concept, that the differences are largely or wholly attributable to genetic factors and hence are biological and physiological (which is only largely true for a few diseases such as the haemoglobinopathies, and partly true for vitamin D deficiency). Equally, the idea based on the ethnicity concept that differences are caused by cultural factors is mostly too readily accepted without scrutiny (it is sometimes true but it detracts attention from the other factors, especially social and economic ones). Here it would be easy to 'blame' modesty as the reason for not sunbathing, but it may be a question of appropriate opportunity, e.g. the availability of some privacy in a private garden or balcony.

Other underlying explanations, such as lifestyle/economic change, migration itself, occupation, poverty, racism, and economic problems, are often inadequately explored. Socio-economic deprivation, in particular, is an important and underestimated explanation for differences in disease among minority groups. This analysis will be developed in the context of inequalities in the next chapter, and in the context of causal research in Chapter 9.

5.2.8 What services are available and how should they be adapted for minority populations?

Since the primary influence of a health needs assessment is on health care (in its broad sense), and in the case of minorities mostly on adaptation of existing services rather than creation of new ones, we need to find out what services are available and how they have already been shaped to meet needs. Fortunately, information on the services available is usually easy to obtain. What is harder to find is what adaptations have been made to accommodate minority groups and, even more difficult, how successful these have been in improving access, quality of care, and health outcomes.

Reliable data on service utilization analysed by minority group are rare because of the lack of high-quality monitoring, as we have discussed. Even when such information is available it is not easy to judge whether the service is adequate to meet needs.

In addition, guidelines are needed on what should be available, and the standards of care that should be attained. This kind of information might be obtainable from the health service itself or from regulatory or professional standards organizations, or national bodies representing particular conditions, e.g. the British or American Heart Foundation.

As an example, for diabetes the required service provision has been detailed by the charity Diabetes UK. The charity's website sets out the standards of care, including that interpreters are to be available when needed, and gives a detailed list of checks to be made at the annual review. Such guidance can then be checked against what is actually available in the local service. The guidance may need to be adapted for the local migrant, racial, or minority ethnic communities. Table 5.7 gives a checklist of services for the management of heart disease and diabetes. The needs assessor uses such a list and checks out local availability.

Table 5.7 Checklist of required services for management of cardiovascular disease and diabetes

Service required	Availability
Lifestyle management	
Risk factor control	
Prescription for exercise	
Annual reviews for ischaemic heart disease and diabetes	
Dietetics	
Foot care	
Eye care	
Hypertension clinics	
Anticoagulation clinics	
Open access echocardiography	
Open access ECG	
Open access Holter monitoring	
Open access exercise testing	
Emergency cardiology services	
Angiography and percutaneous transluminal coronary angioplasty	
Coronary artery bypass graft	
Carotid endarterectomy	
Renal services (dialysis and replacement)	
Rehabilitation (post-stroke)	
Rehabilitation (post-MI)	

ECG, electrocardiogram; MI, myocardial infarction.

Before reading on try Exercise 5.10.

Exercise 5.10 Questions to guide adaptation of services

- What questions would you ask to help adapt the checklist in Table 5.7 for minority groups?

The kind of list in Table 5.7 needs adaptation for use for minority groups by asking further questions of the kind in Box 5.5. The answers may not be available, but they can be the starting point of on-going discussion and analysis. The analysis needs to be infused with the insights from quantitative data, and supplemented with qualitative information, as discussed below.

In posing such questions the health needs assessment is moving from a public health perspective to the domain of health-care organization, quality of care, and clinical delivery, i.e. organizational and clinical cross-cultural competence. In most multicultural societies services will be dealing

Box 5.5 Questions to guide adaptation of services for ethnic minority populations—examples

♦ Are there issues that are priorities for minority groups that might be missed here? For example, the need for same-sex services in some aspects of rehabilitation, e.g. for exercise. Which minority groups would need such an adaptation?

♦ Are staff aware of differences in clinical presentation or outcome that will require varying responses by ethnic group, e.g. for reasons that are not well understood South Asians, and some other minority groups, are much less likely to develop diabetic complications in the foot but much more likely to develop renal failure.

♦ Are there services prioritized here that are not very relevant to minority groups or that we already know will be ineffective?

♦ Have the staff been trained in competently delivering services to minority groups in ways that take account of their culture and other related matters?

♦ Can staff speak in the preferred languages of the local minority populations? If not, do patients have access to appropriately trained interpreters and translators? Have staff been trained to work effectively with interpreters and translators?

♦ Are there procedures in place to ensure that the cultural or religious requirements of patients are recorded in patient and nursing records and that these are referred to in health-care decisions, e.g. regarding the type of insulin prescribed? (For example pork insulin is not suitable for Muslims.)

♦ Are there mechanisms to ensure that dietetic counselling and advice to minority ethnic patients is consistent with the cultural and religious requirements of the patient and the patient's dietary patterns?

with a range of minority populations, so this becomes a complex exercise that requires generalizable principles, rather than a specific ad hoc response that is tailored rigidly to each minority group. In making adaptations it is highly probable that staff will become more knowledgeable and effective and that some adaptations will benefit the entire population, not just minorities, e.g. simpler translation of materials, pictures rather than words, more involvement of relatives, and perhaps even single-sex rehabilitation services. It is apparent that the process is inherently interesting and poses the kinds of challenges that health professionals like to tackle. Before implementation of change arising from health needs assessment it is important to involve those most affected, listening to their ideas and concerns. This is usually best done by dialogue, although views can also be elicited by quantitative questionnaire methods. In Section 5.3, we consider the role of qualitative methods in refining the health needs assessment.

5.3 What do the public and health professionals think of the service? The role of qualitative data in health needs assessment

To answer the kind of question posed in the section heading requires social science methods rather than epidemiological ones. Health needs assessment requires 'mixed methods'—the blending of quantitative and qualitative methods. For more information on how to do such work readers should consult reference textbooks on field methods in research, such as that by Bowling and Ebrahim (2006), which introduces quantitative and qualitative methods in health research. Mackintosh et al.'s (1998) *Step-by-Step Guide* also has more information on methods in the specific context of health and ethnicity which has been incorporated into this book. These issues are also discussed briefly in the context of research in Chapter 9.

Qualitative research is based on information in narrative, rather than numerical, form and focuses on the meanings that people place upon their experiences. It uses methods that are applied in a rigorous way to systematically study individual and group perspectives. The result is often not only complementary to quantitative research, but powerfully synergistic. Narrative can bring statistics to life and has an unexpectedly large impact. Narrative, unlike numerical data, is easy to relate to and everyone can understand it. The case history material produced by qualitative research can be particularly powerful in influencing politicians, policy-makers, managers, the public, and the media. Most health-care professionals, by contrast, prefer quantitative data, which give information on normative and comparative needs. Even then, they can be influenced by narrative. Narrative may not be qualitative research but simply a story or a case history. One such story that moved me into action, and moves other people too, is about my elderly aunt who came from India to Scotland to stay with her son. I visited her in hospital one afternoon about 20 years ago to find her unresponsive. I spoke to the nurses who said she was asleep. I said I did not think she was. They informed me that she'd been spending a lot of time sleeping but because she spoke no English they found it hard to communicate with her so were unsure about how she was. My aunt, who had diabetes, was in a hypoglycaemic comma and revived after being given a glucose infusion. This simple story has motivated me and others to try to do better in caring for minority populations, especially elders. These stories are anecdotes, but qualitative research can reach a much higher place.

Qualitative methods add a new dimension to health needs assessment by answering the following kind of questions:

* What do the individuals in the minority communities perceive as being their most important health needs? This may be different from the picture from statistics and may bring to attention issues that are not captured by formal databases or structured questions. We can ask why they think as they do, and check their views on those needs prioritized by health statistics.

* What are the experiences of members of minority communities as users of health services? In what ways are the services meeting their needs and how could they be improved.

* How can services for minority groups be evaluated in a way meaningful to them? What kind of evidence would they wish to see? What would make them satisfied that the services were being delivered equitably?

* What are the perspectives of health professionals on the needs of minority groups and on their own ability to deliver services equitably? What problems do they encounter that hinder them in achieving the goal of equity?

* Has the action taken to improve things been perceived as successful by public and professionals? If yes, in what way, if not why not?

These questions help assess felt need and expressed need.

The people and agencies that could help answer such questions include: service users, community representatives, community organizations, people identified as leaders, volunteer networks, local primary health-care/locality teams, secondary health-care providers, service managers, and local politicians. A key step is finding and involving people who either have new information to provide or those who are typical of the group. Whether collecting information by self-completion or interview-based questionnaires, or by focus groups, a reliable and comprehensive (but not necessarily representative) sample of people needs to be recruited. A range of opinion is very important, rather than the average opinion. One potential problem is that gaining access to the views of some people is relatively easy, e.g. those who become identified as community leaders and administrators of community organizations, not least because they speak the host population's language well, are articulate, and are quite easy to contact. These people can be effective routes for reaching a wider group of people, but they can also act as gatekeepers who may even restrict access. One common observation of such gatekeepers is that the minority communities are saturated and fatigued by research or consultation. Yet when investigators do contact ordinary members of the public they may well have never been involved in research and are glad to participate and to be consulted.

Data protection laws restrict access to lists of names and contact details that are held by health authorities, so finding people to study is not always easy. These laws are tight in relation to research, but not so when the data are collected for the purposes of service evaluation and improvement by service staff (or honorary staff) from service users. If resources permit service staff to be trained in data collection and freed up to do it, there is some merit in doing this rather than appointing researchers. Some information on how to access study samples is given in Chapter 9, and if this has been achieved there are two main ways of collecting qualitative data, i.e. semi-open and open style interviewing of individuals, and focus groups. In addition qualitative researchers may use participant observation, i.e. observing directly what is going on, and not relying on self-report. The method of participant observations is rarely used in epidemiology, public health, and health services research but deserves more attention.

5.3.1 Gauging the experiences of members of minority communities as users of health services

While this is a generalization, it is worth remembering that many minority cultures place high value on verbal rather than written discourse. This is not only about literacy, though that obviously matters, especially in immigrant populations where knowledge of both the host population's language and sometimes also the written form of their own language is limited. The value placed on verbal discourse transcends literacy. It may be that verbal discourse permits the building of trust and a personal relationship in ways that written discourse does not. Again as a generalization, and following on from this, response rates can be very high when contact is made verbally and very low when contact is in writing. It is for these reasons that I have emphasized interview-based methods rather than self-completion, written methods of acquiring data. Typically, we need to find out what people think about the service, what problems/concerns they have, and what their experiences have been. These are not the kinds of topics that can be standardized easily, and questions need to be tailored to each enquiry. Translation and cross-cultural validity of questions is a crucial issue, as already discussed above and considered again in Chapter 9. It cannot be assumed either that respondents speak the host population's language (either at all or as their first choice) or, and perhaps even more importantly, that they will necessarily share common assumptions about health and well-being which underlie the questions. For example, the idea that open criticism of professionals and services is welcome and is a means to the end of improving them may not be widely shared and may not be self-evident, as it is to health service managers. Indeed, immigrants may well come from places where this is seen as disrespectful. (In practice, it is difficult to give negative feedback because, contrary to management rhetoric, it is usually unwelcome and causes tensions, no matter who you are.) In devising questions, researchers should beware of using jargon, colloquialisms, and other sayings idiosyncratic to the language of the majority population. It may be more appropriate to adopt a simple descriptive approach to questions to avoid misinterpretation both in the main language and/or in the translation. Even for interviewing it is important that the questions or topic guides are agreed and written down in each language to be used. It is important for translations to be consistent across languages. This simplifying process is likely to benefit everyone, including those in the majority population.

There are basically three types of questions—structured, semi-structured, and open-ended—all of which can be used in self-completion questionnaires or at interview. Structured questionnaires underpin quantitative methods rather than qualitative ones, although they may have a part to play. The advantage of self-completion questionnaires is that people can consider questions carefully in their own time. They may also be less embarrassed about giving details about personal issues or those where some stigma is attached, e.g. contraception, sex, and alcohol. Topics which are not sensitive in one culture may be very sensitive in another. For example, the age of a woman is not usually a sensitive topic in Chinese or South Asian cultures (old age is usually revealed with pleasure as an achievement) but it is in modern European ones (revealed reluctantly). Smoking cigarettes is a very sensitive topic for Sikh men because it is forbidden by religion, but not for most other men.

Interview-based questionnaires or topic-guide-led interviewing allow the interviewer to ask the questions and convey the meanings of questions if they are not fully understood (possibly especially important in a translated language). The interviewer either tape records or writes down the answer for qualitative research (or codes the answer using predefined categories for quantitative research). The interview also has great advantages when the study participants do not read and write the language well, as is sometimes the case with minority populations. However, to gain quality, comparable information, the interviewer must be trained to build rapport equally across the different ethnic groups, and ask the questions in a fairly standardized way. Following this straightforward advice is not easy, especially when a team of interviewers is required or when the work is done on several minority groups, where one interviewer is unlikely to be knowledgeable in all the languages.

Earlier we considered the difficulties in interpreting quantitative data and extracting valid information for health needs assessment. Although this kind of critical edge is seldom emphasized for qualitative work in the field of migration, race, and ethnicity, it is equally important. Getting valid messages extracted from qualitative data in multi-ethnic studies where people may be sampled in various ways, and where a range of translators and interviewers have acquired the data, is problematic. The axiom 'compare like-with-like' is perhaps the best overriding advice in this circumstance.

5.4 **Focus groups**

In recent years, focus group methods have soared in popularity in studies of migrants and racial and ethnic minorities. It may be that the method chimes with both the social aspect of the minority culture, with emphasis on family, kin, and community, or it works because of the existence of minority community organizations. Focus groups are not an easy or cheap option. They are hard to organize and manage, especially when the discussion uses several languages simultaneously, as is often the case. For example, in focus groups of Chinese people in English-speaking countries, even those participants fully articulate in the Chinese languages of Mandarin and Cantonese will intersperse their dialogue with at least occasional words, phrases, and sentences in English, even though the focus group was intended to be conducted in the Chinese languages. The focus group is a core qualitative research method used to gain insight through the interaction of a group. The group is 'focused' in that it involves a collective, directed discussion of chosen themes. Focus groups exploit group dynamics. Exploiting group dynamics is a skilful task, especially when one or a few members of a group dominate discussion or others are reticent.

Focus groups extend the interview-based semi-structured or open questionnaire. People might be grouped according to sex, minority background, professional background, etc., and be asked 'What do you think of local hospital services?'. The people are then encouraged to talk, in their own language if desired, to discuss issues and exchange experiences. Through these discussions rich and vivid stories might emerge of how people have interacted with the health services. As with interviewing, whenever possible the discussion is audiotaped and also noted down. These data are then integrated into the health needs assessment and used to improve health care. Box 5.6 gives an example of how the focus group method can lead to practical understanding (Elliott 1997).

Box 5.6 CHD/diabetes focus group methods and integration of results in planning service changes

Focus groups were used in Newcastle upon Tyne, England to explore CHD and diabetes services for the ethnic minorities. Four focus groups were set up; separate male and female South Asian groups, a mixed sex Chinese group, and a minority ethnic professionals group. Participants were encouraged to talk openly about their experiences, and those of their families, of heart disease and diabetes. The English-speaking facilitator asked the questions, which were interpreted by the community workers assisting the facilitator and the answers were fed back via the community workers to the facilitator. Immediately after the meeting, there was a group discussion between the facilitator and the community workers (the research group) to go over and clarify the main points raised. This discussion was recorded and the results transcribed. The research group met on several occasions to agree the main themes which were emerging from the focus groups. The salient points made were placed under theme headings and discussed and changed until the research group was happy that what was emerging was a true record of what had occurred. Conclusions were that the minorities knew little about their conditions (including preventative strategies) but wanted to know more. All participants had or knew of people who had received inadequate health services. The professionals complained that they often did not have the resources to educate the community properly, e.g. materials were not translated and of those that were, most were not easily understandable by the community. The professionals were often inundated with calls from people who wanted help with other matters, e.g. filling out social security forms.

The focus groups produced vivid first-hand accounts of problems with health care. This material was integrated with an epidemiological health needs assessment and a strategy for change was developed. This work in Newcastle was itself integrated by myself and colleagues with three other projects on the same subject (London, Walsall, Manchester) and presented to a combined local authority and health authority forum called the Newcastle Health Partnership. The recommendations were considered by funding authorities. The end result was a nurse-led primary care-based project on cardiovascular and diabetes risk factor reduction set in inner city general practices in Newcastle with larger than average ethnic minority populations. Given that a service is in place (and hopefully adapted) it is important to know whether it is being used—the topic considered in Section 5.5.

Adapted from Elliot et al, *Taking Heart: Reducing diabetes and cardiovascular disease among Newcastle's South Asian and Chinese communities in Strategy for commissioning services for coronary heart disease and diabetes for ethnic minority populations in England and Wales: lessons from a four-site pilot study*, Departments of Epidemiology and Public Health and Medicine, University of Newcastle upon Tyne, Copyright © 1998, with permission of the authors.

5.5 **Do people from minority populations use the available services well? What is the quality of their interaction with staff? Are the services meeting the need?**

These simple questions may be difficult to answer, partly because there are no objective data and partly because interpretation of the answers is often subjective. Front-line staff in frequent contact with patients may have a wealth of information and views on how current services address the needs of individual patients and minority groups, and these views should be accessed in needs assessment exercises as we considered above. It is likely that the only way to assess how well services are being used is to go to the service provider and examine the records, probably using a medical audit/quality assessment approach, where the quality standard is set in advance and records checked to see whether it is met. This is no easy task and can be very time-consuming. To reiterate, such figures for audit should arise from routine monitoring systems but very often these are not able to provide the necessary data. The number of people from the minority population on the list can be compared with the number expected in the light of the population size (census or registry of population) and the pattern of illness in the population of interest (epidemiological studies). The figures can be judged using existing standards of health care, e.g. it may be that, as a matter of policy, all people with a condition, say a stroke, are to be seen by a specialist stroke service. If there are no such standards then a reference value is needed for comparison—usually in studies of minority groups this is that of the White (or other majority) population, admittedly an ethnocentric method but a time-honoured practical one.

Knowing the numbers of people making use of health services in relation to the numbers expected is, however, insufficient. What we need to know is whether people are using the available services optimally. There are significant differences between different minority groups in uptake of services and the interpretation of these differences is complex. Service uptake may be affected by such factors as age distribution, sex ratio, religion, language, socio-economic status, and patterns of morbidity. To understand differences it is necessary to consider these factors in statistical analyses. Adjustment for age and presentation of data by sex is virtually routine but for other factors a thoughtful and careful approach is needed to produce sensible and correctly interpreted results. Optimal use is not only about the amount, or relative amount, of use, but also about the contact during the health-care encounter and its effect.

Staff in health centres and hospitals should find it helpful in raising the quality of care in all sub-populations to understand the cultural and religious aspects of their patients' lives (and, of course, the socio-economic context). Awareness of how attitudes to illness and treatment differ among different minority groups is also important. For example, some female patients, because of religious or cultural influences, would rather have the option of consulting with, and being treated by, female health professionals. South Asian women in particular prefer to be examined by a female doctor whenever possible, and South Asian people generally tend to select South Asian GPs. What is needed is an approach that marries diversity with equity. This does not mean treating everyone in the same way, regardless of differing needs, rather that health services be adapted to be able to take account of diverse cultures, religions, and health if needed.

Staff should not, however, decide from a person's name, appearance, religion, or self-reported migration staus or racial or ethnic group, what their needs are. Culture is not static but is evolving as social groups respond to their experiences. Culture is dependent on more than ancestral origins, e.g. living and working conditions, and on the broader political, economic, and social scene. The socio-economic structures in which people live shape their values and behaviours in ways that have consequences for health and health care. Factors such as satisfaction with the service (or even reports of others' experiences) or discrimination perceived as racism may affect uptake of services. A low service uptake is not necessarily a sign that the service is not meeting needs, though that interpretation needs to be considered alongside others such as a lower prevalence of disease. Equally, it cannot be assumed that a high rate of utilization of services implies excess demand, since it may be warranted by a higher disease rate or even a lower effectiveness of care during each care episode.

Communication is one of the main barriers to accessing health care. To enable effective communication to take place, health professionals need to be aware of.cultural and social factors that shape people's perceptions and behaviours. Barriers to effective communication between health practitioner and patient include differences in social, status and culture, which are then compounded if the patient does not speak or understand well the language used by most of the staff or other patients. Staff need to remember that even people who are generally fluent in a language may not have the concepts or words needed in health settings, e.g. a hormone, pituitary gland, the spleen etc. (Those who have learned a foreign language will appreciate this well.) Some questions that address issues concerning the quantity and quality of care for minority groups are given in Box 5.7.

If problems are identified they should be followed up more systematically. An advisory group could be formed comprising GPs, community members/groups, allied health professionals, secondary health-care providers, and other interested parties. The purpose of this group would be to provide direction in the formulation of the needs analysis, links to organizations and groups within the community, and to ensure that all members of the community are represented in the

---

Box 5.7 Some questions to guide assessment of quality of care

- How physically accessible are services (e.g. public transport, disabled access etc.)?
- Is the timing of clinics and nature of appointment systems suitable?
- Are the privacy and dignity of the patient and the patient's carers respected?
- Is consideration given to the individual needs of the patient and the patient's carers?
- Are cultural and religious requirements recognized and catered for?
- Are dietary requirements recognized and provided for?
- Are difficulties in communication responded to and catered for?
- Is there access to a professional bilingual and/or advocacy service?
- How appropriate is the available patient information about services?
- Is there access to written information regarding service provision in community languages?
- Is account taken of a patient's preferences to consult and be examined by a male or female nurse/doctor?
- Do patients have access to complaints and suggestions procedures?
- Is appropriate physical and personal care available to meet individual cultural/religious requirements?

development and subsequent recommendations formulated. The effectiveness of the changes made needs to be assessed. Unfortunately, too often there is little immediate or obvious impact. In Chapter 8, I will examine policy formulation and impact, particularly with a view on what helps successful implementation.

5.6 How can services for minority groups be evaluated?

One of the early checklists for evaluation, *Checklist. Health and Race: a starting point for managers on improving services for black populations*, was prepared in 1993 by Yasmin Gunaratnam of the Kings Fund Centre, London. It gave guidance on how to ensure that the health needs assessment process identifies the specific needs of local ethnic minority populations. It also provided the framework for a strategy for active community participation in service planning and review and for ethnic monitoring in service provision. A more up-to-date and comprehensive toolkit for evaluation of progress in the ethnicity and health field has been developed by the National Resource Centre for Ethnic Minority Health in Scotland. These and other tools will be considered in more detail in a strategic and policy context in Chapter 8.

Change can be shown by clinical/medical audit. For example, if a service audit has been undertaken, it should be repeated to assess if there is any improvement in the service, e.g. uptake of cardiac rehabilitation services by the minority ethnic community. This will allow researchers to see the effect—has any change taken place and if so has this change been evaluated and found to be worthwhile? Such audits can help release resources for change, as illustrated in Box 5.8.

Audit is a powerful and under-utilized process for evaluating change, and yet it is seldom perceived as an integral part of the process of health needs assessment. I am pleased to record that a series of large-scale audits have reported that the kind of problems identified in Box 5.8 are now largely a matter for the past in the UK.

5.7 A synthesis of knowledge accrued from service-level research and evaluation

In Section 5.2.6 I gave an overview of what epidemiological studies of migrant, racial, and ethnic minorities have shown. Given the diversity of populations and contexts, that overview was, necessarily, general. To do the same for this latter part of the needs assessment process seems necessary,

---

Box 5.8 Example of improving standards by audit

An audit of diabetes services was conducted in Newcastle. This project sought to compare the quality of both GP and hospital diabetes services for the South Asian population with that of the general population. Preliminary results suggested that neither group was receiving the optimum level of care but that for the South Asian population the situation was much worse. This study complemented earlier work in the area which examined levels of CHD and diabetes in the community and looked at users' views of services for these diseases. As a result of the findings Newcastle and North Tyneside Health Authority provided funding for community linkworkers to be employed with a specific remit to support CHD and diabetes care.

but is it not an impossible task? Even in attempting the impossible some useful, generalizable insights tend to emerge.

Across the world we have now accrued, collectively, a massive amount of experience on how to meet the needs of minorities, and this can be considered as three broad streams. First, there is a do-nothing or do the minimum stream, the second is setting up separate services, and the third is to adapt available services, also sometimes knows as the mainstreaming approach. In truth, in all societies, all three approaches are applied at different times and for different groups. At present the third stream is the one commanding support.

Some grand-scale examples of separate services are available, one of them being the American Indian Health Services (for Native American people). This service is long established. The health and health care of Native Americans is generally relatively poor, notwithstanding this service. Such grand-scale separate services are most commonly seen in support of indigenous peoples or other highly distinct groups such as Roma/Gypsies, often living in residential segregation, especially in rural areas.

By contrast to the grand schemes, which are few in number, there are innumerable small-scale services, often set up as projects on short-term funding to meet a deserved short-term need or to demonstrate efficacy of the concept. These have a chequered history. Most run out of funds long before the job is done or evaluated. Some are clearly shown to be successful at meeting needs and may either continue as projects or be absorbed into the mainstream of services.

These kinds of projects are an integral part of the migration, race, and ethnicity scene that will continue. There is one migrant group for whom they are of especial importance—undocumented migrants, especially in countries such as European ones where national health-care systems dominate. There, private care is difficult to access and expensive and 'ad hoc' projects are necessary because the mainstreaming approach below may not work, either because of lack of a clear health-care policy or a lack of trust by potential users.

Generally, health needs assessments favour the adaptation of mainstream, existing services to meet the general and specific needs of minorities. Most national laws and policies also support this approach. Conceptually, this view is strong, but making concrete and effective change in large, existing systems is a high-level challenge, especially in financially constrained times. We will discuss this further in Chapters 7 and 8.

While the amount of qualitative research and evaluation done in most localities is small—and much consists of local reports that are not openly published—worldwide there is a large literature, and to some extent the findings are consistent: minorities tend to be more satisfied with services than one might expect but definitely want better and respectful communication and tailoring of services in specific ways that relate to their culture or health outlook. On these accounts the demands of minorities are not great.

These kinds of views are supported by numerous studies showing there is considerable utilization of services by minorities, especially primary care and emergency room services. The consistent exception tends to be dental care, which often requires some fee-for-service. Surprisingly, the uptake of some preventive services, especially for children, e.g. immunization, tends to be high, while cancer screening rates tend to be low. It is of interest that these kinds of observations are being reported in the United States, Canada, several European countries, Australia, and New Zealand. Even when service uptake is equivalent, the outcomes may not be, and this is a matter of importance. Is this an inequity, caused by an inferior quality of service, or is it a matter of patients' preferences or biology? These are the new kinds of challenges that arise as data become available, and they require new, higher-order health needs assessment. We will return to these issues in later chapters.

5.8 **Conclusions on health needs assessment for minority populations**

This chapter shows that migration status, race, and ethnicity can be of practical use in the process of health needs assessment, and equally that the process is important to minorities. Effective consultation and involvement of minority groups in establishing clear objectives for collecting information and for agreeing how such information will be used is clearly desirable and important. In this way continuing (and not ad hoc) dialogue between health-care providers and local minority ethnic communities can occur. In practice, however, health needs assessments may be largely office-based statistical exercises.

Health needs assessment is a means of synthesizing information for policy, planning management, and service delivery purposes. It is a means to an end—better services and better health—not an end in itself. There are at least three reasons why some needs assessment projects may fail. First, there is a lack of understanding of what is involved and how to do it. Second, there is lack of resources or commitment. Third, there is a failure to integrate the results with planning and processes to produce change. Partnership with patients and community organizations seems like a way to reduce the risk of failure. With the increasing availability of data, and the interest and involvement of numerous public and charitable organizations in data collection and interpretation (Box 5.9), there is an increasingly solid platform for health needs assessment. Whatever we do, and whatever the needs assessment shows, there are bound to be tensions because of conflicting values, preferences, assessed needs and resource constraints.

The different models for meeting needs, e.g. separate services, special projects, and integrated approaches, introduced in section 5.7, will be considered further in Chapter 8.

Multi-ethnic societies need to be conscious of the wider effects on society of meeting needs by service adaptation. As discussed in Chapter 4, the response to rising racial and ethnic diversity is, initially at least, usually a negative one, with a tendency to blame the minority populations for innate or cultural effects that underlie their health problems. In such a phase, setting up specialist

---

Box 5.9 Some sources of data for health needs assessment

- Organizations with responsibility for census and other national demographic data. Organizations set up to collate, synthesize and publish information usually public health agencies or charitable foundations focusing on diseases.

- Local government offices (town hall or civic centre). Local population data analyses are usually based on national data sets but sometimes on local censuses or surveys.

- Organizations that are responsible for the health of defined populations, e.g. health and social care authorities.

- Epidemiology and public health departments in higher education institutions—for the latest research on minority groups internationally, nationally, and locally.

- Organizations responsible for health education and health promotion.

- Community organizations, particularly in undertaking consultations, and qualitative research or service evaluations.

- Services themselves through their diversity monitoring systems and quality improvement and audit programmes.

services may well be resented. However, spurred by rising global and national movements for universal human rights in the late 20th century, and the changing population structure now requiring more young and economically active citizens, many countries are changing their stance on immigrants. Equity of health status and health care has become a central focus in this changed world and health needs assessment is one of the tools needed to achieve this.

The following principles of needs assessment are important to minority health:

1. Avoid the piecemeal approach to tackling minority health needs whereby so-called ethnic-specific topics are tackled one by one. An overview is needed and it must be balanced.

2. Base the needs assessment on ranks of causes using case numbers and disease rates.

3. Refine understanding by looking at comparative indices, which will focus attention on inequalities and inequities.

4. Interpret the quantitative data in the light of the qualitative findings.

5. Draw causal hypotheses based on differences with care, and with due emphasis on social and economic deprivation as explanatory factors. Compare like with like.

6. Beware that inferences of biological differences between groups may be particularly prone to error and misinterpretation, and may harm the standing of minority groups. Even if there are biological differences these should not be interpreted as indicating superiority or inferiority.

7. Make a judgement, preferably in consultation with the minority populations concerned, on how the data can be best used to improve the health and health care of the population, majority and minority groups alike. This requires an understanding of the services already available.

8. Minority ethnic groups must not be excluded from, or inhibited from using, major public health and health-care initiatives even if segregated or special services are set up (and equally, others should not be excluded from the special services).

9. The needs of minority groups should be met simultaneously with the rest of the population, not deferred until some later date and handled as a separate matter.

10. All public health policies and plans should make explicit how the needs of minority groups are to be met. The details of how these are to be met in practice should not be relegated to secondary documentation.

The implementation of these principles in relation to national policies is discussed in Chapter 8. In Chapter 6, on inequalities, and Chapter 7, on priorities, I consider some of the issues that underpin the policies.

5.9 **Summary**

A health needs assessment is a systematic, comprehensive overview of both quantitative and qualitative data on a population or subgroup of the population. Its purpose is to help to create or adapt policies, strategies, and services to improve population health and health care. Health needs assessment in relation to migrant, racial, and ethnic minority groups is sometimes problematic because of a lack of data, particularly at local level and at the level of subgroup detail that is required. In addition to lack of data there may be lack of time, funds, expertise, and means to implement findings. Health needs assessment, particularly at the local level, is often limited to qualitative studies or consultations. For national studies, data from administrative databases recording broad categories of migration status, race, or ethnicity, or proxies for ethnic group such as country of birth, may need to be used. The limitations of such data need to be understood to reduce the risk of making poor decisions.

Needs assessment for minority populations should start by examining the actual level of health states, disease patterns, and health-care utilization within each group. This is the absolute risk approach. The findings can then be compared with other minority and majority groups. In most instances the standard comparison is with the White population. This is done for ease, habit, ethnocentrism, availability of data, the policy and political leverage of the approach, or statistical power. An alternative conceptual approach, but one that is rarely used, is to set the standard comparison against the group with the most desirable level of the health indicator under study. These comparative approaches comprise the relative risk approach. Qualitative data enrich and help validate the quantitative analysis by giving needs assessors access to opinions, perceptions, beliefs, attitudes, self-reported behaviour, and case histories.

Health needs assessments have shown that commonly held views on the needs of minorities are often erroneous, e.g. levels of immunization are sometimes high not low, life expectancy may be greater than in the population as a whole, and health education materials may bear little relation to disease patterns, etc. Having said this, some generalizations also tend to hold: needs vary by group; minority groups are better off in health status and even health care in some respects and worse off in others; service quality, including for preventive health issues and face-to-face communications, is usually worse for minority groups; and the articulated needs of minority groups focus on communication, information, religious requirements, dietary preferences, and informed consent. Needs assessment is an important way of influencing the development of services and improving the health and health care of minorities and contributing to the health of the entire population.

References

Aspinall PJ (2010) Concepts, terminology and classifications for the 'mixed' ethnic or racial group in the United Kingdom. *Journal of Epidemiology and Community Health* 64: 557–60.

Bowling A (1997) *Measuring Health: a review of quality of life measurement scales.* Buckingham: Open University Press.

Bowling A, Ebrahim S (2006) *Handbook of Health Research Methods: investigation, measurement and analysis.* Maidenhead: Open University Press.

Elliott B for the Newcastle Strategy Group (including RSB) (1997) Taking heart: reducing diabetes and cardiovascular disease among Newcastle's South Asian and Chinese communities. In *Strategy for Commissioning Services for Coronary Heart Disease and Diabetes for Ethnic Minority Populations in England and Wales: lessons from a four-site pilot study.* Newcastle upon Tyne: Departments of Epidemiology and Public Health and Medicine, University of Newcastle upon Tyne.

Gill PS, Kai J, Bhopal RS, Wild S (2007) Black and minority ethnic groups. In Raftery J (ed.) Health Care Needs Assessment. The Epidemiologically Based Needs Assessment Reviews, pp. 227–389. Abingdon: Radcliffe Medical Press Ltd. Available at: http://www.birmingham.ac.uk/research/activity/mds/projects/HaPS/PHEB/HCNA/chapters/index.aspx

Gunaratnam Y (1993) *Checklist. Health and Race: a starting point for managers on improving services for black populations.* London: King's Fund.

Hunt S, Bhopal R (2004) Self-report in clinical and epidemiological studies with non-English speakers: the challenge of language and culture. *Journal of Epidemiology and Community Health* 58: 618–22.

Mackintosh J, Bhopal RS, Unwin N, Ahmad N (1998) *Step-by-Step Guide to Epidemiological Health Needs Assessment for Ethnic Minority Groups.* Newcastle upon Tyne: Department of Epidemiology and Public Health, University of Newcastle upon Tyne.

Marmot MG, Adelstein AM, Bulusu L (1984) *Immigrant Mortality in England and Wales 1970–78.* London: HMSO.

Rawaf S, Marshall F (1999) Drug misuse: the ten steps for needs assessment. *Public Health Medicine* **1**: 21–6.

Senior P, Bhopal RS (1994) Ethnicity as a variable in epidemiological research. *British Medical Journal* **309**: 327–9.

Stevens A, Raftery J (eds) (1994) *Health Care Needs Assessment: the epidemiologically based needs assessment reviews.* Oxford: Radcliffe Medical.

Unwin N, Harland J, White M, Bhopal R, Winocour P, Stephenson P, Watson W, Turner C, Alberti KGMM (1997) Body mass index, waist circumference, waist–hip ratio, and glucose intolerance in Chinese and Europid adults in Newcastle, UK. *Journal of Epidemiology and Community Health* **51**: 160–6.

Other sources and further reading

Bhopal RS (1988) Health care for Asians: conflict in need, demand and provision. In Equity. A Prerequisite for Health. Proceedings of the 1987 Summer Scientific Conference of the Faculty of Community Medicine *of the Royal Colleges of Physicians of the United Kingdom in Collaboration with the World Health Organization.* London: Faculty of Community Medicine, Royal College of Physicians.

Bhopal RS and Donaldson LJ (1988) Health education for ethnic minorities: current provision and future directions. *Health Education Journal* **47**: 137–40.

Hawthorne K (1994) Accessibility and use of health care services in the British Asian Community. *Family Practice* **11**: 453–9.

Jones DS (2006) The persistence of American Indian health disparities. *American Journal of Public Health* **96**: 2122–34.

Madhok R, Bhopal RS, Ramaiah RS (1992) Quality of hospital service: an 'Asian' perspective. *Journal of Public Health Medicine* **14**: 271–9.

Madhok R, Hameed A, Bhopal RS (1998) Satisfaction with health services among the Pakistani population in. Middlesbrough, England. *Journal of Public Health Medicine* **20**: 295–301.

Murphy J, Clawson N, Allard M, Harrison D, Gocke, P (1981) Health Care Provision for the Asian Community. Working Paper No. 45. Manchester: Department of Social Administration, University of Manchester.

NAHA (1988) *Action not words.* Birmingham: NAHA.

Raleigh VS (1994) Public health and the 1991 census: non-random underenumeration complicates interpretation. *British Medical Journal* **309**: 287–8.

Chapter 6

Inequalities, inequities, and disparities in health and health care by migration status, race, and ethnicity

Objectives

After reading this chapter you should be able to:

- Understand why inequalities by migration status, race and ethnicity are inevitable.
- Appreciate the scale of such inequalities in a number of countries.
- Be able to differentiate between differences, inequalities, and inequities (or disparities).
- Appreciate the importance of these inequalities both to medical and health sciences, and to clinical and public health practice.
- Be able to discuss the strengths and weaknesses of several strategies for tackling such inequalities.

6.1 What are health inequalities and why are they inevitable by migration status, race, and ethnicity?

It is self-evident, intuitive, and common knowledge that each individual's risk of illness or death is variable, and often unpredictable. Each individual is unique and this even applies to identical twins, though less so because here only their environment differs. So we understand and accept that one person may have a much higher risk of a disease than another. It is less intuitive, but true, that this also applies to different population groups. Why does a disease or health problem, say a heart attack, premature death, or poor perceived health, occur more commonly in one group of people than another? This question lies at the heart of the debate on inequalities in health. While the observation of population-level differences in health is ancient, and is in the writings of Hippocrates in Greece about 2000 years ago, scientific pursuit of their causes and the development of actions to counter them are relatively recent and accelerating developments.

Before reading on look at Exercise 6.1.

Exercise 6.1 Inequality, difference, and variation

- What is meant by the word inequalities? What undercurrents are there to this word in industrialized countries such as the UK, the United States or The Netherlands? How does the meaning differ, if at all, from difference or variation?
- What kinds of inequalities are pursued in current research and which are not?
- Can you think of actions either in the past or in the present focused around health inequalities that were not driven by the desire to reduce the gap?

Inequality is difference, variability, and unevenness. Differences can be a result of many factors. The words variation and difference are quite objective and here have no specific associated interpretation. In the context of health and health care, by common usage, the term 'inequalities' is usually used to refer to those differences where social and economic factors are thought to be relevant in causation. Such inequality is considered undesirable in modern, democratic, egalitarian states. This was not always the case. In the times of slavery and Empire and their aftermath the idea of equality would have been alien to many people. The perpetuation of inequalities has been a goal of some societies, e.g. South Africa based on apartheid (see Chapter 4), India where occupation and social status were linked to caste and lineage, and of course the racist Nazi state in Germany (see Section 6.3.5). These are only a few examples of societies in which the focus on inequalities was not their reduction through compassionate interventions but their sustenance or even their exacerbation. In modern times, notwithstanding the rhetoric of equality, virtually all economies are structured to create economic inequality.

Most attention to inequalities in health, at least in European countries, has focused on wealth, sometimes measured as income, but since this is sensitive information more often it is measured indirectly by location of residence or by an indicator of earning potential and social status, such as occupation. There is no logical reason why those who are looking at inequalities in the health field should not, say, focus on inequalities between men and women, by age group, or by migration status, race, or ethnicity instead. Some work has been done on such inequalities, but not nearly as much as on those thought to be a result of socio-economic factors. In the United States, until recently, emphasis on race-based inequalities (currently termed disparities) exceeded that on wealth-related ones, although race was recognized as an important indirect indicator of wealth differentials. (The historical importance of race in the United States was discussed in Chapters 1 and 4.)

Inequality by migration status, race, and ethnic group is, potentially, a powerful tool both for scientific analysis and for social action in the field of health. For example, why, in comparison with the British population as a whole, is diabetes so common (two to five times higher in various studies) in people who originate in India but live in industrialized countries, and why is colorectal cancer relatively uncommon in the same population (about half the rate)? Interestingly, diabetes and colorectal cancer share some risk factors, e.g. obesity. Answers to these questions should hold important information about the causes of disease and should benefit all populations, because results are likely to be generalizable. The potential value of research tackling such questions is enormous, but in practice the potential for knowledge gain has been hard to realize, and it has been hard to take public health actions to reduce inequalities; in these examples, by reducing diabetes in Indians and reducing colorectal cancer in British populations.

Before reading on, reflect on the questions in Exercise 6.2.

Exercise 6.2 Genesis of migration status, racial, and ethnic inequalities in health and health care

- ◆ Why are such inequalities in health and health care inevitable?
- ◆ List five to ten broad factors that are important in generating health, preventing disease, and prolonging life.
- ◆ Are any of these factors closely related to migration status, race, and ethnicity?
- ◆ Which of these factors are potentially changeable within our lifetimes?
- ◆ What are the consequences, positive and negative, for health inequalities by migration status, race, and ethnicity?
- ◆ What are the consequences for trying to explain, as opposed to describe, such inequalities?

Health status, disease occurrence, and mortality patterns in populations are sculpted by factors such as wealth, environmental quality and protection, diet, behaviour, occupational and domestic stresses, and genetic inheritance. Varying exposures to these and other factors in different minority groups over long (in some instances evolutionary) timescales generates differences, as shown in Box 6.1 and Figure 6.1.

In the model in Figure 6.1 five major influences acting over long time periods are circled at the top. Taking them from the right, first we have genetic changes, which relate to the biological concept of race. Genetic changes occur differentially in different places and have lasting consequences, e.g. northern Europeans have through natural selection over some thousands of years lost much of the pigment in their skins, with the resultant high rates of skin cancer when they emigrate to sunny climes such as Australia. Then we have social changes that also occur locally and will also have long-lasting influence, e.g. in attitudes to the consumption of alcohol. These influences relate to culture and hence the concept of ethnicity.

The third and fourth influences are environmental, changing either the way humans interact with each other or other living things or with the natural environment. Clearly, long-settled groups have a long multigenerational history of living in particular environments, including interacting with differing patterns of microbes. These environments have shaped their physiology, biochemistry, body shape, and possibly immune systems too. For example, cool climates lead to a stockier build and warm climates to longer and leaner limbs. The final influence in the figure is human discoveries, including how to manipulate the environment, whether drugs or tools that permitted more efficient farming or manufacturing of goods. These factors are also related to the wealth of places. These influences differ from place to place, and hence the health of populations in different places begins to vary. When populations migrate they carry the historical and current impacts of these influences with them. In their new environments, a complex process of change is inevitable. Differences between places in environmental and socio-economic circumstances both drive, and arise from, migration. Differences can be perpetuated by the geographical and socio-economic segregation that is so common following migration.

Immigrants tend to settle in areas where there is cheap housing, and to take on poorly paid jobs. Such fundamental differences in culture, biology, and the socio-economic and physical

Box 6.1 Major factors generating or influencing health inequalities by migration status, race, or ethnicity

- Culture, e.g. taboos on tobacco, alcohol, contraception, etc., many of them generated by religious and spiritual beliefs that differ between populations.
- Social, educational, and economic status, e.g. knowledge of biology and causes of ill-health, languages spoken and read, qualifications that are recognized, and occupational opportunities.
- Environment before and after migration, e.g. climate, housing, air quality, etc.
- Lifestyle, e.g. behaviours in relation to exercise, alcohol, diet.
- Accessing, and concordance with, health-care advice, e.g. willingness to seek social and health services and adhere to advice, and use of 'complementary/alternative' methods of care including the health systems of the country or origin.
- Genetic and biological factors, e.g. birth weight, growth trajectory, body composition, genetic traits and diseases, etc.

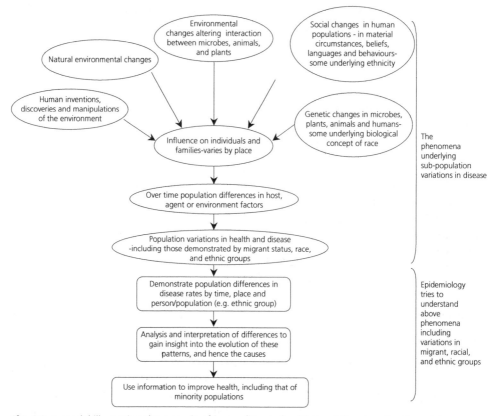

Fig. 6.1 A model illustrating the genesis of inequalities in health in relation to migration status, race, and ethnicity and how epidemiology tries to understand them.

Adapted from Bhopal RS, *Concepts of Epidemiology*, Figure 10.1, p. 350, Oxford University Press, Oxford, UK, Copyright © 2008, with permission from Oxford University Press.

environment, all closely linked to migration, race, and ethnicity, must lead to inequalities in health. It would be rather extraordinary if they did not. Some of these differences are captured in Box 6.1.

Socio-economic factors are profoundly important in causing, explaining, and countering health inequalities. The WHO Commission on Social Determinants of Disease, established in 2005, places especial (but by no means exclusive) emphasis on socio-economic factors, and calls for rebalancing in the structural drivers of health inequalities, i.e. in power, money, and resources. It is obvious, even from the most cursory examination of the issues, that these structural drivers are of the utmost importance to minorities, for almost everywhere they are concentrated disproportionately amongst those who are relatively disadvantaged. When economic hardship hits a nation, they are hit hardest. There may, surprisingly, be some difficulties in demonstrating the association between socio-economic status and ill-health in minority groups, particularly in the period following migration, for reasons that are discussed below.

Try Exercise 6.3 before reading on.

> ### Exercise 6.3 Inequalities, socio-economic status, and minority health
>
> ◆ Would you expect there to be important inequalities by occupation-based socio-economic grouping in minority groups?
> ◆ Why?
> ◆ If such inequalities did not occur why might that be so?
> ◆ What measures other than occupation-based ones would you use to study the association, in minority groups, between ill-health and socio-economic status?

There is a long-established and almost universally applicable link between better socio-economic status and better health. There is no reason, in principle, to expect that the link between high socio-economic status, high-level occupation, and better health outcome would not exist in minority groups. Socio-economic group (or traditionally, social class) measured by occupation, however, may be a poor measure of social status and access to resources in the period following migration, as well-educated people in minority groups may need to hold low-skilled, low-paid jobs, and immigrants who are apparently in the managerial classes may be in small businesses which are often struggling financially and involve low income and long and hard working hours. Some people in business, who may well have little education, will be doing well financially. (The main exceptions to the disruption of the link between education/skills and occupation are those immigrants who are selected on the basis of special skills for jobs where there is a shortage of qualified candidates in the recipient country.) The relationship between educational, occupational and social status, income and wealth, and health may well be disrupted by these kinds of changes. Over time, however, these relationships would be expected to be re-established. Williams et al. (1998) wrote an important theoretical paper explaining why migration disrupts the usual relationship and how it is re-established through change in patterns of behaviour, environment, biochemistry, physiology, and then clinical change. In long-established minority populations the importance of socio-economic factors is demonstrable. Other more direct and immediate indicators of socio-economic status, e.g. educational qualifications, ownership of household goods or a car, might give a truer picture in the early stages of migration. Area-based indicators, often based on postcode (zipcode) of residence are very popular as indictors of socio-economic position (area information coming from censuses), but they do not work well in studying minority health. While the residential patterns of long-settled majority populations might be shaped by socio-economic factors, e.g. the professional classes live in expensive neighbourhoods, the residential patterns of minorities are more complex, reflecting preferences to live in certain neighbourhoods where people similar to themselves live. This point is discussed in more detail in Section 6.4.

Cultural factors are also of great importance in generating health inequalities but decline in influence as health-related behaviours change across generations. Usually, there is a convergence of the minority populations towards the behaviours of the majority, which in relation to health-damaging behaviour is unfortunate.

The processes by which health inequalities occur, and the actions that are effective in narrowing them, need to be understood in the context of minority health. Each specific health inequality is likely to have its own genesis; unfortunately for public health there is no general explanation. For example, group inequalities in risk of skin cancers such as melanoma are likely to have a biological basis relating to skin colour (hence relating to race), while inequalities in stroke need to take account of many factors including behaviour, biochemistry, physiology, culture, health care, economic circumstances, and the presence of other diseases; and all these need consideration over the life-course, or even across generations. Fortunately, the powerful forces causing inequalities are amenable to change, and quickly—certainly over a lifetime. The main exception to this is genetic influence. Genetic factors are dominant in generating inequalities in a small number of diseases, e.g. the haemoglobinopathies, and contribute importantly in others, e.g. diabetes. Of course, an interplay of genetic and environmental factors underlies most specific diseases. One of the most contentious factors underlying inequalities is racism. It is by no means the sole or even dominant cause, but it has special importance and is given prominence in this chapter (Section 6.3).

Health inequalities across migrant, racial, and ethnic groups are complex and rapidly changing phenomena, and are only partially understood—a state that is unlikely to change greatly, because population sciences are not easily able to decipher such complexity. Worthwhile, if imperfect, public health actions are possible with incomplete knowledge based on sound general principles. Some such actions are considered in Chapter 8 while the scale of health inequalities across migrant, racial, and ethnic groups is considered in Section 6.2.

6.2 What is the scale of health inequalities by migrant status, race, and ethnicity?

Before reading on, try Exercise 6.4.

Exercise 6.4 The scale of inequalities across migrant, racial, and ethnic groups

◆ Estimate using the percentage scale (where 100% is the value for the population as a whole) the difference in the relative occurrence across minority groups of the following health conditions in industrialized wealthy nations such as Australia, the United States, the UK, and The Netherlands: tuberculosis, prostate cancer, lung cancer, CHD, suicide, road traffic accidents.

◆ Assume that the value for the group with the lowest occurrence is 100%, then state, as a percentage, the value in the group with the highest rate, e.g. 300% indicates three-fold variation.

The danger of emphasizing differences has been discussed but, nonetheless, inequalities in specific outcomes are surprisingly wide. For most of the specific conditions listed in Exercise 6.4 the variation would be at least three-fold and often much bigger. For infectious diseases differences are known to be exceptionally large, even 20-fold or more for diseases such as tuberculosis. Inequalities in cancers can also be very high, perhaps reflecting differences in exposure to causal factors, sometimes known (e.g. lung cancer and smoking) but often unknown (e.g. prostate cancer). Most surprising, perhaps, is inequality in non-cancerous chronic diseases. Some sample data are given in Table 6.1.

We do not usually see such big variations with most epidemiological variables. Variations of this magnitude, or even greater, are seen in international comparisons by country. Such international variations are, of course, partly reflected in the variations in migration status, race, and ethnicity we are considering. In minority groups some diseases are more common, others less common; the balance in terms of overall mortality and morbidity can, surprisingly enough, be hard to predict, and is certainly not always worse, particularly in populations that have migrated relatively recently. Quite often, overall rates are close to the population average or lower.

Table 6.1 Extent of variations in mortality by migrant or ethnic group: examples in men in England and Wales, The Netherlands, and Canada

Condition	England and Wales[1]		Netherlands[2]		Canada[3]	
Diabetes						
Highest	Bangladeshi born	670	Suriname born	5.29	Not reported	
Lowest	Chinese born	85	Turkish born	1.72		
Variation		788%		308%		
Ischaemic heart disease						
Highest	Bangladeshi born	151	Suriname born	0.93	South Asian origin	320.2
Lowest	Chinese born	44	Moroccans	0.40	Chinese origin	107
Variation		343%		233%		299%
Lung cancer						
Highest	Whole population of England and Wales	100	Turkish/Antillean/ Aruban born	0.68	European origin	129.5
Lowest	Pakistani born	34	Suriname born	0.38	South Asian origin	22.1
Variation		294%		179%		586%

Source: Data from (1) Gill et al, Health Care Needs Assessment: Black and Minority Ethnic Groups, in Raftery J. Abingdon (Ed) *Health Care Needs Assessment. The epidemiologically based needs assessment reviews, Third Edition*, pp. 227–389, Radcliffe Medical Press Ltd, Abingdon, UK, Copyright © 2007; (2) Bos et al, Ethnic inequalities in age- and cause-specific mortality in the Netherlands, *International Journal of Epidemiology Association*, Volume 33, pp. 1112–19, Copyright © 2004 International Epidemiological Association; and (3) Sheth et al, Cardiovascular and cancer mortality among Canadians of European, south Asian and Chinese origin from 1979 to 1993: an analysis of 1.2 million deaths, *Canadian Medical Association Journal*, Volume 161, pp. 132–8, Copyright © 1999 Canadian Medical Association. All rights reserved.

Migration may alter or exaggerate inequalities, e.g. population-level inequalities in diabetes have been increased by migration of South Asian, African Caribbean, and other groups to afflu- ent industrialized societies. This is an example of the contradiction of the general expectation of convergence of disease patterns following migration, because the migrants' levels of diabe- tes greatly exceed those of the receiving population, i.e. overshooting rather than converging. In long-settled minorities, and particularly in populations that have been displaced by colonists or enslaved, however, there is generally a health deficit and this can be very large. African Americans and Native Americans in the United States, Maoris in New Zealand, and Australian Aborigines are among groups that fit this generalization. Some general points on such populations were made in Chapter 4 in the discussion of Australia's response to ethnicity and health. The New Zealand Maori populations also show a huge health deficit, though possibly it is the most empowered of the world's indigenous populations.

The causes of inequalities are, as already stated, complex and difficult to disentangle even with careful and prolonged research. Of the numerous inequalities the one that has been studied most carefully of all is that between Black African Americans and White Americans. African American men live for 7–8 years less on average than White American men and this number has varied a little over the last 100 or so years, sometimes reducing, sometimes enlarging. The deficit arises from excess mortality in many causes, but particularly from chronic diseases such as CHD and stroke, and is partly explained by income differentials. This inequality increased over the 20th century, even in the face of improvements in civil rights in the 1960s leading to political and social equality. In the last 20 years the United States has made intensive policy and service-level efforts on this front and some reduction in inequality has occurred. Interestingly, immigrants of Black African or Caribbean origin in the United States have substantially longer life expectancy than US-born African Americans. Since official statistics often combine these groups, some of the African American/White American gap may be disguised. A legacy of slavery followed by a long period of open racial discrimination is proving hard to overcome but the existence of an intensive effort for improvement and some tangible success is encouraging. Economic status, social conditions, and social status are changing for African Americans with the rise of affluence, although far from uniformly. This kind of change ought to improve health status and reduce inequalities in the long run. Unfortunately, the worldwide economic recession since 2008 is hitting the poor harder than the rich and a temporary setback may follow. Indeed, in the UK levels of unemployment have risen most sharply in young Black men. Interventions to reduce health inequalities do not seem to have had much success, in that the inequalities seen in socio-economic indicators have proven resistant to change. So examples that narrow racial and ethnic inequalities are especially noteworthy.

In 2002 the Institute of Medicine published a landmark report: *Unequal Treatment: confronting racial and ethnic disparities in health care*. It promoted the use of the word disparities (which means difference, or inequality, or variation); this became widespread in North America and has also spread internationally. The Institute of Medicine defines disparity in a special way, i.e. a difference that arises neither from patients' preferences nor clinical need. In essence, there is an element of unfairness or injustice. This nuanced meaning is also seen in much writing on inequalities in health in Europe, where often inequality is not simply interpreted as a difference. In Europe the word inequity has been promoted, as this means unfairness and lack of even-handedness in treatment. The word inequity has not, however, become the standard terminology (possibly because it is unfamiliar and technical or perhaps because it sounds very similar to inequality). In usual usage, inequity, inequality, and disparity have almost identical interpretations. The issue of unfairness, in the health arena, is most sensitive in relation to health services.

Inequity in health care for minorities has been widely studied, and the detailed work in the United States on African Americans and White Americans has proven insightful. African Americans receive less health care, at least for high-technology procedures, than White Americans. This is at least partly explained by the financial burden of health insurance, which cannot be met by poor and especially unemployed people. African Americans are, compared with the US population as a whole, relatively poor with high levels of unemployment. Recent research has shown that hospital services for cardiovascular diseases in places where there is a large African American population are not as good as those where White Americans live. Given that the United States is highly geographically segregated by race and ethnicity this is important. The US experience over the 20th century, in which there has been great difficulty in narrowing inequalities, teaches us that racial and ethnic health inequalities may worsen even though they are closely studied and are socially and politically deplored, and notwithstanding excellent policies. The causes of Black/White health disparities in health status and health care in the United States are clearly complex. Racism is one of the proposed explanations. In countries other than the United States, which has confronted the problem of racism relatively openly, there are usually also concerns about the potential role of racism, though these are often not deeply or openly explored. Naturally, this is highly controversial, with many people, particularly politicians, unwilling to admit that racism could be important in health. Reviews of racism and health consistently show clear associations between perceived racism and ill-health, whether it be in relation to mental health (the most clear-cut case) or physical health status such as raised blood pressure. While the interpretation of data on this topic is not straightforward, a causal relationship is perhaps the most compelling explanation—even though the causal pathway is likely to be complex. I will consider in Section 6.3 why it is necessary to look into the history of racism in science and medicine to help overcome one's own and others' disbelief about the potential importance of present-day racism, to generate the moral drive for action, to provide insight into how the powerful groups in society may abuse data on racial differences, and to learn that individuals and institutions act according to the expectations of their times.

An emphasis on disease differences (often quite unrelated to unfairness) that is so fundamental to the analysis required in science has spilled over to the arenas of health policy and management, where it is not always appropriate. Because the overriding interest of scientists, and of scientific journals, is on extracting insights into disease causation from data on differences, by way of hypothesis generation and hypothesis testing, the presentation of data generally emphasizes relative risks using summary measures which compare one population with another. Such presentations, understandably given their purpose, under-emphasize disease numbers or rates. (The principles were discussed in Chapter 5.) Such research may then be used in making policy on disease priorities. Uncommon diseases which are, nonetheless, more common than in the general population may receive emphasis at the expense of common diseases which have comparable or lower frequency. For example, lung cancer in populations of Indian origin rarely receives attention, yet it is the commonest cancer in men of Indian origin. One outcome is that health education for Indian-origin populations about smoking, the principal cause of this disease, is not given due priority. Attention to specific differences (inequalities) can paradoxically worsen general health inequalities. This matter is considered in more detail in Chapter 7.

6.3 Perpetuation and augmentation of ethnic health inequalities: the potential role of racism

Try Exercise 6.5 on racism before reading on.

Exercise 6.5 Racism

◆ What do you understand by the term racism?

◆ What kind of racism can you envisage in a health-care setting?

◆ In what way might information on differences in health in relation to migration status, race, and ethnicity worsen racism?

6.3.1 Defining racism and assessing its importance

Racism is the belief that some races are superior to others. This is used to justify actions that create, perpetuate, or deepen inequality by favouring the supposedly superior groups over others. In practice, as was done by the House of Lords in the UK, the definition of race is broadened to include ethnicity, religion, and other similar characteristics, including being foreign, i.e. migration status, so that discrimination on such grounds is also covered under laws against racism. Various kinds of racism are discussed later in this chapter.

While racism is not usually based on research evidence, it can both be initiated and made more potent by research. Paradoxically, differences potentially caused by racism can then be used to justify it; e.g. if the rate of homicide is high in a particular migrant, racial, or ethnic group, or performance in IQ or school tests is poor, perhaps as a result of racism leading to economic deprivation, this information can be used to make claims about the inferiority of such a group. In this way further racism is (falsely) justified and a vicious cycle is created. For more general health inequalities arguments might be based upon pseudo-Darwinian-type notions of survival of the fittest, as illustrated by the following quotation:

> By the turn of the century, Darwinism had provided a new rationale for American racism. Essentially primitive peoples, it was argued, could not be assimilated into a complex, white civilization. Scientists speculated that in the struggle for survival the Negro in America was doomed. Particularly prone to disease, vice, and crime, black Americans could not be helped by education or philanthropy. Social Darwinists analyzed census data to predict the virtual extinction of the Negro in the twentieth century, for they believed the Negro race in America was in the throes of a degenerative evolutionary process.
>
> The medical profession supported these findings of late nineteenth- and early twentieth-century anthropologists, ethnologists, and biologists. Physicians studying the effects of emancipation on health concluded almost universally that freedom had caused the mental, moral, and physical deterioration of the black population.
>
> Brandt (1978)

Some people deny that racism is commonplace in modern, industrialized, multi-ethnic societies, but research shows it is very important. In the 1990s, in a national representative survey in the UK by the Policy Studies Institute (Modood et al. 1997), 20–26% of the White participants (p. 159) admitted at interview to prejudice against Asian, Caribbean, or Muslim ethnic minorities. In truth, the figure is likely to be larger, for some people do not give publicly unacceptable answers at interview. Surveys also show that negative attitudes towards immigrants and immigration are commonplace, and have recently become commoner, though negative attitudes are less common in younger generations. While racism is perceived to be a pervasive problem that is being brought under control, the suggestion that a health-care system is racist is hard to accept by health professions governed by ethical codes emphasizing their humanitarian duties.

While racism in health care is often evoked as an important explanation for inequalities, empirical research demonstrating this is surprisingly hard to find, interpret, and act upon. Much anecdote and analysis, however, puts racism at the hub of ethnic and racial disparities in health and health care. A rapid rise in ethnic minority populations in many cities, easy international travel, pressures increasing migration from developing countries, the presence of undocumented migrants, and a rise in the number of refugees are among factors fuelling tensions in health and welfare services in the 21st century.

When research implies that genetic factors are the cause of group differences in health status, minorities may be portrayed and perceived as biologically weak. In these circumstances biology and medicine may become the servants of racism. We have already discussed in Chapter 1 the potential harms of the race concept. Racism can cause death and despair in ways that are, with the exception of disease epidemics, almost unparalleled in human history, as in the massacres in Nazi Germany, Bosnia, Serbia, and Rwanda. Racism can be compounded by other forms of discrimination, e.g. on the basis of religion, sex, or disability. Antiracism activity, therefore, sits squarely in the wider arena of the struggle against oppression. A historical perspective is useful in shedding light on what is happening and what could happen, and provides a sound basis for thinking through the arguments for and against positive discrimination. The following account builds upon the foundation laid in Chapter 1, and will be considered again in the context of research in Chapter 9.

6.3.2 **Historical racism**

Thinking about different human populations and trying to interpret differences is not a new or modern phenomenon. For example, amongst many comparisons, Hippocrates contrasted the feebleness of the Asiatic races with the hardiness of the Europeans. Seemingly, his concept of race was of human groups shaped by ancestry in different geographical conditions, especially climate, which he saw as a powerful influence on character. It appears that intrinsic and fixed genetic, biological differences were not the point of emphasis. The following quotation from Montagu (1997) illustrates the kind of thinking found in earlier eras.

> From the earliest times, the emotional attitude that one's own ethnic group, nation, or culture is superior to others, has been a concomitant of virtually every culture. Within any society, in earlier times, men might be persecuted or made the object of discrimination on the grounds of differences in religion, culture, politics, or class, but never on any biological grounds such as are implied in the idea of racial differences.
>
> Montagu (1997, p. 59), reproduced with permission from AltaMira Press.

This emotional attitude is described as ethnocentric. The scientific idea of races as distinct species of human beings (polygeny), which was against the teachings of most religions including Christianity, gave way to the idea of races as biological subspecies of a single human species (monogeny) in the 18th century (see Chapter 1). In the 19th century differences in anatomical, physiological, behavioural, and health status by race were avidly sought. The central tenet of racism, that some races are superior to others, was widely believed, seen as self-evidently true, and vigorously supported by influential scholars and researchers in the 19th century (for more details see Chapter 9). Genetics undermined the biological concept of race in the 20th century and Nazi racism generated the widespread disgust that fatally undermined ideas of a master race and its refinement through eugenics. In Section 6.3.5 I introduce Adolf Hitler's views on race and health as an example, admittedly extreme, but still informative, of why racism is, and must remain, a central health issue.

Remarkably, although the concept of race is now considered to be based on a few physical features (such as colour and facial features) that are of little direct importance to health, but which serve important social and political purposes, the idea of a biological basis for health differences by race and ethnicity remains strong. The resurgence of the biological race concept is already evident, and there is new genetic research that is re-exploring old territory with novel methods. Some of it is perpetuating the traditional racial classifications (see Chapter 9).

According to Krieger et al. (1993) much research has supported, albeit unwittingly, the four assumptions needed for racism: distinct races, racial features linked to other important attributes, the differences between races being genetic, and the view that some races are superior to others. Krieger et al.'s charge is that racism is important because it leads to socio-economic inequalities, which underlie health inequalities; and that there are unexplained inequities in health care, including treatment for heart disease, renal failure, bladder cancer, and pneumonia. These inequities, at least in part, are inferred to be a result of racism.

I believe that few health professionals and researchers are racist, and that most hold humanitarian, antiracist views. We all are, however, products of our societies and are shaped by them. Scientists and policy-makers of the 19th century, when the prevailing attitude was that White races were superior and had a right (indeed responsibility) to subordinate coloured people, probably did not perceive their views and actions as immoral and would have justified them as in the interest of society and all racial groups. We should learn from the mistakes of our predecessors. The current thinking is that the basis of inequality is complex and we need to demonstrate and quantify the specific effect of racism so that rational action can be taken. In the meantime there is a reluctance to concede the possibility that racism is important. In time, will this viewpoint be judged in the same harsh way we judge 19th-century thinking? Will our successors judge current health care to be racist, and our institutions to be trapped by the prevailing ethos of *our* times? Will they judge that knowledge about racism was more than ample to justify action?

As the research record does not permit an unequivocal quantitative answer to the question of whether current inequalities in health and health care are created and maintained by racism, should we do more research until its distinct contribution becomes clear, or should we accept the consensus of scholarly and political analysis as the basis for action? The answer is unclear. Some question the value of researching racism, while others advocate that racism is researchable and should be researched.

In Britain, empirical research evidence which directly supports the case for racism being important to the health and health care of ethnic minority groups is rare except for discrimination in health-care employment and training. This was discussed in a wider context in Chapter 4, and will be considered in Chapter 8.

The United States leads, by a very long way, in the examination of inequalities in health care by ethnic group, as illustrated in Section 6.3.3.

6.3.3 Differences between Black (African American) and White patients in the management of disease in the United States

Numerous studies have documented that in the United States the intensity of activity relating to medical care for White patients exceeds that for non-White, especially Black, patients (Geiger 1996).

The consistent and repeated findings that Black Americans receive less health care, particularly using expensive new technology, than White people is becoming an indictment of the United States' health-care system. The disparities have been observed across geographical areas and times and are not simply due to differences in socio-economic circumstances, but are undoubtedly strongly influenced by the capacity to purchase medical insurance in the United States and by where you live.

A study by Escarce et al. (1993) was typical of the genre (for others see Section 6.3.4). They examined 32 procedures and found that White patients were more likely to receive 23 services while Blacks were more likely to receive seven. Four main hypotheses were considered: different disease patterns; differential contact with physicians, especially specialists; financial and organizational barriers, e.g. caused by the fact that government health-care support schemes Medicare and Medicaid still require patients to pay some costs; and patients' preferences. The authors emphasized the possibility that physicians managed their patients differently on the basis of race.

In Chapter 8, we will briefly examine some of the policy documents that review the evidence, and the recommended responses.

The literature on disparities in the management of heart disease by race in the United States is large and difficult to interpret. The studies focus on the quantity, not quality, of care and one study examining outcomes, by Peterson et al. (1997), does not evoke a sense of inequity, unlike those which only examine quantity of care. The increasingly common interpretation that racism has a part to play surely has some truth in it, but how much? Can the distinctive contribution of racism be disassociated from the many interacting factors, including patients' preferences? For example, one kind of explanation of the findings on medical care procedures which links historical racism to the current disparities is this: that due to the legacy of racism Blacks distrust invasive diagnostic and therapeutic procedures which inhibits them accessing care and accepting it even when offered. In this climate of distrust, physicians may be inhibited from advising invasive procedures.

If so, even if patients' preferences are judged to be partially responsible for the disparities, racism will not be exonerated. This explanation is over-simplistic because, given the opportunity, African Americans are enthusiastic users of the United States' health-care system. In a recent systematic review (Shah et al. 2012) we showed that African Americans continue to have much lower survival after cardiac arrest—even after so much research and policy on this and related topics.

Bringing health and health-care inequalities to public attention, however, has risks, as we now discuss.

6.3.4 Inequalities, stigma, and the social standing of migrant, racial, and minority ethnic groups

Before reading on, do Exercise 6.6.

Exercise 6.6: Potential of harm from portraying inequalities related to migrant, racial, or minority ethnic group

- Consider the inherent dangers of publicizing inequalities related to migration status, race, and ethnicity.
- Consider the dangers in relation to: public standing of these minority populations, priority-setting, policy formulation in health care, the type of research done, and media portrayal.

The misperception that the health of migrant, racial, and minority ethnic groups is poor, as opposed to different (in some ways better, in some ways worse), can augment the popular belief that minorities are a burden, particularly on health-care systems but also on society generally. The perception is at least partially false, and some migrant groups, especially men, as shown in Table 6.2, show a healthy migrant effect. There are variations by disease cause but overall SMRs hover around the average for the population of England and Wales.

By contrast, variations in specific diseases are very considerable, as we have already discussed in association with Table 6.1. The perception of poor health amongst such minorities arises from a focus by researchers and planners on those differences where there is an excess of disease in the minority population, while often ignoring differences were there is little difference or even a lower risk of disease. In fact, for many causes morbidity and mortality rates are lower in minority groups and this is especially true in countries which have highly selected immigrants and where immigration is from afar.

Most research studies (including most of my own) are based on the comparative paradigm, and present data using the majority, non-migrant (often European-origin White) population as the standard against which to compare minority groups. Attention is then focused on those diseases which are more common in minority groups than in the White population, thereby displacing such problems as cancer and respiratory disease, which are also very common but less so than in the comparison White population (Gill et al. 2007). Cancers are, indeed, one of the central priorities of migrant, racial, and minority ethnic groups even though they are, overall, usually comparatively less common as we shall discuss in Chapter 7.

Racial prejudice is fuelled by the selective emphasis of facts, particularly in the more popular mass media, which generally portray migrant, racial, and ethnic minorities as inferior and the majority as superior. Infectious diseases such as AIDS and tuberculosis are a common focus for such publicity. Researchers and public health practitioners cannot be responsible for the negativity

Table 6.2 Standardized mortality ratio for all causes of death by country of birth and sex in the age group 20–69 (20+ years for Wild 2007)

Country of birth, first author, and date of publication	Sex	
	Male	Female
Indian subcontinent/India		
Marmot (1984)[1]	99	111
Balarajan (1990)[2]	106	105
Wild (1997)[3]	106	100
Wild (2007)[4] (India only)	96	104
Caribbean/East Indies		
Marmot (1984)[1]	95	131
Balarajan (1990)[2]	79	105
Wild (1997)[3]	77	91
Wild (2007)[4]	102	98
Africa/West Africa		
Marmot (1984)[1]	133	144
Balarajan (1990)[2]	109	114
Wild (1997)—West Africa[3]	113	126
Wild (2007)—West Africa[4]	117	121

[1] Mortality in the period 1970–2.
[2] Mortality in the period 1979–83.
[3] Mortality in the period 1989–92.
[4] Mortality in the period 2001–3.

of some media reportage, but they should be aware that their data may well be used to damage the standing of the populations they are studying. Researchers and policy-makers, however, have a responsibility to provide an overview and not to overstate problems.

In grappling with these difficult issues, we should heed two great historical lessons. First, the study of health and health-care differences by migrant, racial, and ethnic group will be distorted by the prevailing ethos in society. If society is racist, the study of migrant/racial/ethnic difference will also be racist, in effect if not in intent. Second, the act of seeking differentials by migrant, racial, and ethnic group, while important for reducing inequities in health status and health care, poses a potential danger to the people studied, for the outcome is dependent on the interpretation and use of the data. While racist attitudes and behaviours persist, the danger of abuse of research for racist purposes will remain. A supreme example of these lessons is the abuse of Binet's test of intelligence, designed to select children for special educational attention but used in the 1920s as a tool for immigration control and for the demonstration of racial inferiority and superiority (see Gould 1984).

6.3.5 Racism: some lessons from the views of Adolf Hitler

We forget historical lessons at our peril. One lesson that should never be forgotten is of racism in Nazi Germany. This example provides a strong motivation to fight racism. Hitler's views were published in his book *Mein Kampf* (volume 1 was published in 1925) to widespread acclaim and support, acting as an inspiration to much of the German public, and the German medical profession in particular. Hitler clearly tried to build his case upon science, albeit in retrospect poor science. If the modern world were free of racism, nationalism, and other forces leading to harsh inequality and directed cruelty, there would be no reason to reflect on Hitler's views. Sadly, this is not the case, and there are many signs that racism as a component of right-wing political policy is making a comeback, partly as a result of Islamophobia following the al-Qaeda attacks in New York in September 2001 and partly because of the economic crisis since 2008. Echoes of Hitler's views, albeit much softened, are abundant in the mainstream media, e.g. arguments based upon the need to increase the cultural cohesion of society, the danger of diluting national traits by immigration, and subtle versions of the concepts of cultural and racial superiority.

Readers can access a succinct review by Silver (2003) on the central role of the medical profession—'the staunchest supporter of the Nazi regime'—in the euthanasia of psychiatric patients, the imposition of sterilization and other policies of eugenics, race medicine, marriage laws, killing of children regarded as defective, experimentation in concentration camps and on prisoners, anti-Semitism, and the attack on academic and professional standards. Some of the key points mentioned in Silver's article are shown in Table 6.3.

After decades of resistance, in 2012 the German Medical Association admitted the guilt of the profession and of its leaders, fittingly in Nuremberg. Hitler built upon a rich legacy of racism in medicine and science, much of it developed in Germany but also the tradition of eugenics fostered in the United States (see Chapter 9). The economic, social and political circumstances that allowed Hitler's policies to flourish could return, and at the time of writing (2013) right-wing, anti-immigrant political parties are gaining support.

Table 6.3 Key events relevant to the medical profession, race science, and racism in Germany

1905	Racial Hygiene Society formed in Berlin
1931	Prospective marriage partners of SS troops checked by a physician for racial purity over five generations
1932	20 institutes of racial hygiene and 10 journals in existence in Germany
1933	13 000 Jewish physicians in post. Jews forbidden from publishing in German books and journals, and German doctors forbidden to quote works of Jews. Jewish students restricted to 1.5% of total. 6% of doctors have joined Nazi league
1933	Euthanasia becomes policy
1935	Marriage or sexual intercourse between Jews and citizens of German blood prohibited
1935	Widespread medical experimentation with focus on eugenics, with Dr Joseph Mengele as a leader in Auschwitz
1937	4200 Jewish physicians in post
1938	Most Jewish doctors decertified
1945	45% of doctors had joined the Nazi Physicians League (6% in 1933). 7% of doctors were SS members compared with 0.5% of the population

6.3.5.1 Hitler on racial admixture

Race science flourished in Germany in the early 20th century. According to Silver (2003), Hitler's policies were influenced by such work. Hitler drew his arguments against the sexual mixing of races from the natural world (Hitler 1992). His analogies refer repeatedly to animals. He believed that such mixed unions were deleterious because they reduced the superior breed. Hitler's denigration of mating between human racial and ethnic groups, as if they were different species, was scientifically wrong. His idea that the offspring of unions of mixed race/ethnic group are inferior does not fit with genetic and evolutionary theory favouring outbreeding to inbreeding, or what gardeners refer to as 'hybrid vigour'. Hitler was simply wrong.

The philosophy that Hitler promoted wanted subordination of the inferior and weaker. he wrote, 'in a bastardized and niggerized world all the concepts of the humanly beautiful and sublime, as well as all ideas of an idealised future of our humanity, would be lost forever' (Hitler 1992, p. 348). Hitler's extreme language on mixing of the races marked the emotional foundations of his arguments, despite their being presented as ostensibly scientific.

6.3.5.2 Hitler on the superiority of the Aryan race, and the exploitation of inferior groups

Hitler attributed everything worthwhile in human culture to the Aryan race. While stating that it was idle to argue which race started human culture, he then claimed that it was the Aryan, without whom the 'dark veils of an age without culture will again descend on this globe' (Hitler 1992, p. 348). His thesis was that the contribution of Aryan people stimulated foreign people to achieve. When they reproduced with the Aryans, however, according to Hitler, their new-found advances collapsed, with the degradation of the master race and the subjugated race alike.

Racial commissions would be required, Hitler wrote, to issue settlement certificates in newly acquired territories, after the individual's racial purity was established. Hitler proposed that evaluation of race be done on individuals using blood tests; such evaluations are now being done with DNA as permitted by the new genetic technologies (see Chapter 9).

6.3.5.3 Drawing lessons from Hitler's legacy

The truism that those who forget history are bound to repeat is one that applies to racism. Hitler's goal of creating a superior society is shared by most political leaders, and many of his means, e.g. nationalism and control of occupational opportunities, reproduction, and immigration, are components of the political armamentarium of (especially) right-wing politics. Eugenics in its open form, by scientists and leading thinkers, is currently out of favour but its return is a likely accompaniment to the genetic revolution. Only open and flagrant racism remains unacceptable in mainstream politics, but that is because it is illegal in most societies. Knowing the effects of Hitler's views should stiffen the resolve of health professionals and researchers to combat racism. They should ensure their professional and learned societies have constitutions and policies that will empower them to resist, rather than assist as in Nazi Germany, a future racist state. As we will discuss in Chapters 8 and 9, some ethical codes for conduct in research and the medical profession are already in place, so the ground is prepared.

6.4 **Racism, ethnocentrism, and equity in service delivery**

6.4.1 **Types of racism in health care**

Try Exercise 6.7 before reading on.

Exercise 6.7 Racism, ethnocentrism, and equity

- Why might migrants and patients from minority racial and ethnic groups get worse care in a health setting?
- What kinds of racism can you see?
- What experiences of racism can you recount, either from personal experience or based on the experience of close friends or relatives?

Health services may offer a poorer service to migrants and minority racial and ethnic groups for the following five broad reasons:

1. Entitlement to health care is either not equal or, if it is, managers and staff are either unaware of that or unwilling to implement official policy. Virtually everywhere in the world the entitlement of legally settled migrants and minority racial and ethnic groups is equivalent to that of the majority. This entitlement may not result in equal care. The same is not true for undocumented migrants, and there may also be restrictions in practice, if not in law, on asylum seekers, and especially those who fail in their claim to asylum and hence are not given refugee status.

2. An individual member of staff treats the patient unequally because of racial prejudice. (Of course racial prejudice can also be exhibited by patients against staff.)

3. The policies of the service are based on the needs of the majority population and not those of the minority populations, thus creating inequity. Health services are planned and managed largely by members of the majority population, often on the basis of an implicit, rather than explicit, understanding of the needs and preferences of the users of the service. However, there is also a class bias and people from poorer, less articulate groups are likely to receive poorer quality (though not quantity of) care.

4. The specialist resources required to meet the needs of minority groups simply do not exist even though they are recognized by policy-makers.

5. Employment practices in the service are discriminatory.

There is evidence that all five of these forces are in action and contribute at least in part to the now well-established general finding that even when health care is, in theory, available to minorities it is sometimes not there in the quantity and often not of the quality that might be expected. A series of studies indicates that undocumented migrants find it very difficult to access services, even those they are entitled to. Entitlement is usual for primary care, emergencies, pregnancy, and for certain communicable diseases. For asylum seekers entitlement is usual but the quality of the service delivered may be suboptimal, especially when they are being held in detention centres. For settled minorities, access to and utilization of most health services is mostly adequate but with higher than expected use of emergency services and lower than expected use of services such as dental care and cancer screening. In Europe, unlike the United States, recent studies indicate that settled minorities do have access to most high-technology hospital interventions, overturning findings from some decades ago. On-going concerns focus especially on services where there are insurance payments or fees to be met directly by the users, the quality of interaction where there are linguistic or cultural barriers, and preventive services. Given this context we can consider the issue of racism.

There are various kinds of racism (hence the use of the word racisms by some writers), including the following:

- *Direct racism.* This occurs where people are treated less favourably because of their migration status, race, ethnicity, religion, etc. Most people equate racism with this type of action, and in modern societies such racism is both abhorred and illegal. When it occurs there may be high-level controversy and media interest. Direct racism is increasingly only seen either in war, during communal tension, gang fights, in public gatherings such as football matches, and as sporadic incidents which are sometimes serious, such as murder. Day-to-day discourse may utilize racist ideas in humorous ways, but mostly it has gone or been suppressed. Importantly, health-care systems do not tolerate direct racism.

- *Indirect racism.* Services are provided, on the face of it, equally to all people, but the form in which they are provided favours some groups. It may not be obvious. Moreover, it may not be perceived as a problem. For example, provision of information by health professionals only in English indirectly discriminates against those who cannot understand or read this language.

- *Institutional racism.* The concept further develops indirect racism but as applied to organizations, and is extremely controversial, not least because of its great challenge. Institutional racism is defined in the Macpherson report as:

> *The collective failure of an organisation to provide an appropriate and professional service to people because of their colour, culture or ethnic origin. It can be seen or detected in processes, attitudes and behaviour which amount to discrimination through unwitting prejudice, ignorance, thoughtlessness and racist stereotyping which disadvantage minority ethnic people.*
>
> Macpherson (1999, para. 6.34, p. 8), licensed under the Open Government Licence v.1.0

The Macpherson Report was commissioned in response to the racist murder of Stephen Lawrence in London, and the inadequate investigation of this by the Metropolitan Police. The inadequacy was explained as being due to institutional racism.

Some people are baffled by institutional racism, while others may pretend to be, possibly as part of the process of denial. A simple example would be the failure of the health-care system to make accurate diagnoses because it fails to provide the training and facilities (e.g. interpreters) to achieve communication of sufficient quality between patient and doctor to take a detailed medical history. Sceptics may still wonder why such practices are wrong, and might argue that not knowing the local language is not a problem for the service but for the minority populations. There is a kernel of sense in that argument and it is wise for minorities to maximize their local language skills. While counter-arguments are usually couched in terms of social justice, morality, ethics (particularly beneficence), and rights, increasingly the argument is being made on good business and professional practice, focusing on meeting the clinical needs of the patient as a valued customer in an efficient and effective way and the essential needs of the professional. Interpreting services are a perennial target of attack and controversy, and calls for their abolition are common and sometimes successful, as recently happened in The Netherlands. We will discuss this again in Chapter 8, in the context of developing health-care strategy.

Ethnocentrism (see Section 1.5.3) may well underlie indirect and institutional racism, because it may lead to inappropriate assumptions and perceptions about the needs and ideal behaviour of people from minority groups that are based on the experience of the health professionals in serving, and being acculturated in, the majority (usually White) population. Practitioners, policy-makers, the general public, and politicians may also feel that their own (ethnocentric) way is the correct or even ideal one, and that minority populations ought to conform to it, at least in the local context. Interactions between health professionals and minority users are, of course, shaped by social conventions, whether real or perceived. It may be that White people of European origin cannot see the advantages that they have in comparison with non-White people.

Explanations offered for the inability of professionals to deliver an equitable service have included the social distance between them and their minority patients, the gap of culture and communication between practitioners and patients, and the complexity of the problems of many minority patients, particularly as they relate to social and economic deprivation. Fundamentally, however, most professionals can only reflect the social mores of the times—a minority of them will be spearheading a process of change. Racism is mostly deplored but still prevalent in most societies and it affects health-care systems and their staff (and, of course, their patients).

6.4.2 **Personal experiences of racism**

As a child born in India to Indian parents (who migrated to the UK in 1955) but raised from the age of 2 years in Glasgow, Scotland, being called 'darkie' or 'Paki' was a daily event when I was in primary school in one of the poorest areas of the city. When I was 17 I was offered, by telephone, a summer job selling household goods door to door, a much-coveted opportunity for earning some money for a schoolboy. When I reported for work next day the offer was abruptly withdrawn. A senior manager had overridden the person who employed me (to his obvious embarrassment). Although unspoken, I knew and he knew that the company perceived that a brown skin was a disadvantage for a door-to-door salesman. At university some much-loved friends (including my roommate) regularly enjoyed racial banter at my expense, e.g. 'you're a black bastard Jindi [my nickname]'. Their intention was humorous and (probably) was not to hurt me, but it did hurt, and as time went on the banter destroyed some close friendships. I regret I did not have the strength to combat it at the time.

The house I had surveyed as a middle-ranking doctor in training in a middle class neighbour-hood in Glasgow was withdrawn from sale after I put my offer in, to the embarrassment of the estate agent. It turned out a neighbour had objected to the sale to a coloured person.

My aunt was left in diabetic coma all day in a prestigious teaching hospital because the nurses could not communicate with her and so left her 'to sleep' (a mix of negligence and institutional racism).

I have also heard a great deal of racism from people of my own ethnic group, i.e. Indians, and this has been directed at a range of others including White British, Jewish, and African communi-ties. No group is free of racism but racism with power is the cause of larger-scale problems.

These are relatively minor matters compared with some experiences of racism, such as mob lynching and racist murder, but they are on the same spectrum. My experiences are not unique, and they may have lasting consequences

I have preferred in my life to emphasize the thousands of positive interactions rather than the relatively few negative ones. Certainly, in schools, university, and in employment I have had huge support from teachers and colleagues, which far outweighed any racism. I am proud to be a British and Scottish Indian, and to work to create an even better society than the excellent one we already have. No doubt I have been guilty of racism, though I have consciously tried to avoid it in my life.

Nonetheless, I now see that I have been somewhat complacent throughout most of my life. Until about 1990 I refused to use the word racism in my writing and in my lectures, believing that its use did more harm than good. I hear others say racism is an ugly word and concept, and I understand them. Injustice, harassment, and prejudice on the basis of colour, religion, culture, migration status, or ancestry are even uglier and not tolerable. In retrospect, I ought to have been ready to confront these problems earlier, even in small ways.

6.4.3 Using migration status, race, and ethnicity to combat racism and reduce inequalities (disparities) in health and health care

Migration status, race, and ethnicity are clearly important in many ways, including the development of identity, belonging, and social relations, and are, naturally, the focus of racism. Trying to remove race and ethnicity from the mindset in multicultural societies is both impossible and, even more importantly, self-defeating. One conundrum we face is that a denial of difference is not a solution, partly because the social and service norms and policies are based on the needs of the majority, usually 'White', population. The resulting ethnocentric (Eurocentric) approach can be adjusted only after awareness of the issues is raised, and an analysis based on examination of differences is available. Such an analysis requires data by migration status and racial or ethnic group (for ethnic monitoring), and this requires classifications, which in turn requires acknowledging the importance of migration status and the concepts of race and ethnicity. Such data may be used to accentuate differences and provide the potential for abuse. So, we need a governing principle to help us progress.

I believe that the concept of equity provides the core ethical principle that we need. Try Exercise 6.8 before reading on.

Exercise 6.8 Equity, inequity, equality, and inequality

◆ What is the difference between equality/inequality (or disparity) and equity/inequity (or disparity)?

◆ Why might the concept of equity/inequity be more fitting in the context of minority health than inequality?

◆ Consider whether any of the following is an inequity: (1) the lower prevalence of smoking in women of Chinese origin compared with women of White European origin seen within a number of countries; (2) the higher rate of colorectal cancer in White people than in South Asians, even in the same country; (3) the lower life expectancy of African Americans than White Americans in the United States.

There is a general vocabulary used that discusses differences, but the words are commonly interpreted variably. The Glossary gives my understanding of the commonly used terms. In epidemiology and public health, differences are usually called variations and that is a synonym (disparities is potentially another synonym). Differences could also be called inequalities, which is, in fact, also a synonym. However, there is a long-standing use of this word indicating that the difference under study is neither inevitable nor just. The majority of work on inequalities comes from a socio-economic perspective. It is surely true that if socio-economic inequalities were changed health inequalities would also change, so in that respect the use of the term inequalities in this way is understandable. Exactly the same point applies to the word disparity that we discussed earlier. The only drawback is that not everyone will understand the nuance of injustice in the use of the words inequality and disparity, especially if they rely on dictionaries. By contrast the word equity means fairness and in line with the principles of justice, and inequity means the opposite.

An equitable service would meet equal needs equally, but this requires a diversity in the organization of services, to ensure uniformity in access, use, and quality at the point of delivery. An equal service, in the sense that everyone got exactly the same service, would not be equitable. For example, if a health professional gave all patients exactly the same amount of time, say 10 minutes, the service would be equal but inequitable. Some patients with complex problems, such as depression, may need 20 minutes, while others with simple problems, say the common cold, may need 4 minutes. In other words, the nature of the service should be tailored to meet the need, so it is equitable rather than equal. The principle in relation to meeting the needs of different ethnic groups is exactly the same. In international law one of the most important rights is that of non-discrimination on a number of grounds including race, ethnicity, and other characteristics such as nationality. The law only permit discrimination when there are objective reasons, including the need to rectify an imbalance. Achieving equity is, therefore, both an ethical imperative and compatible with the law on non-discrimination.

The extra challenges identified by studies of access and quality of care are usually well within the scope of the service. Improvements in services for minority groups often benefit the whole population, for many issues are common to all, e.g. the desire for health professionals and carers of the same sex for intimate (e.g. genital) examinations, and the wish for hospital food that is tasty and variable. Meeting the health-care needs of minority groups needs to be seen as a key responsibility of the service, not a chore or the patients' problem. Sometimes, in adaptations there will be some extra costs and management efforts required but these tend to be modest and bring savings in return.

Not every inequality is an inequity. It is hard to argue that ethnic variations in the prevalence of smoking are inequitable. There is no intrinsic injustice in the relatively low prevalence of Chinese women smoking compared with White women in European and North American settings. There would potentially be injustice, and hence inequity, in variable access to smoking cessation services by migration status or ethnic group. I can see no injustice in variations in colorectal cancer rates. There would potentially be an injustice if there was differential access to colorectal cancer prevention or treatment services. The words differences or variations are good in these circumstances, though inequalities and disparities are commonly used, simply through custom and the perception they attract more attention and interest. By contrast, I perceive a serious injustice in major differences in life expectancy in different migrant, racial, and ethnic groups, because these are almost certainly a result of other social injustices. By contrast with differences in life expectancy by migrant group, race, or ethnicity, it is hard to claim that the greater life expectancy of women compared with men is unjust, at least until we have a better understanding of the causes. At present, the causes are thought to be largely hormonal and biological or related to chosen lifestyles. Some of the sex variation may be a result of occupational hazards which may be inequitable.

Fairness in employment is a fundamental component of equity in health service delivery. Fair and open practices are needed for selecting people for study or employment, assessment of performance, disciplinary procedures, service on strategic decision-making bodies, career progression, and rewards. Talent and ability have no racial, ethnic, or cultural exclusivity. Migrants have demonstrated their talents across the globe, sometimes to the perceived detriment of local populations who may find it harder to compete for jobs. Health services across Western Europe, North America, and Australasia are major employers of migrants and have special responsibilities in fair non-discriminatory employment practices. International laws are extremely strong on human rights and non-discrimination and put strong emphasis on health and health care. International law takes precedence over national law. Most countries are signatories to international law. These laws are of great importance to migrant, racial, and ethnic minorities.

To create equitable services, however, needs more than legislation; it needs winning over the hearts and minds, and particularly the consciences, of service providers and managers. Guidance from professional bodies needs to be combined with national and international human rights and non-discrimination legislation to promote change. The professions of medicine, nursing, and public health should be in the vanguard of the historical and global struggle against inequality, injustice, and racism. Strategies for doing this will be discussed in Chapter 8.

Section 6.5 considers a more technical matter: assessing the role of socio-economic factors in inequalities, using an example around CHD. I have chosen this as it is an area in which I am particularly interested.

6.5 The role of socio-economic position in variations in health by migration status, race, and ethnicity: the example of CHD in South Asians in the UK

There are many factors contributing to the kinds of variations in health status we have considered in this chapter. Their causes are likely to be context and population specific. Nonetheless, there are two general explanations that are invoked or perceived as important. The first is genetic and as a result of biological differences. It is a scientific cliché for research to conclude that 'these differences may be genetic'. Though a popular explanation, it is rarely shown to be correct. This kind of explanation has already been considered and will be again in Chapter 9. The second common explanation is that the differences are 'merely' a result of variable socio-economic circumstances. This kind of explanation is also plausible and attractive and deserves careful evaluation. To illustrate the wide range of issues raised I am only considering CHD in South Asians in the UK, as the full topic requires a book in itself.

The background to this explanation is that those with socio-economic disadvantages such as poverty, unemployment, or low educational attainment tend to have worse health than those who are not so disadvantaged. CHD is one of many diseases where this association is consistently found. (There may be a short period of time, in the early years of a CHD epidemic, when the more advantaged groups have more CHD, but even if this is true it is not a lasting pattern.) Why might this be so? We can set aside the role of chance and study bias for the purposes here—both are unlikely anyway. The following seem relevant:

1. Those with CHD become disadvantaged as a result of their disease. This type of 'reverse' causation reasoning may apply to some people but is not considered an important explanation in this context.

2. The life circumstances of socio-economically disadvantaged people lead directly to CHD (possibly through stressors such as lack of control at the workplace or depression). For minorities, those in poorer circumstances may be faced with more stressors such as racism.

3. The life circumstances of socio-economic disadvantage lead to behaviours that are risk factors for CHD, e.g. more cigarette smoking or poor quality diet.

Assessing the role of these kinds of explanations is difficult, both conceptually and technically. The time-honoured but over-simplistic statistical approach is to examine what happens to the disease inequalities after adjustment for available indicators of socio-economic position. So, typically, the relative risk might be 1.5, i.e. 50% excess. The question is whether this will be changed (attenuated) towards the no difference relative risk of 1.0 after adjustment. If so, a typical interpretation would be that the ethnic difference was explained by socio-economic factors. By implication, we do not then need to invoke migration status, racial, or ethnic factors. If the difference is not attenuated, the typical interpretation might be that the difference is not explained by socio-economic factors and therefore other explanations are required. By this reasoning socio-economic factors are being treated as confounding factors (see Glossary). Confounding factors are association with both the outcome (CHD) and the variable under study (migration status, race, or ethnicity). Confounding factors are not, by definition, on the causal pathway between the variable under study and the outcome (though in our context, this requirement may not be met).

With this background we can now consider the case in question, i.e. the comparatively high rates of CHD in South Asians in the UK (and indeed in many other South Asian communities across the world). South Asians in the UK, especially Bangladeshis and Pakistanis, rather than Indians, are socio-economically disadvantaged compared with the White population. It is an obvious and reasonable question whether this disadvantage explains their high risk. If so, as socio-economic advancement occurs we would expect the differences to diminish.

Marmot et al. (1984) reported on immigrant mortality in England and Wales based on mortality by country of birth in years around the 1971 census; they showed that social class, based on occupation, and CHD mortality rates were unrelated in those born in the Indian subcontinent. If social class were the explanation we would expect CHD to be higher in people of lower social class born in the Indian subcontinent, i.e. those in semi-manual and manual occupations. In this study people born in the Indian subcontinent had a 15% excess of CHD mortality compared with those born in England and Wales, but the excess was not related to social class. Others, including McKeigue et al. (1989), reported that economically deprived (Bangladeshis) and better off (Indians) South Asian communities were at similarly high risk. If socio-economic factors were especially important we might have expected more disease in Bangladeshis than in Indians. The assumption was that socio-economic factors were not important, at least at this stage of the evolution of the CHD epidemic. This assumption fitted with the idea that CHD emerges in high-income groups first and the observation that the CHD epidemic in India is affecting those in groups with a higher economic status. The inference was that the epidemic in South Asians was at an intermediate stage where it was in balance in groups with lower and higher economic status. The view was that social and economic deprivation had not been an important determinant of the excess of CHD in South Asians. There are several plausible reasons why the expected association between socio-economic deprivation and higher CHD rates in South Asians was not seen. Obviously, the first reason is that it did not exist. If it did exist, however, it is possible that the indicators used to assess socio-economic status were not appropriate, or were in themselves insufficient. One powerful reason, discussed in detail by Williams et al. (1998), was that migration had disrupted the usual pattern of social stratification. It is a commonplace observation that after emigration some people with advanced education end up doing manual and other unskilled jobs, while others who did such jobs in the country of origin end up running a successful business. On this basis, given that the usual social stratification is likely to occur after settlement following migration, Williams et al. (1998) predicted that 'an inverse association between social class and coronary heart disease will emerge eventually in South Asians'.

Analysis by Harding and Maxwell (1994) of UK mortality data by country of birth for men aged 20–64 years around the 1991 census years, showed a social class gradient in all ethnic groups, with the highest SMRs in men in manual classes. For men born in the Indian subcontinent the overall SMR was 150, i.e. 50% higher than in the standard population. The SMR ranged from 132 in those in social classes I/II combined, to 223 in social classes IV and V combined. Taking social class into account statistically did not remove the difference between the men born in the Indian subcontinent and the standard population. The authors concluded that social class was an important factor for studying inequalities within the South Asian population. Social class did not, however, provide an adequate explanation for mortality differences between the population born in the Indian subcontinent and the standard population. Some indicators of social and economic circumstances are used because they are easily available or have been found to work (i.e. show associations) in other populations. Measures of social position based on occupation, education, or postcode (zipcode) of residence are examples. They have repeatedly been shown to be excellent for discovering and describing socio-economic inequalities. Nonetheless, they might not work for migrant, racial, and ethnic minorities. Perhaps other more direct measures would be more pertinent.

Nazroo (1997, 2001) found that the prevalence of self-reported CHD, assessed in a national cross-sectional survey in 1993/4, was associated inversely with the standard of living. In a statistical model, most of the excess in prevalence of self-reported CHD in Indians, Pakistanis, and Bangladeshis was removed after adjustment for an index of standard of living. Nazroo reported substantial differences between these three South Asian groups. For diagnosed heart disease or severe chest pain the overall odds ratio for Indians and African Asians (South Asians who were born/lived in Africa prior to immigration to the UK) combined was 0.95, which was, surprisingly, lower than for the White standard population, but after adjustment for standard of living it was 0.78 (95% CI = 0.6–1.01), i.e. much lower than in the White population (even though the 95% CI includes 1.0). Nazroo emphasized the comparatively low adjusted prevalence of CHD in Indians and the differences between the Pakistani/Bangladeshi and Indian subgroups of the South Asian community. He also emphasized the difference in the socio-economic standing of the three South Asian populations, with Indians being comparatively affluent, and Pakistanis and Bangladeshis relatively poor. Finally, he demonstrated that there were sizeable disparities in income between minority ethnic and majority (White) populations within the same social class grouping. These studies are consistent with the two alternative views that in the 1960s/1970s social/economic inequalities did not exist among South Asians but emerged later and that inequalities were missed for lack of sensitive indicators. The selection of potential indicators of socio-economic position and the demonstration of their cross-group validity is an important issue that has recently been studied. While the construction of an index of living standards, possibly based on reported possession of durable goods, is a promising approach, the problem is that these kinds of data are not routinely available so cannot be used in the analysis of existing large, national data sets. As there is no theoretical stance, to my knowledge, to guide our decisions the quest for valid indicators is an empirical one.

Amongst others, Bhopal et al. (2002) explored these ideas using data from the Newcastle Heart Project, a detailed, population-based cross-sectional study, designed to ascertain the prevalence of disease and risk factors. We used three measures: social class divided into manual and non-manual groups, educational status, and a composite measure based on the components of the Townsend score, an area-based index of socio-economic deprivation. These three measures capture slightly different aspects of someone's socio-economic position in society. Social class is an indicator of current or recent access to both income and social status. Educational level reflects, in particular, social standing in childhood and early adulthood, and is linked to earning power and social status. Education as an indicator of social standing is particularly important where education is not compulsory and is not free. The Townsend score is a reflection of the level of material wealth in the population in the area where a person lives. These kinds of measures are in widespread use in research on health inequalities.

The hypothesis under test was that socio-economic factors are associated with CHD and diabetes and their risk factors across the four ethnic groups studied, i.e. Indians, Pakistanis, Bangladeshis, and White Europeans. Williams et al. (1998) predicted that inequalities emerge with settlement. If so, in the population under study inequalities by socio-economic factors should be greatest in ethnic groups which have been settled for longest, i.e. Indians (42% moved to the UK before 1962) and Pakistanis (44% moved before 1962) and least in the most recent migrants, i.e. Bangladeshis (23% moved before 1962).

Mostly, as expected, lower socio-economic position was associated with more cardiovascular disease and diabetes and their risk factors in White Europeans but the pattern was less clear in the South Asian groups. We showed that social class, education, and Townsend deprivation score were more consistently associated with disease and risk factors in Europeans than South Asians combined; in Indians than in Pakistanis and Bangladeshis; and in women than in men. The European pattern of inequalities was partly established in South Asians, but different in different South Asian populations. We concluded that the emergence of socio-economic gradients in diseases and risk factors requires a mix of time, acculturation, and socio-economic advancement, and is influenced by factors such as sex, religion, and place of origin.

While their work was not on CHD, Kelaher et al. (2009) examined the possibility that conventional socio-economic and asset indicators might not be equally valid across all ethnic groups. They pointed to three reasons for this: (1) surveys asking the questions might have different response rates and be prone to response bias; (2) there might be cultural and social differences in economic priorities/opportunities; (3) within socio-economic strata there might be differences between ethnic groups in their assets. They provided evidence within their survey data, and recommended education as potentially the most effective indicator for across-ethnic group studies; but they also suggested including other variables such as car ownership, and more subtle indicators such as ability to loan money to family/friends. This sets the stage for describing the work done on establishing appropriate indicators within the Scottish Health and Ethnicity Linkage Study (SHELS).

SHELS consists of computer linkage of data from the 2001 Scottish census to a wide range of data on health status and health-care utilization (see Section 3.6.3 on linkage). Among the outcomes studied were a range of cardiovascular diseases. We included the first case of cardiovascular death or hospital admission in the period from 2001 to 2008. We were interested in whether the variations we found by ethnic group would be substantially reduced by adjustment for socio-economic factors. We developed a method for selecting appropriate and valid cross-ethnic indicators. We extracted eight such potential indicators from the census. We set the following criteria for variables that would be good indicators for examining socio-economic confounding. First, the indicator should be associated with both the factor under study (ethnic group) and the outcome (CHD). This is, indeed, a fundamental requirement—otherwise confounding cannot occur. Second, the direction of association between disease and indicator should be the same in each ethnic group. In other words, if the indicator (say higher education) was associated with a lower level of CHD in one ethnic group, it should not be associated with higher CHD in any other ethnic group. Where an indicator had several levels (e.g. our area indicator had five levels—quintiles) the association would, ideally, be linear across these levels. Finally, the inclusion of the variable in a statistical model where the indicator was used for socio-economic adjustment should alter the risk ratio. In line with Kelaher et al. (2009) we found the variable 'highest education of the individual' best met these criteria. Some variables were extremely inconsistent in the direction of association in different ethnic groups. Like Kelaher et al. we were able to show that sometimes inclusion of other indicators modestly improved the 'explanatory' power of the model. [In separate work we showed that education is a good variable for exploring potential confounding for CHD but not for other outcomes such as mental health (car ownership and housing tenure were better) or cancers (no indicators were satisfactory).] Even after adjustment for education, however, ethnic variations in CHD remained, and in some ethnic groups they were larger than before adjustment. In this context, ethnic variations could not simply be attributed to socio-economic factors. While it is possible that our eight indicators were not the right ones, the alternative explanation, that other socio-economic factors are more important in explaining these variations, seems unlikely. The questions of why socio-economic variables may have different effects in different populations in different settings and times is one open for research. It fits squarely within modern thinking about the study of different facets of inequality simultaneously, i.e. at their boundaries ('intersectional-ity' being the technical term used).

This kind of research is relevant to developing broadly based strategies for tackling inequalities, the topic of the Section 6.6.

6.6 **Strategies for tackling inequalities by migration status, race, and ethnicity in health and health care**

Before reading on do Exercise 6.9.

Exercise 6.9 Strategies to reduce inequality and inequity

♦ What strategies can you conceive of for tackling inequalities by migration status, race, and ethnicity in the health setting?

♦ Which facets of the underlying concepts of race and ethnicity, or the migration experience, might be amenable to change?

♦ What problems/conditions would you tackle first?

♦ How could relative and absolute risk approaches be used to devise a strategy?

I propose that strategic thinking in this field of inequalities needs a major adjustment of the usual research-led health paradigm which typically extols migration status, race, and ethnicity as keys to unlocking the secrets of disease causation. We need to see them as the means of assessing inequality, and guiding policy and practical action for improving population health, of minorities and the majority alike. Adding to causal understanding is, I propose, a bonus and not the primary goal. In this regard, migration status, ethnicity, and race become like indicators of social and economic status where expectations of causal understanding are tempered but their importance is still recognized. There are two separate but overlapping strategic outcomes—better health care and improved health status.

Box 8.5 (chapter 8, p 242) gives a ten-point outline used in the work of a health authority (NHS Lothian Health Board) serving a population of 650 000 people in the east of Scotland, of whom about 4% were from minority ethnic populations. This plan summarized the development of my ideas, influenced by a wide range of academic and service documents, studied over about 20 years. Examination of this 13 years later (it was proposed by me in about 2000) offers many insights in relation to the pace of change in the field.

I find this plan chimes with current strategies and policies. The only new point of emphasis is that the plan is generalizable to migrant, indigenous, and racial minorities—and could be generalized to other groups, e.g. the disabled, albeit with minor modification. The most straightforward strategic goal is an equivalent quality of health care for the entire population. This will require monitoring for equity in the quality of health care. All documents on health and health-care policy and service development/implementation should contain background information on, and a plan for, inclusion of minority populations. The key is to ensure that meeting the needs of minority groups is an integral part of the mainstream health-care and public health function. This principle is very hard to enact. Developing policy and services is a difficult task even without these complexities. Equality impact assessment of policies and plans provides a way to ensure that the needs of specific populations are articulated explicitly. There is resistance to this, and in 2012 the UK government announced it was proposing to withdraw the requirement for equality impact assessment. The Prime Minister, David Cameron, was reported to say that skilled civil servants don't need such tools to ensure their policies attend to equality. The question then is, why were they deemed necessary in the first place? Even now, policies are typically drafted without equality issues being given due attention.

Guidance on the health care of populations should promote actions to ensure the inclusion of minorities, and this issue should be a high priority for anticipated investments, i.e. in business planning. Information systems should be redesigned to produce health information, automatically, by minority group. In addition there should be an exploration of the potential for unlocking data already available by the retrospective addition of minority status codes (see Chapter 3).

Health-related literature available nationally, providing information and advice on both available services and on the health of minority populations, should be summarized and utilized more widely. Minority populations require health education/health promotion and service-related information to be adapted and either translated or conveyed face-to-face by interpreters/advocates. Minority populations, elders in particular, need high-quality translation, interpretation, and advocacy services to ensure high-quality communications in health care.

Culturally sensitive services are needed, and the highest priorities here will be:

- appropriate food in institutional care (hospital and long stay);
- advice that is meaningful in the cultural context in which it is to be implemented;
- facilities to pray and perform appropriate ablutions in inpatient facilities;
- choice of the gender of the health professional for, in particular, examination of the reproductive tract;
- sensitive and appropriate support in relation to the dying and the recently deceased.

Training is needed for all staff involved on the issues of migration, race, ethnicity, and health, including population size and structure; living circumstances and lifestyles; languages spoken and read; religions, both in terms of their tenets and as practised; and the implications of all this for modification of care. Equal opportunities policies will need to lead to sufficient employment of minorities for the service to have, within the workforce, the role models and insights to serve multi-ethnic populations. This may require proactive recruitment of staff with particular language skills or cultural understanding.

Principles concerning the causes, consequences, and control of inequalities derived from the general body of research, although largely on White populations, are highly likely to apply to minority groups. Failure to apply the general knowledge and general principles we already have while awaiting new research evidence specific to minorities, an ideal that would take several decades and hundreds of millions of pounds, is likely to be damaging. The challenge is to adapt general policies appropriately.

Health policies need to place emphasis on integrating primary care, social services, public health measures, and hospital care. They need to be based on sound data that are interpreted with care to achieve a robust understanding of priorities. Data do not, on their own, help people make coherent policy, and for this a set of social values is needed to guide their interpretation. The key value is equity—equal service for equal need. This value needs to permeate society and services, such that researchers, policy-makers, and practitioners are united in their common perspective and goal.

Health and health-care initiatives need to build on the work of community organizations, academic researchers, and the NHS. Community organizations are often well placed to highlight minority populations' experience of health and illness. They are likely to perceive health in the broad way that is usually favoured in public health, to include issues like poverty, housing, employment, discrimination, and violence. These perspectives are particularly valuable when combined with the insights of academic researchers examining patterns of disease and access to service provision by specific population groups.

The diversity of the population is very important in health and health-care policy and delivery. Migration status, race, and ethnicity should be considered as important elements of diversity alongside gender, age, religion/spirituality, sexuality, disability, and so on. There is, of course, diversity both within and between groups. For example, Pakistanis, Bangladeshis, and Indians differ in respect of religion, spirituality, and language. They also have differing patterns of disease and disability. Even within a group that is relatively homogeneous, e.g. Pakistanis, there is considerable diversity. Heterogeneity of migrant, racial, and ethnic groups is a massive problem for effective policy and practice, but needs to be accounted for as best as possible. Lumping disparate groups together can mislead policy and planning, e.g. as shown earlier South Asians collectively have a low prevalence of smoking but Bangladeshi men, a subgroup of South Asians, have an extremely high one (Table 3.1).

Effective strategies acknowledge that people from minority groups continue to experience racism in their daily lives, and this affects their mental and physical health. Refugees are likely to have suffered physical or mental problems, possibly even torture, in their place of origin, and may be particularly sensitive to the experience of racism in their receiving country.

The problem of inequity and inequality in the health and health care of minority groups has defied easy solutions. The explanation is not simply a lack of knowledge, interest, or even money. Paradoxically, by focusing on differences, inequalities can widen, as will be illustrated in Chapter 7 with a theoretical example. This approach has been historically harmful, and in recent decades unhelpful. The better approach, which was examined in some detail in Chapter 5, is to focus first on the important problems and diseases. Then, if necessary, refine the sense of priority using the relative approach. In this way important matters such as cancer and respiratory disease will not be ignored, as often happens. This would also avoid the piecemeal approach to tackling so called minority health issues. There are so many differences that it is difficult to find a logical way to make a selection. CHD, stroke, cancer, haemoglobinopathies, and respiratory diseases including tuberculosis would, however, find their place on any list of priorities to reduce ethnic inequalities in health status. Further discussion on priority setting is in Chapter 7, and on the development of strategic responses in Chapter 8.

6.7 **Conclusion**

Inequalities in health and health care by migration status and racial and ethnic group are abundant but their underlying causes, and the contribution of racism, is a complex and much debated matter. Arguably, the major cause of inequalities in health, and even more of inequalities in access to health care, is inequality in wealth. This is the stance taken by the WHO's Commission of the Social Determinants of Health. Minority groups generally find it difficult to overcome inequalities in wealth, partly because creating wealth takes time and opportunity, and partially because of racially discriminatory actions and policies that limit opportunity. Racial discrimination in the fields of employment (including health services) and social security is well documented. Minority groups do not always (particularly in the period after immigration) have worse health than the ethnic majority. There are differences in specific health outcomes. The same applies to the utilization of health services. Almost invariably, however, they have comparatively lower quality of health care and less use of fee-for-service health care. The difficulties are not in demonstrating differences, but in interpreting their meaning and using them to benefit the population.

One major explanation, which has had insufficient attention, is the role of socio-economic status. On arrival in their new country most migrants tend to hold unskilled low paid jobs. This legacy may be passed to their children (though there are many exceptions). Overall, minority communities have more than their share of unemployment and low-paid work. Minorities are hardest hit when the economy falters and may become scapegoats for economic difficulties in the nation. Much, though by no means all, of the health disadvantage associated with minority groups may not result from their migrant status, racial, and cultural background itself, but from their socio-economic disadvantage. Their health status for specific health outcomes may be comparable to that of the lower social classes in the majority population, and the solutions to health problems may in some ways be similar. Putting the issue on the political agenda is a necessary but not sufficient step. Inequalities may remain or even widen in the face of both political interest and research—the most clear-cut example being the Black/White disparity in life expectancy in the United States. This is almost certainly because wider economic and social policies are increasing inequality. The link between economics and health has been particularly well shown in relation to the mortality of Maori people in New Zealand (Tobias et al. 2009).

While general inequalities, e.g. overall high death rates, are probably unjust, specific inequalities may not be. For example, one group may have a high rate of heart disease but low cancer rates. Another group may have high cancer rates but less heart disease. Overall, the mortality or disease rates may be very similar. The differences between the two populations in cancer and heart disease would be inequalities but not necessarily inequities. Specific inequalities are, of course, important in helping set priorities and guide research.

General inequalities, such as life expectancy, have social, public health, clinical, and scientific implications. They challenge the health-care system to adapt policies to take into account the migration, race, and ethnic dimensions. Heterogeneity of minority groups and their health status and health-care needs is a challenge for effective policy. Policies can, however, articulate general principles that apply to heterogeneous populations using the concept of equity.

Inequalities by migration status, race, and ethnicity in health and health care pose a formidable challenge to research. The challenge arises from a mixture of underlying causal complexity, rapid changes in circumstances, and the methodological difficulties of collecting valid, timely data across a range of minority groups. These research issues will be discussed in more detail in Chapter 9. Accompanying the challenges is the promise of important advances, particularly in the epidemiological understanding of the causes, consequences, and control of diseases. The potential for understanding causes has been difficult to realize; this is not a cause for despair, but for reflection on and correction of expectations. Public health research describing ethnic variations in health and health care is also valuable because it directs priorities, strategies, and resource allocation, as considered in Chapters 7 and 8. Such research brings evidence to bear on preventative care, health promotion, and health care for ethnic minority populations.

6.8 **Summary**

Health status, disease occurrence, and mortality patterns in populations are sculpted by factors such as wealth, environmental quality, diet, behaviour, and genetic inheritance. Most of these factors are directly or indirectly related to migration status, ethnicity, and/or race; therefore, it is unsurprising that there are stark health inequalities by migration status, race, and ethnicity. The questions of interest are why they occur and what needs to be done to narrow them. Specific health inequalities are likely to have their own causes. For example, ethnic inequalities in risk of skin cancers such as melanoma are likely to have a biological basis relating to skin colour, while inequalities in stroke need to take account of many factors, including health care, cultural, economic, and biological matters over the life course.

The concept of inequity, as opposed to inequality, is central to policy and strategy. Inequity implies an inequality that is unfair or unjust (disparity is the equivalent word in the US context). Some inequalities are unjust, e.g. those arising from inadequate access to knowledge or services, and these form a primary target for action, particularly if effective interventions are available. Other inequalities, e.g. the differences in the rate of skin cancer, are not always unjust. They nonetheless pose a major challenge to understanding and a focus for science and services. Inequalities are demonstrable using virtually all classifications of migration status, race, and ethnicity, and are usually sharpened by taking account of population heterogeneity and examining men and women separately. The differences such groups are often large, particularly for specific conditions, e.g. prostate cancer, and less so for general measures of health, e.g. life expectancy. Even where such inequalities have been carefully studied and actions to reverse them are proposed, they have mostly not been greatly narrowed and sometimes have widened.

Inequalities by migration status, race, and ethnicity are of value in generating research questions for the health and medical sciences, and in guiding health policy and service delivery. They could help set new more demanding target, e.g. in many countries in Europe, North America, and Australia the target for CHD mortality could be set as the value for the Chinese population, and that for bowel cancer as that of the South Asian population.

Clinical services need to be adapted to counter health inequalities. Monitoring of health status, and use and outcomes of services, is necessary to achieve this. One of many dilemmas is the choice of which of the many inequalities to tackle. Selecting the priorities based on high relative risks associated with relatively rare specific conditions may increase inequalities overall. Strategies that reduce inequalities in common outcomes may offer the best option.

References

Balarajan R, Bulusu L (1990) Mortality among immigrants in England and Wales, 1979–83. In **Britton M** (ed.) Mortality and Geography: a review in the mid 1980s, pp. 103–21. London: HMSO.

Bhopal RS (2005) Hitler on race and health in Mein Kampf: a stimulus to anti-racism in the health professions. *Diversity in Health and Social Care* 2: 119–25.

Bhopal R, Hayes L, White M, Unwin N, Harland J, Ayis S, et al. (2002) Ethnic and socio-economic inequalities in coronary heart disease, diabetes and risk factors in Europeans and South Asians. *Journal of Public Health Medicine* 24: 95–105.

Bos V, Kunst AE, Keij-Deerenberg IM, Mackenbach JM (2002) Mortality amongst immigrants in the Netherlands. *European Journal of Public Health* 12: S41.

Bos V, Kunst AE, Deerenberg IMK, Garseen J, Mackenbach JP (2004) Ethnic inequalities in age- and cause-specific mortality in the Netherlands. *International Journal of Epidemiology* 33: 1112–19.

Brandt AM (1978) Racism and research: the case of the Tuskegee Syphilis Study. *The Hastings Centre Report* 8(6): 21–9.

Escarce JJ, Epstein KR, Colby DC, Schwartz JS (1993) Racial differences in the elderly's use of medical procedures and diagnostic tests. *American Journal of Public Health* 83: 948–54.

Fischbacher C, Brin G, Bansal N, Pearce J, Bhopal R (2011) Which measures of socio-economic position perform most consistently across ethnic groups? Retrospective cohort study using census data linkage. *Journal of Epidemiology and Community Health* 65(Suppl. 1): A73.

Geiger HJ (1996) Race and health care—an American dilemma? *New England Journal of Medicine* 335: 815–16.

Gill PS, Kai J, Bhopal RS, Wild S (2007) Black and minority ethnic groups. In Raftery J (ed.) Health Care Needs Assessment. The Epidemiologically Based Needs Assessment Reviews, pp. 227–389. Abingdon: Radcliffe Medical Press Ltd. Available at: http://www.birmingham.ac.uk/research/activity/mds/projects/HaPS/PHEB/HCNA/chapters/index.aspx

Gould SJ (1984) *The Mismeasure of Man*. London: Pelican Books.

Harding S, Maxwell, R (1994) Differences in mortality of migrants. In Drever F, Whitehead M (eds) Health Inequalities, pp. 108–21. London: Office for National Statistics.

Hitler A (1992) *Mein Kampf* (trans. R. Manheim). London: Pimlico.

Institute of Medicine—Committee on Understanding and Eliminating Racial and Ethnic Disparities in Health Care (2002) *Unequal Treatment: confronting racial and ethnic disparities in health care* (ed. Smedley BD, Stith AY, Nelson AR). Washington, DC: National Academies Press.

Kelaher M, Paul S, Lambert H, Ahmad W, Smith GD (2009) The applicability of measures of socioeconomic position to different ethnic groups within the UK. *International Journal for Equity in Health* 8: 4.

Krieger ND, Rowley DL, Herman A (1993) Racism, sexism and social class: implications for studies of health, disease, and wellbeing. *American Journal of Medicine* 9(6) (Suppl.): 82–122.

Marmot MG, Adelstein AM, Bulusu L (1984) *Immigrant Mortality in England and Wales 1970–78*. London, HMSO.

Macpherson WH (1999) *Report on the Stephen Lawrence Inquiry*, Cm 4262–1. London: HMSO.

McKeigue PM, Miller GJ, Marmot MG (1989) Coronary heart disease in south Asians overseas: a review. *Journal of Clinical Epidemiology* 42: 597–609.

Modood T, Berthoud R, Lakey J, Nazroo J, Smith P, Virdee SBS (1997) *Ethnic Minorities in Britain: diversity and disadvantage*. London: Policy Studies Institute.

Montagu A (1997) *Man's Most Dangerous Myth—the fallacy of race*. Lanham, MD: AltaMira Press.

Nazroo JY (1997) *The Health of Britain's Ethnic Minorities: findings from a national survey*. London: Policy Studies Institute.

Nazroo JY (2001) South Asian people and heart disease: an assessment of the importance of socioeconomic position. *Ethnicity and Disease* 11: 401–11.

Peterson ED, Shaw LK, DeLong ER, Pryor DB, Califf RM, Mark DB (1997) Racial variation in the use of coronary-revascularization procedures—are the differences real? Do they matter? *New England Journal of Medicine* 336: 480–6.

Shah KS, Shah AS, Bhopal R (2012) Systematic review and meta-analysis of out-of-hospital cardiac arrest and race or ethnicity: black US populations fare worse. *European Journal of Preventive Cardiology*. doi:10.1016/S0735-1097(12)61908-1

Sheth T, Nair C, Nargundkar M, Anand S, Yusuf S (1999) Cardiovascular and cancer mortality among Canadians of European, south Asian and Chinese origin from 1979 to 1993: an analysis of 1.2 million deaths. *Canadian Medical Association Journal* 161(2): 132–8.

Silver JR (2003) The decline of German medicine, 1933–45. *Journal of the Royal College of Physicians (Edinburgh)* 33: 54–66.

Tobias M, Blakely T, Matheson D, Rasanathan K, Atkinson J (2009) Changing trends in indigenous inequalities in mortality: lessons from New Zealand. *International Journal of Epidemiology* 38:1711–22.

Wild S, McKeigue P (1997) Cross-sectional analysis of mortality by country of birth in England and Wales, 1970–1992. *British Medical Journal* 314: 705–10.

Wild SH, Fischbacher C, Brock A, Griffiths C, Bhopal R (2007) Mortality from all causes and circulatory disease by country of birth in England and Wales 2001–2003. *Journal of Public Health* 29: 191–8.

Williams R, Wright W, Hunt K (1998) Social class and health: the puzzling counter-example of British South Asians. *Social Science and Medicine* 47: 1277–88.

Other sources and further reading

Anonymous (1989) Contemporary lessons from Nazi Germany. *Institute of Medical Ethics Bulletin* February: 13–20.

Ayanian JZ, Udvarhelyi S, Gatsonis CA, Pashos CL, Epstein A (1993) Racial differences in the use of revascularisation procedures after coronary angiography. *Journal of the American Medical Association* 269: 2642–6.

Bhopal R (1997) Is research into ethnicity and health racist, unsound, or important science? *British Medical Journal* 314: 1751–6.

Bhopal RS (1998) The spectre of racism in health and health care: lessons from history and the USA. *British Medical Journal* 316: 1970–3.

Bhopal R (2001) Racism in medicine. *British Medical Journal* 322: 1503–4.

Bhopal RS and Donaldson LJ (1988) Health education for ethnic minorities: current provision and future directions. *Health Education Journal* 47: 137–40.

Bos V (2005) *Ethnic Inequalities in Mortality in The Netherlands and the Role of Socioeconomic Status.* Rotterdam: University Medical Center.

Bos V, Kunst AE, Garseen J, Mackenbach JP (2005) Socioeconomic inequalities in mortality within ethnic groups in the Netherlands, 1995–2000. *Journal of Epidemiology and Community Health* 59: 329–35.

Council on Ethical and Judicial Affairs (1990) Black–white disparities in health care. *Journal of the American Medical Association* 263: 2344–6.

Davey Smith D, Chaturvedi N, Harding S, Nazaroo J, Williams R (2000) Ethnic inequalities in health: a review of UK epidemiological evidence. *Critical Public Health* 10: 375–408.

Dominguez-McNeilly M (1996) Perceived racism scale. *Ethnicity and Disease* 6: 154–66.

Dressler WW (1991) Social class, skin colour, and arterial blood pressure in two societies. *Ethnicity and Disease* 1: 60–77.

Gamble VN (1993) A legacy of distrust: African Americans and medical research. *American Journal of Preventive Medicine* 9: 35–8.

Gornick ME, Eggers P, Reilly TEA (1986) Effects of race and income on mortality and use of services among Medicare beneficiaries. *New England Journal of Medicine* 335: 791–9.

Hannan EL, Kilburn H, O'Donnell JF, Lukacic G, Shields EP (1991) Interracial access to selected cardiac procedures for patients hospitalised with coronary artery disease in New York State. *Medical Care* 29: 430–41.

Jeffreys M, Stevanovic V, Tobias M, Lewis C, Ellison-Loschmann L, Pearce N, et al. (2005) Ethnic inequalities in cancer survival in New Zealand: linkage study. *Research and Practice* 95: 834–7.

Krieger N, Sidney S (1996) Racial discrimination and blood pressure: the CARDIA study of young black and white adults. *American Journal of Public Health* 86: 1370–8.

Kushnick L (1988) Racism, the National Health Service and the health of black people. *International Journal of Health Services* 18: 457–70.

La Veist T, Wallace J, Howard D (1995) The color line and the health of African Americans. *Humboldt Journal of Social Relations* 21: 119–37.

Lawrence D (2002) Which diseases contribute to life-expectancy differences between races? *The Lancet* **360**: 1571.

Lorant V, Bhopal RS (2011) Ethnicity, socio-economic status and health research: insights from and implications of Charles Tilly's theory of durable inequality. *Journal of Epidemiology and Community Health* **65**: 671–5.

Lowry S, Macpherson G (1988) A blot on the profession. *British Medical Journal* **296**: 657–8.

Marmot M, Allen J, Bell R, Bloomer E, Goldblatt P (2012) WHO European review of social determinants of health and the health divide. *The Lancet* **380**: 1011–29.

McKeigue PM, Richards JDM, Richards P (1990) Effects of discrimination by sex and race on the early careers of British medical graduates during 1981–87. *British Medical Journal* **301**: 961–4.

McManus IC, Richards P, Winder W, Sproston KA, Styles V (1995) Medical school applicants from ethnic minority groups: identifying if and when they are disadvantaged. *British Medical Journal* **310**: 496–500.

McNeilly M, Robinson E, Anderson N, et al. (1995) Effects of racist provocation and social support on cardiovascular reactivity in African American women. *International Journal of Behavioral Medicine* **2**: 321–38.

Olshansky SJ, Antonucci T, Berkman L, Binstock RH, Boersch-Supan A, Cacioppo JT,et al. (2012) Differences in life expectancy due to race and educational differences are widening, and many may not catch up. *Health Affairs* **31**: 1803–13.

Osborne NG, Feit MD (1992) The use of race in medical research. *Journal of the American Medical Association* **267**: 275–9.

Parker H (1997) Beyond ethnic categories: why racism should be a variable in ethnicity and health research. *Journal of Health Service Research and Policy* **2**: 256–9.

Singh GK, Hiatt RA (2006) Trends and disparities in socioeconomic and behavioural characteristics, life expectancy, and cause-specific mortality of native-born and foreign-born populations in the United States, 1979–2003. *International Journal of Epidemiology* **35**: 903–19.

Smith R (1987) Prejudice against doctors and students from ethnic minorities. *British Medical Journal* **294**: 328–9.

Stronks K, Ravelli ACJ, Reijneveld SA (2001) Immigrants in the Netherlands: equal access for equal needs? *Journal of Epidemiology and Community Health* **55**: 701–7.

Warren R (1993) The morbidity/mortality gap: what is the problem? *Annals of Epidemiology* **3**: 127–9.

Chapter 7

Principles for setting priorities for the health and health care of migrants and racial and ethnic minorities

Objectives

After reading this chapter you should understand:

- That setting priorities is a crucially important but very difficult activity.
- That data on health status can guide priority-setting within the broader framework of social values, available resources, cost-effectiveness, and individual preferences.
- That quantitative data can be used to derive understandings of absolute (or actual) and relative health states.
- That focusing only on differences between minority and majority populations can deflect attention from other priorities and exacerbate inequalities.
- The merits and limitations of a framework for setting priorities based on a set of standards for the population as a whole, and health information based on actual and relative measures.

7.1 Introduction to priority-setting in the context of migration, race, and ethnicity

Before reading on, try Exercise 7.1.

Exercise 7.1 Priority-setting

- Why is priority-setting necessary: (1) in general, for all populations and (2) when considering the needs of migrant, racial and ethnic minorities?
- Why is it difficult, and particularly so in relation to minority groups?

Priority-setting is a process for making rational choices, given options. It is an all-important activity which, in the context of health care in particular, has received insufficient honest debate, analysis, and research, partly because of its close (and entirely understandable) connections with rationing. Rationing implies restriction of the supply of a service or goods, usually through sharing, sometimes on the basis of allocation of a fixed and limited amount. This tends to be politically unacceptable, particularly in rich countries, not least because it is unpopular with the public. Rationing is associated with difficult times, whether in war, emergencies, or natural or economic disasters. It is contrary to the currently popular philosophy of freedom to choose and the freedom to spend our money as we wish.

In a static or shrinking health-care economy the need for a rational and just means of priority-setting becomes glaringly obvious, especially when new, better interventions become available and are to be implemented. Something else will need to be deprioritized, perhaps even stopped. Even where the health-care economy is growing, however, priority-setting is important, especially to guide new expenditures but also for review and analysis of existing expenditures. Without a fair process, decisions will be ad hoc and swayed by the biases of powerful individuals and groups. Priority-setting is important, and some see it as inseparable from rationing, itself a job for politicians. Rationing in health and health care is still not acceptable, but it is nonetheless widely practised, especially in relation to some migrants. In many countries undocumented migrants are allocated limited rights (rationing), usually to emergency care and sometimes primary care (especially for pregnant women and children). Asylum seekers usually have full access, as do refugees (asylum granted), but those whose leave to remain is refused usually find that their access to services declines with time. Where privatized health care prevails, migrants and settled racial and ethnic minorities may find they have less access because they cannot afford health insurance or fees. These are important issues, but they are small in scale compared with the prioritization of general services.

Health-care systems have priorities that are dictated by the disease and health patterns of the whole population and population subgroups, and the political expectations and explicit standards of public services, the general public, and the users of services. These priorities include the prevention and management of disease, the promotion of health, health education, reduction of inequalities in health, high-quality health care, cost-effective and value for money services delivered within budget, and respectful, sensitive, and equitable services that win public support. Such ambitious and wide-ranging priorities are virtually universal (at least in affluent countries), and though the phraseology and emphasis change, they are found in every important health-care policy document. The emphasis changes from place to place and time to time, e.g. inequalities and inequities are high on the international health agenda at the moment (see Chapter 6 for a discussion of the overlaps and distinctions between inequalities and inequities).

Are these the right priorities for minority migrant, racial, and ethnic groups? Are there others that are more important to minority health but are not on the list? Are there nuances needed for minority groups, such that the priorities need modification or a change of emphasis? These are the key questions for this chapter, which focuses on the principles and methods for answering them, rather than the answers themselves. We need also to ensure that minority groups are not bypassed when priorities are implemented, either because the priorities are not the right ones or because they are not being applied, perhaps because managers and health professionals perceive them to be inappropriate or even lacking endorsement or validity for and by minorities. There is one central issue that drives our analysis of priorities: in what ways are the health and health-care needs of minority groups similar to, and yet different from, the majority population that the health service has evolved to serve? This question relating to needs, the topic of Chapter 5, provides the link between needs assessment and priority-setting. Having made this link, of course, actions need to be taken, and that is the topic of Chapter 8.

Whether in research, policy, or health care, the choices for actions to improve the health of minority groups are virtually limitless, especially in complex, multicultural societies. Social values are important in priority-setting and in the context of migration, race, ethnicity, and health the most important are the values of equality and equity and these, in turn, are based on human rights. Fortunately, most countries subscribe to international human rights laws, though a few do not. Others do not implement the laws. Antimigrant views and prejudices against some racial or ethnic groups are amongst the blocks to speedier progress.

A historical analysis shows a shift away from over-emphasizing differences, which are relatively small for most health-care and general health status situations though often large for specific diseases, to similarities, which are surprisingly large (see Chapters 4 and 5). In Chapter 5 I introduced the needs assessment by Gill et al. (2007), which showed that many of the needs in the population as a whole also apply to the main minority ethnic groups in the UK. In particular, the emphasis on the prevention, treatment, and long-term care for cardiovascular diseases, cancers, mental health, and other health problems of modern societies is appropriate for the majority and minorities alike. A few diseases and problems that tend not to figure greatly in the priorities of health services were also found to deserve a place in the context of minority ethnic health, e.g. the haemoglobinopathies and tuberculosis. A focus on these specific needs, however, should not be at the expense of the main priorities, but in addition to them. This general principle may not apply to specific migrant groups, e.g. young migrant workers, especially seasonal workers who are returning to their normal country of residence. Their needs and priorities may revolve around occupational health problems or the health problems arising from poor living conditions. For some asylum seekers, the top priority may be mental health care.

The idea of special or additional priorities can easily be misinterpreted—as an extra or bonus that minorities enjoy at the expense of the majority. This is usually wrong. The majority population (usually White in Europe and North America) is also an ethnic group that has special needs, e.g. cystic fibrosis is much commoner in White ethnic groups, and for reasons relating to age distribution so is senile dementia, a very costly health problem. Furthermore, if young migrants need more of one service, e.g. occupational health, they will be likely to need less of another, e.g. cancer services, which are mostly used by older age groups.

The need for a balanced and considered approach to needs assessment as a prelude to priority-setting was illustrated in Chapter 5 (Section 5.1.2) by the example of stroke and CHD in the African Caribbean population in the UK. I showed that neglecting CHD in favour of stroke would miss the bigger problem and run the risk of the African Caribbean community losing its relative advantage in regard to CHD over the population as a whole (thereby repeating what happened to African Americans in the USA). This general principle will be illustrated later.

Like the population as a whole, minority groups need services that are respectful and sensitive, but they have additional concerns because the services were not set up with their needs in mind, as discussed from a historical perspective in Chapter 4. This poses particular demands on health services, e.g. language support, which is perennially controversial. In Chapters 4–6 we discussed some of the required service delivery responses, and we will consider strategy and policy in Chapter 8. We continue here with the role of epidemiological thinking.

7.2 The epidemiological underpinnings of priority-setting in the context of the health of minorities

Before reading on do Exercise 7.2.

Exercise 7.2 Information for priority-setting

- What kind of information would you need to set priorities?
- What kind of information is generally available on the health of minority migrant, racial, and ethnic groups? What is usually missing?
- How will you proceed despite the missing information?

Priority-setting is a complex and incompletely understood activity. Epidemiological concepts and data underpin priority-setting, but decisions on consumption of resources are always heavily influenced by economics and politics (Figure 7.1 and Table 7.1).

Table 7.1 places equal emphasis on the epidemiological and medical aspects of the problem (frequency, effects, causes, treatment) and the wider social factors. While there is still a shortage of epidemiological and clinical data by migrant, racial, and ethnic group status the need for such information is increasingly accepted and information systems are being developed (see Chapters 3 and 8). Most information from the general population will apply to minorities, though this may not be so for the effectiveness, and even more so the cost-effectiveness, of interventions. Cost-effectiveness data come from clinical trials and it is extremely rare for these to report by minority group (see Chapter 9 for a fuller discussion). While interventions based on drugs and

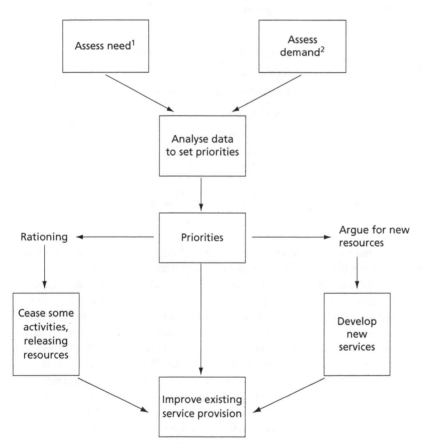

1 Using demographic, lifestyle, sociological, economic, and epidemiological data

2 Using the views, and patterns of past behaviour especially service use, of professionals, pressure groups, patients and the public.

Fig. 7.1 The place of priority-setting in relation to the need for, demand for, and provision of services.

Adapted from Bhopal, Getting priorities for healthcare, p. 58 in Rawaf and Bahl, (eds) *Assessing Health Needs of People from Minority Ethnic Groups*, Royal College of Physicians, London, UK, Copyright © 1998, with permission from the Royal College of Physicians London.

Table 7.1 Some characteristics of problems given high priority*

(A) Epidemiological and clinical factors	
The problem is:	Common
	Severe in its effects
	Long-lasting
	Communicable, especially if it occurs as epidemics
	Externally, or iatrogenically, acquired
	Affects young people
	Treatable/curable especially if this is cost-effective
	Preventable
(B) Social, economic, and political factors	
The problem is:	Of high public and political interest
	Economically important
	Lobbied for by pressure groups
	Free of stigma
	Socially acceptable
	Of interest to health professionals

* Problems which do not have these characteristics, or have opposite characteristics, are given low priority.

Adapted from Bhopal, Getting priorities for healthcare, p. 59 in Rawaf and Bahl, (eds) *Assessing Health Needs of People from Minority Ethnic Groups*, Royal College of Physicians, London, UK, Copyright © 1998, with permission from the Royal College of Physicians London.

procedures are likely to have similar effects, and hence cost-effectiveness, across most subgroups of the population, this is not true for health promotion or screening interventions.

As the minority populations have increased in size, public and political interest has increased, albeit sometimes in negative ways. Whether positive or negative, the issues arising have moved higher up the agenda for debate or action. It is helpful to minorities that a great number of health-care staff, at every level, are themselves from minority backgrounds. This leads to an intrinsic interest, helped by the genuine and rising interest of researchers, health-care planners and professionals, and managers in doing their best to improve the health of minorities.

The kind of information in part B of Table 7.1 is not usually available by migration status, race, or ethnic group and methods to collect it are not well developed. For example, we do not know whether epilepsy has more stigma associated with it in Chinese, African, or Pakistani populations than in White or Arabic ones. Nonetheless, informed judgement may help us on these matters. The high priority given in health-care systems, at least in affluent countries, to a diverse set of conditions such as heart disease, diabetes, obesity, childhood leukaemia, child abuse, and Legionnaires' disease, can be understood in the context of the characteristics in the table. The relatively low priority for mental retardation, sexually transmitted diseases, suicide, and senile dementia can also be understood.

The example of Legionnaires' disease is interesting: it is a rare pneumonia, but it is externally acquired and sometimes a consequence of demonstrable negligence on the part of industries, government agencies, and hospitals. If so, compensation may be payable to the sufferer and the adverse publicity may be very damaging to the organization responsible. The disease can occur in outbreaks that cause panic and receive major media coverage. In principle it is preventable, and usually it is curable. In contrast to its small contribution to the burden of disease it is a high priority. By contrast, mental retardation is not curable and rarely gains publicity unless it is caused by medical negligence. It is self-evident that the people affected are not well placed to argue the case for a higher priority, although their relatives and friends may do so. In relation to its massive public health impact this problem is often given low priority. These factors help us understand why some issues come to prominence and others do not.

It can be puzzling to people in the field of migration, race, ethnicity, and health that arguments for screening and good-quality treatment for specific conditions such as haemoglobinopathies have been difficult to win. By contrast, for another rare genetic disease, cystic fibrosis, similar arguments have been easy. The difference does not lie in the factors in part A of Table 7.1 but in part B. Haemoglobinopathies occur mainly in minority groups while cystic fibrosis occurs mainly in White populations. There is simply more public, professional, and political pressure to do something about cystic fibrosis. Fortunately, leaders in the migration, race, ethnicity, and health arena have argued the case for haemoglobinopathies and these services have gained more priority. Indeed, a national service for screening for sickle cell disease has been developed in England. However, the consequences of such developments are not always for the better, as the following quotation about the experience in the United States demonstrates:

> *The National Sickle Cell Anaemia control act, enacted by the USA Congress on 16 May 1972, called for mandatory screening for the sickle cell trait in all people who were 'not of the Caucasian, Indian or Oriental race' and marks the start of a screening programme that is held up as the benchmark for failure. The act had a serious effect on the lives of USA citizens of African descent; in some states marriage licences were not issued to those of African descent unless the sickle cell test was taken, in others a test was a condition of entry to school. The presence of the sickle cell trait could lead to loss of employment, increased insurance premiums, inappropriate medical therapy, delay in adoption of children and sometimes problems in the revelation of 'non-paternity'.*
>
> Bradby (1999, p. 303), reproduced with permission of Cambridge University Press.

The achievement of a priority needs to be well motivated and followed up by excellence in its implementation, not be allowed to be detrimental to those whom it is intended to benefit.

The entire field of migration, race, ethnicity, and health research can be considered in the light of part B of Table 7.1. All the factors in part B are of relevance, but I would draw special attention to the role of pressure groups and freedom from stigma. As minority groups have won positions of status and power their voices have been heard. This, combined with laws and policies that promote work on migration, race, ethnicity, and health, and place it in the wider framework of equalities and equity, has freed the entire field of stigma—it is a field one can be proud to work in that is no longer on the margins of research and the professions. Within many new and recent health policy documents, in contrast to those of 20 or more years ago, there is an emphasis on, or at least reference to, the health and health care of minority groups. Scarce resources of time, energy, and (new) funds may need to be found and applied to maximize the benefit of such policy statements. As funds are scarce, choosing between alternatives is invariably necessary. Setting priorities for minority health populations given limited resources is an exacting challenge because they are extremely heterogeneous, and their disease patterns and lifestyles are both incompletely understood and changing rapidly within and between generations. What principles should guide us here?

The decision to offer (or not to offer) a service is based upon a judgement of the needs of a community. Such judgements may be subjective and based on past experience or common sense. Since few senior decision-makers are from the minority communities the judgements based on such subjective appraisal may be inappropriate due to a lack of necessary insights. Of course, even people from the minority communities are unlikely to have the knowledge required to make valid and objective judgements on priorities. Their judgements should be supported by assessed needs as reflected in data on the community.

The importance of accurately interpreting data on disease patterns of minority ethnic groups is crucial to the characteristics in part A of Table 7.1. (In Chapters 3 and 5 we discussed how priorities may be skewed by misinterpretation.) It is important to attend to the factors in part B. For those working in the field there is a huge challenge in (1) maintaining migration, race, ethnicity and health as a priority generally in competition with other matters and (2) deciding priorities within this theme. First I will provide an overview of past decision-making processes in the field of migration, race, and ethnicity, and then offer an approach for the future that is founded on epidemiology.

7.3 Analysis of past approaches in selecting priorities in the fields of migration, race, ethnicity, and health

Past approaches to priority-setting in the field of minority health can be examined in four ways: analysing the nature and emphasis of past initiatives; analysing the nature and emphasis of current initiatives; reading the scientific and professional literature; and assessing the opinions of decision-makers and providers. For illustration, I focus on South Asians in the UK, the topic I know best, but one that yields generalizations that apply, to a great extent, to other populations and settings. An examination of UK literature shows sparse recognition of the health of South Asians, with the earliest reports of conferences appearing in the 1960s.

My first formal analysis was done in the 1990s. I found that there was no agreed prioritization, or process for it, on the part of the NHS and that past approaches were largely tactical rather than strategic. The tactics had been based on interested professionals or community organizations grasping opportunities, themselves usually arising from the perspective that there were distinct, 'ethnic minority group problems' to be solved. For instance, national attention in the UK in the late 1960s through to the early 1980s was aroused by problems such as rickets in Asians. Much professional, research, policy, and media attention was devoted to this and similar problems in the 1960s and 1970s. It would be wrong to imply that this kind of issue was not important then, and it remains important even now as it has not been resolved (in December 2012 there were media headlines telling us that rickets was becoming more common in the UK). The interesting question is how did this, and similar problems, come to gain such prominence over others? Other problems gaining early attention on the UK included the use of kohl/surma, an eye cosmetic that adorned my (and many other South Asians') eyes in my childhood, and traditional health remedies. There were fears (reasonably founded) that surma and some traditional remedies contained lead and other metals that were hazardous. Such examples drew attention to the culture of minority ethnic groups as a prime consideration in their health.

The 1980s Mother and Baby Campaign run by the Department of Health in England, although long over, remains to this day one of the biggest ever national initiatives concerning minority ethnic issues in the UK—its emphasis was also around culture and communication. The scientific literature in the 1970s mirrored the issues to which the health service was devoting attention, with emphasis on a number of diseases and health problems, particularly nutritional and infectious ones. Tuberculosis, for example, received some attention and publicity. The views of professionals seem to have been deeply influenced by the focus of the scientific literature. In gaining national attention, these matters became top priorities; they were obvious things that were concerning clinicians. They stood out because they were either rare, preventable, somewhat exotic, and hence interesting, or transmissible from person to person and hence a threat to the whole population. We can be glad that attention was paid to them because it helped those who were affected directly, but also helped indirectly the minority populations as a whole by opening the door to a wider range of inquiry and action on the spectrum of health needs. This kind of opportunity is important if we are to make progress. For example, in many countries now the specific issue of female genital mutilation (or female circumcision) is attracting attention and has become a priority. This provides a platform from which to work on a wider range of issues. But how has focus on these issues matched quantitatively demonstrable health needs?

At the same time as attention was being given to matters such as rickets and surma (the 1960s and 1970s), 45.3% of deaths of men born in the Indian subcontinent but dying in Britain were due to cardiovascular or cerebrovascular disease, as shown in the second column of Table 7.2 (an extract from Table 5.7); the corresponding figure for women was 29%. Yet until the 1980s this fact went largely unnoticed (the report by Marmot et al., *Immigrant Mortality in England and Wales 1970–78* was published in 1984, although Tunstall Pedoe and colleagues had published an influential article in 1975 showing that Asians in east London had higher rates of heart attack than the population as a whole). These were the first UK data but they supported similar observations from other countries, including South Africa and Singapore.

The landmark publication on immigrant mortality by Marmot et al. (1984) placed heavy emphasis on relative mortality experience, and the tables therein gave rankings based on SMRs. I have discussed in Chapters 3 and 5 the importance of examining data using numbers of cases and actual rates. The analyses based on SMRs may have made it difficult to see the priorities as clearly as a focus on actual numbers and rates of deaths might have done. We can see a mismatch between the focus and concerns of the health service and quantitative demonstrated health problems.

While some health education material had been specifically adapted for minority ethnic groups, up to 1987 none of those items in the catalogues of the Health Education Authority (England) concerned heart disease, as shown in an analysis published by me and Donaldson (Bhopal and Donaldson 1988). In 1987 information was available for England's ethnic minorities on a wide range of other matters including lice infestation, the dangers of spitting, and even colostomy. The emphasis of health education, however, was on birth control, infant care, and feeding. In the 1990

Table 7.2 Deaths (by rank order of number of deaths) in male immigrants from the Indian subcontinent aged 20 and over (total deaths 4352)

Cause	SMR*	No. of deaths	% of total
Ischaemic heart disease	115	1533	35.2
Cerebrovascular disease	108	438	10.1
Bronchitis, emphysema, and asthma	77	223	5.1
Neoplasm of the trachea, bronchus, and lung	3	218	5.0
Other non-viral pneumonia	100	214	4.9
Above five causes	—	2626	60.3

* Standardized mortality ratio compared with the male population of England and Wales, which was by definition 100.

Adapted from Marmot et al, *Immigrant mortality in England and Wales 1970–78: Causes of Death by Country of Birth (Studies on Medical and Population Subjects)*, p.132, HMSO, London, UK, Copyright © 1984, licensed under the Open Government Licence v1.0.

Health Education Authority catalogue four of 179 items concerned heart disease. Clearly, at that time the impact of epidemiological data in influencing priority interventions was modest, at least in relation to health education. Understanding the underlying basis for this gap between need, as reflected in epidemiological data, and provision, as reflected in health education materials, and the implications of such gaps for future strategy, is of great importance in priority-setting.

Public health practitioners such as health educators are to a large extent 'demand-led'. Their work is partly and sometimes largely determined by the requests made to them by other health professionals, particularly health visitors, and by the officers of the health authority or health-care facilities such as hospitals or primary care centres. In addition, most health education departments will have their own priorities, sometimes following the community development model, which emphasizes social improvement, rather than the medical model, which puts emphasis on causes of death and disease. Thus, health education interventions for migrant, racial, and ethnic minorities may be generated by health professionals who see a specific clinical problem which requires a solution, rather than as a response to a comprehensive appraisal of the health education needs of a community. While this approach may result in satisfactory delivery of services for the majority community, the culture and health of which most health professionals have considerable knowledge, it may not suffice for minority communities because of a lack of knowledge about them.

Demand for health education services may also come, directly or indirectly, from individual members of the public, community groups, and politicians. Being less vocal, less well-organized in terms of groups, less familiar with the health services, and even less knowledgeable about health and disease, the minorities' own demands for health education may be very limited. Migrants, in particular, may not be familiar with the kinds of diseases that are common in their new homeland. Professionals' demands may relate to recent published research and the resultant reports in the media and popular magazines, which often highlight differences. Minority communities are likely to be less likely to encounter or absorb such reports, for reasons including lower education, poorer command of the local language, and less use of mainstream media.

Ideally, in making service improvements judgements should be informed by appropriate indicators of health status, choices of which will depend on the objectives of the service. In terms of health education services, the needs are defined by what the community knows about health, what it ought to know, what its current health status is, what improvements in health status can realistically be achieved, and what the most effective interventions are.

There are no routinely collected data in the UK (and possibly elsewhere) on the population's health beliefs, knowledge, and attitudes disaggregated by country of birth, race, or ethnicity and we rely upon ad hoc surveys. In the case of minorities, the few data that exist indicate that their knowledge on a range of health issues, particularly the causes and prevention of ill-health and on the value of medical procedures, is low. An illustrative study is that by Rankin and Bhopal (2001) showing the extremely limited knowledge about heart disease and diabetes of Indians, Pakistanis, and Bangladeshis in north-east England. The low knowledge base is sometimes hard to build on, especially in people who have not studied biology and the local language. Basic ideas like an artery, a gland, or cholesterol are difficult to discuss in any circumstances but extremely so when dealing with people whose first language is not the same as that of the speaker. Many medical words cannot be translated, and even if they can the correct term found by learned translators may be unfamiliar to professionals and public alike.

The message from the above analysis is that a strategic approach to priority-setting, based on agreed principles, is essential. The strategic approach should meet needs, based on an analysis of the circumstances and health status of minority groups, and not merely focus on those matters where the differences between the minority and majority groups are obvious. In short, as discussed in Chapter 5, absolute and not relative needs should dominate our priority-setting strategy.

Table 5.3 showed the key causes of death, first ranked on the SMR, a measure of relative excess or deficit of deaths, and then the actual number of deaths. The patterns are quite different. The former pattern guides, primarily, research, the latter services and priority-setting.

In setting priorities, the perceptions, opinions, and attitudes of decision-makers are important, as reflected in part B of Table 7.1, though they are hard to gauge objectively. Sometimes, these are fully in alignment with the positive pro-minority proclamations of equality and human rights laws and policies, but often they are not. In the assessment of priority needs, one issue always stands out: the enhancement of the quality of communication between minority populations and health professionals. Communication refers to more than the exchange of words and encompasses mutual respect, under-standing of life circumstances and culture, clear use of language, and empowerment of the individual to say what they want and ask questions without fear or inhibition.

Some quantitative research has evaluated the impact of interventions that improve communi-cations, e.g. interpreters, link workers, and patients' advocates, though it is modest in relation to the importance of the matter. There is a great deal of consultation and qualitative research which provides useful information, though of a different kind. This body of work supports the prioritiza-tion, on first principles, of services to improve communication. Most, if not all, health authorities in multi-ethnic societies have either implemented interpretation and translation schemes or have aired the issues as a prelude to doing so. This basic requirement of good communication-enhancing services for minority patients as a fundamental aspect of quality health care is not a universally ingrained, high-quality, routine part of health services. In some countries nationally agreed stand-ards require such services, e.g. the United States (see Chapter 8).

Other basic issues such as correct recording of names, the availability of hospital food that is suitable for religious or cultural requirements, and the opportunity for examination by a health professional of the same sex (at least for intimate examinations) have yet to be attended to in most health services, despite being deemed of high importance in consultation on priorities.

The problems include: a failure to agree priorities; too much of a focus on specific 'ethnic' health issues at the expense of larger-scale problems which are shared by the whole population; and insufficient quality (and in some places even availability) of basic services which, in general opin-ion and research, are high priorities, e.g. communication services. A set of principles, some of which are offered below, are required to make progress.

7.4 Towards a set of principles and standards for setting priorities in relation to migration, race, ethnicity, and health

Try Exercise 7.3 before reading on.

Exercise 7.3 Standards and priorities for migrant, racial, and minority ethnic groups

Using the population as a whole as a guide to standards and priorities for migrant, racial and minority ethnic groups

- What principles can you think of to help us set priorities?
- What are the strengths and limitations of using existing public health priorities for the population as a whole and applying them to minority groups?
- What are the strengths and weaknesses of using existing quality of care standards for the population as a whole in setting standards for minorities?

There should be a fundamental principle behind priority-setting for minority groups. One principle might be that the priorities are those issues where available interventions would provide maximum benefit for the specific minority group. This is an approach advocated in health economics and it has an appealing logic that is easy to grasp. It is an approach that requires a great deal of research to implement. Health economics also emphasizes that such interventions need to be cost-effective. Another principle is to prioritize those issues where actions will improve the health of the minority ethnic group either to the level of the population as a whole or to that of another minority group, perhaps the one with the best health. This principle prioritizes equality and equity. The usual principle, however, sometimes unfortunately, is to prioritize those issues which will allow minorities to aspire to the standard of health of the White or majority population. The latter is a pragmatic approach and one that fits in with the way societies work. Integrating the three approaches meets the twin goals of maximizing health and tackling health inequalities.

Quantitative and qualitative data by minority group on health status, service utilization, and quality of care are sparse, but the data that are available need to be utilized carefully to help apply these principles. In contrast, information on cost and effectiveness of interventions as applied to specific minority groups is rarely available—posing a formidable challenge to future research but making decisions on health economic grounds nigh impossible at present.

The main advantage of applying existing national priorities include the following: (1) no further thought or analysis is required, (2) the decision would be uncontroversial, at least from the point of view of the authorities, and (3) actions to deliver the priorities could occur simultaneously in majority and minority populations. The limitations include the following: (1) the existing priorities may be the wrong ones or important nuances may be overlooked, (2) the crude use of priorities in this way may convey a degree of thoughtlessness, especially to the minority populations, and (3) opportunities to improve the set of priorities through comparative analysis for minorities and majority alike may be missed.

The same kind of reasoning can be applied to quality of care standards. We will be considering such standards in Chapter 8. In Section 7.5 we will look at the effects of using general priorities within the field of cancer.

From a public health perspective, the idea of taking general health priorities as the starting point for minority populations too is a good one, for the pattern of health problems in any geographical or social context either is similar or becomes similar over time. Scotland's public health strategy prioritizes the health of children, dental/oral health, sexual health, CHD, cancer, mental health, and accidents and safety. It would be hard to argue that that is not an excellent starting point for setting priorities for any subgroup of the population.

If we accept national priorities and standards to be a starting point, pending refinement for minorities, we might then extrapolate this to a range of needs as in Box 7.1.

The principles which are encapsulated in the needs in Box 7.1 are these: acceptance of national standards as the aim for health care of migrant, racial, and minority ethnic groups; emphasis on basic needs, irrespective of similarities or differences between minority and majority populations; and emphasis on quality of service rather than specific conditions.

The key principle for implementing a programme of work associated with given priorities is integration. Action is required at international, national, regional, district, service provider, and community levels. The policies, strategies, and action plans at each level need to be harmonious. Chapter 8 examines how this can happen. In Section 7.5 we look at the use of epidemiological data around a specific example—cancer.

Box 7.1 National priorities and standards in relation to some needs of minority populations.

1. Clinical care of a quality equal to national standards:

   (a) equal access to and quality of advice and facilities

   (b) equal respect from carers

   (c) equally clear and effective communication

   (d) equally suitable and culturally appropriate accommodation, facilities, and services such as food

   (e) equally effective clinical diagnosis, therapy and advice.

2. Preventive care/health promotion of a quality equal to national standards:

   (a) equal access to appropriate range of information/advice

   (b) equally effective communication

   (c) equally acceptable and relevant information

   (d) focus on common and preventable diseases/health problems

   (e) focus on matters perceived as important by minority groups

   (f) equal efforts to involve the community.

7.5 Setting priorities in multicultural societies using epidemiological data: the example of cancer

Before reading on try Exercise 7.4.

Exercise 7.4 Prioritizing health issues for minority populations using data

- In terms of setting priorities, what are the strengths and weaknesses of each of the relative risk and absolute (or actual) risk approaches?

- What is the danger in prioritizing conditions on the basis of the difference between minority and majority populations?

- Similarly, what is the danger of prioritizing without regard to such differences?

For relative risk you may wish to reflect on the SMR. The value for this in the reference population is 100. For absolute rates you may consider numbers of cases and incidence rate of mortality or cancer registration. These terms are defined in the Glossary.

Since the ultimate objective of public health, including health education and health-care services, is to improve health and control illness and disease we can try to identify priority needs on the basis of the common causes of ill-health as reflected in morbidity and mortality statistics.

Epidemiological data on disease frequency, causal, and other risk factors, the effectiveness and cost-effectiveness of interventions, and the population's characteristics clearly play a key role in identifying needs and setting priorities. This section focuses on Bhopal and Rankin's (1996) review of published epidemiological data on the frequency of cancer in UK minority ethnic populations which aimed to illustrate how to answer two key questions vital to the theme of this section:

1. How common is cancer in these populations?
2. Which cancers deserve special attention in terms of policy, prevention, service provision, causal research, and health services research?

In the course of this section we will reflect on the questions raised in Exercise 7.4. Then I will present an overview of recent advances in this context. The principles of the approach outlined here, and possibly many of the conclusions, ought to be internationally generalizable.

Bhopal and Rankin identified studies that provided information on cancer frequency in a defined population and permitted analysis of a range of cancers, following the approach advocated in Chapter 5 on health needs assessment, as follows:

◆ total cancer cases;

◆ rankings of cancer (top seven) by frequency of occurrence;

◆ overall SMR;

◆ rankings of cancer (top seven) by excess risk as indicated by the SMR/cancer standardized registration ratio (SMR/SRR) or the proportional mortality/registration ratio (PMR/PRR)—see the Glossary.

Measures of relative frequency were converted to percentages for easy comparison when required.

The largest studies were based on mortality data, and focused on populations born in the Indian subcontinent (South Asian) and Caribbean, with some data on African-born populations. There were major limitations of the data which made interpretation and utilization for priority-setting awkward, as outlined below.

1. The studies by Marmot et al. (1984), Balarajan and Bulusu (1990), and Grulich et al. (1992) were based on the country of birth code on the death certificate. The country of birth does not accurately identify racial or ethnic origin, as we have already discussed. For example, many people of White ethnic origin were born and lived in British Empire or Commonwealth countries and returned to Britain following the independence of their country of residence. Marmot et al. (1984) also used a names analysis to identify the South Asian group within the population in the Indian subcontinent.

2. Accurate denominators (population at risk) were not always available, making the calculation of accurate disease rates and SMRs impossible, particularly between census years.

3. The assignment of ethnic origin used various approaches, e.g. names analysis for South Asian populations. Two studies based ethnicity on information from medical records or asked doctors to assign it, and one study gave no information on how ethnicity was assigned. In general the categories for ethnic categorisation were extremely broad. Grulich et al. (1992) reported data on East and West Africans, but in other studies there was no differentiation of population by subregion.

4. The numbers of cases in several studies were very low, particularly those based on regional cancer registry data. The precision of the estimates of frequency is low in these studies and especially so for rarer cancers.

5. The study of Powell et al. (1994) used data that were also used in the studies by Muir et al. (1992) (71% of cases) and by Stiller and McKinney (1991) (20% of cases), which means that the three studies on children were not independent.

Even given these limitations, progress in selecting priorities and, more importantly, creating a logical way of doing so was made.

7.5.1 **Populations of South Asian and Caribbean origin**

Tables 7.3 and 7.4 set out some of the data. Cancer was shown to be a common and important cause of death and morbidity in the minority groups reported on, causing about one-sixth of all deaths. Generally, cancer was less common in these ethnic groups than in the usual reference UK-born, predominantly White, population (SMR = 100 by definition), with the overall SMR mostly being in the range 50–80 for South Asian and Caribbean populations but about 100 in African populations (indeed, higher in West Africans and lower in East Africans).

Table 7.3 illustrates, using data on South Asians, how published data can be used to provide an overview of the importance of cancer overall, and for top-ranking cancers. Clearly, a strategy focused on the commonest cancers captures a much higher proportion of all cancers (here 53–69%) than one focused on the cancers which are relatively common in relation to the reference population (14–32%).

Table 7.4 summarizes data from Balarajan and Bulusu (1990) on populations of Caribbean origin. The commonest seven cancers, which include lung cancer, stomach cancer, and leukaemia, accounted for about 70% of cancers. In this group four of the cancers which were common in terms of number of cases were also relatively common in comparison with the standard population, i.e. stomach, lymphatic, prostate, and liver cancer.

For women the seven commonest cancers contributed 67% of cancers, and the ranking was dominated by cancers of the reproductive tract (breast, cervix, and ovary). The cancers ranking highest on SMRs were uncommon, but those of the lymphatic system, oesophagus, cervix, and stomach appeared on both sets of rankings.

7.5.2 **Interpreting patterns of cancer to help set priorities**

The methodological limitations of the data, as discussed above, need to be borne in mind in reaching conclusions. Patterns based on rankings, particularly when substantiated by several studies, are probably sound, even where there is uncertainty about the precision of rates and ratios arising from the difficulty of measuring accurately the numbers of cases and the population at risk. Clearly, these disease data need to be interpreted alongside information on the lifestyle and behaviour of migrant, racial, and minority ethnic groups, and their access to effective services. Nonetheless, they provide the starting point for in-depth analysis.

The sense of priority gained from this analysis differed from earlier publications. Earlier work had emphasized that cancer was relatively uncommon in minorities and had, effectively, deprioritized it, though interest was focused on those cancers that were much commoner than in the population as a whole, e.g. of the nasopharyngeal tract and of the liver. First, cancer was unequivocally shown to be a key cause of death and morbidity in the minority groups considered. The comparative lack of attention given to cancer in the past, and the perception even amongst some informed observers that cancer is not a key issue for minority ethnic groups, was not justifiable. Certainly, the statement by Karmi and McKeigue (1993), two leading UK scholars in this field, that 'Although cancer is one of the key areas . . . in the Health of Nation's white paper, it is not especially relevant to ethnic groups in the UK' was demonstrably untrue. Their bibliography of research on ethnic health identified only a few papers on cancer. Hopkins and Bahl (1993) made no reference to cancer research or services in their book on access to health care, and only one item on cancer was listed in a 1990 Health Education Authority publication listing health education materials. In his comprehensive book, Smaje (1995) had discussed the scientific literature on cancer and minority ethnic groups in Britain in under two pages (of 151, and so fewer than the ten pages on mental health and three on diabetes) noting that although relatively

Table 7.3 Cancer in adult South Asian men (mortality) and men and women combined (cancer registration): example of an overview for needs assessment

Author	Total cancer cases (overall SMR or SRR)	Cancer as % of all mortality or morbidity	Top seven cancers (% of all cancers)	Top seven cancers on SMR or SRR (as % of all cancers)
(A) Mortality				
Marmot et al. (1984)	722 (SMR = 69)	16.6	69	30
Balarajan and Bulusu (1990) (20–69 years)	1183 (SMR = 59)	15.6	68	32
(B) Cancer registration				
Donaldson and Clayton (1984)*	251 (SRR not stated)	Unknown	53	14

SMR, standardized mortality ratio; SRR, standardized (cancer) registration ratio.
* Male and female data combined by Donaldson and Clayton (1984).
Reproduced from Bhopal R., and Rankin J., Cancer in minority ethnic populations priorities from epidemiological data, *British Journal of Cancer*, Volume 74, Supplement XXIX, pp. S22–S32, Copyright © 1996, with permission from Nature Publishing Group, a division of Macmillan Publishers Limited. All Rights Reserved.

Table 7.4 Cancer experience of men of Caribbean origin aged 20–69 years: top seven cancers based on actual (A) and relative (B) frequency

								Total	Total of top seven	Top 7 as % of total
(A) Neoplasm ranked by actual frequency										
	Trachea, bronchus, and lung	Lymphatic	Stomach	Prostate	Pancreas	Liver	Colon			
No. of cases	151	116	108	54	41	39	29	744	538	72
SMR	35	135	116	175	77	317	43			
(B) Neoplasm ranked by relative frequency										
	Liver	Prostate	Lymphatic	Gall-bladder	Stomach	Buccal cavity and pharynx	Colon			
SMR	317	175	135	118	116	78	43	744	370	50
Number of cases	39	54	116	7	108	17	29			

Adapted from Bhopal R., and Rankin J., Cancer in minority ethnic populations priorities from epidemiological data, *British Journal of Cancer*, Volume 74, Supplement XXIX, pp. S22–S32, Copyright © 1996, with permission from Nature Publishing Group, a division of Macmillan Publishers Limited. All Rights Reserved. Source: Data from Balarajan R and Bulusu L, Mortality among immigrants in England and Wales, 1979-83, pp. 103-201, in Britton M (Ed), *Mortality and Geography*, HMSO, London, UK, Copyright © 1990.

little attention has been given to cancer research, cancer is a major killing disease in minority ethnic groups and its incidence is likely to increase. The Bhopal and Rankin (1996) paper was presented at what was, to my knowledge, the first UK conference on cancer in minority ethnic groups, held in 1995.

Second, in this analysis cancers such as those of the lung, breast, cervix, stomach, and leukaemia emerged as among the highest priorities. Previously, in the context of migration, race, ethnicity, and health, these cancers remained in the shadows, while others, such as those of the liver and the oropharynx, came to prominence. The reason for the marked shift in perspective was simply that previous analyses had been comparing cancer patterns in minority groups with the majority population using the relative risk approach alone. In the context of setting priorities such an approach alone is inappropriate, yet as it is so deeply rooted the alternative and more appropriate method of focusing on actual numbers of cases (or disease rates) is rarely used. The variations between populations are, however, useful as an adjunct to disease frequency (absolute risk) data in refining the picture of health and health-care needs, and for generating hypotheses. Given this, principles for priority-setting for minorities in the field of cancer were generated by Bhopal and Rankin (see Table 7.5) and applied as discussed below.

Policy-makers need to note that cancer is important in migrant, racial, and ethnic minorities, and need to address the issue, especially as such populations have traditionally had a young age structure but are now ageing too. As cancer occurs more commonly in older people this will become increasingly important. UK national policy documents and national initiatives on cancer, unlike those on CHD, have not properly addressed the needs of minority populations. One potential explanation for this might be that the needs of minorities are perceived to be so different that priorities, principles, and initiatives for the general population are deemed by planners to be unsuitable for minority groups. This perception is, however, wrong. The analysis above has

Table 7.5 Principles of priority-setting in the context of cancer in migrant, racial, and minority ethnic groups (edited version)

Policy	Base on actual frequency
	Refine on relative frequency
	Incorporate migration, race, and ethnic dimensions into national policy
Prevention	Primary focus on common cancers with avoidable risk factors
	Base on population-attributable risk (see Glossary)
Care	Common cancers are most important
	Clinical awareness of rarer cancers which are relatively common in minorities
	Education and awareness of unusual clinical history
Access, quality, and outcomes research	Focus on cancer as a whole
	Relative versus actual frequency is unimportant
Causal research	Focus on cancers where causes are obscure and ethnic variations (relative measure show excess or deficit) provide a hypothesis or model for testing

Adapted from Bhopal R., and Rankin J., Cancer in minority ethnic populations priorities from epidemiological data, *British Journal of Cancer*, Volume 74, Supplement XXIX, pp. S22–S32, Copyright © 1996, with permission from Nature Publishing Group, a division of Macmillan Publishers Limited.

demonstrated that common cancers in minority populations should be tackled as part of existing national initiatives which prioritize such cancers.

Priorities for prevention need to be founded on the concept of population attributable risk, whereby both the prevalence of risk factors and the risk of cancer are considered, to derive an estimate of the potential amount of cancer in the community that could be prevented by an effective strategy. Based on this concept, cancers for which the causes are known and can be tackled by prevention or treatment, those which are common, and those which are much commoner in people with known and reversible risk factors should get higher priority. Priorities for prevention are likely to lie within the top-ranking cancers. On this basis, for example, for South Asian men the priorities might be cancer of the lung, oesophagus, liver, and buccal cavity. For South Asian women cancer of the breast, lung, cervix, liver, and oropharynx stand out. For men of Caribbean origin cancer of the lung, liver, and colon are amongst top contenders, and for women those of the breast, cervix, colon, lung, and liver. For men of African origin cancer of the lung, liver, colon, oesophagus, and oropharynx (East Africans) are potential priorities. For women of African origin the priorities include cancer of the breast, colon, and oropharynx (East Africans).

In the clinical setting the pattern of disease in the population is less important, as each case will be diagnosed and treated individually. Doctors are more likely to see cancers which are in the top ranks on the basis of actual frequency, not relative frequency. However, doctors' perceptions about the patterns of disease are likely to be based on the scientific literature and will influence the process of diagnosis. For example, if there were a misperception that cancer of the lung is rare in South Asians and this diagnosis was not considered in investigating a lung mass (in favour of, say, tuberculosis) delay in diagnosis could occur. Alternatively, investigation and accurate diagnosis of a liver mass might be hastened by a high level of awareness of the relative frequency of liver cancer in some minority groups, most notably of Caribbean and African origin. A knowledge of cancer patterns by migration status and racial and ethnic group is potentially of value in the clinical setting. However, the benefits can be overstated, and the dangers of false generalization overlooked. As the patterns of disease and risk factors are so complex, it would be a difficult task to adequately educate all doctors about all the minority groups. While an epidemiologist or public health practitioner can look the data up, the clinician needs to have an intuitive and internalized knowledge that can be used in the consultation with patients and their families. Clinicians need to be aware of unusual presentations of cancers in minority populations.

There is a paucity of research on access to, the quality and effectiveness of, and outcomes of health care in relation to cancer services. The priority here is a focus on cancer as a whole. The rare cancers deserve as much attention as the common ones for problems are more likely to arise with these.

The demonstration of usually large variations in disease experience in population subgroups provides enormous opportunity for the development and testing of hypotheses about the causes of cancer (see Section 7.5.3). The fact that certain cancers are common in minority ethnic populations may permit epidemiological studies that would otherwise be impossible, because the assembling of a case series of rare cancers may become practical, e.g. oropharyngeal cancer studies may be possible in East London, where oral tobacco and betel leaf with areca nut are chewed commonly, especially by the large Bangladeshi population. Finally, hypotheses about disease causation (developed outside the context of the health research arena) might be explored using the migration/race/ethnicity/health model. For sparking off high-quality research we need to have unanswered questions, disease variation, testable hypotheses, and the resources and will to pursue the hypothesis until valuable observations have been made or the hypothesis is discarded. Many authors have proclaimed the potential value of ethnic variations in cancer, yet research rarely proceeds beyond the description of variation, which is insufficient to provide valuable causal insight. In the analysis by Bhopal and Rankin (1996), as in others, interesting variations deserving priority attention were demonstrated, including:

- the low SMR/SRR for many cancers including those of the stomach and colon in South Asians;
- the high SMRs for liver and oropharyngeal cancers in several minority groups;
- the high SMRs for prostate cancer in West African and Caribbean populations, but the low SMRs for South Asian and East African populations; and
- the surprisingly high SMR for lung cancer in South Asian women who report insignificant levels of smoking.

Priorities for policy, prevention, clinical care, and research need to be analysed and stated separately. Research priorities will continue to be largely guided by relative frequency, but priorities in policy, prevention, and clinical care need to pay more attention to the actual, not relative, frequency of cancers.

Figure 7.1 illustrates how data may influence the provision of services. The goal is to modify, develop, or even remove services. This is done within a context of setting priorities, whether this is explicit or implicit. The priorities themselves are based on the values of those in decision-making positions and are influenced by two sets of complementary data: on needs and what are often described as demands. These two sets of information are brought together to set priorities which are used for modifying, or developing anew, health services. In relation to cancer we see a tension between a muffled voice from demand and a clear need from quantitative data analysis. The tensions need debating in the priority-setting process. In Chapter 8 we will consider how such data and debates can be turned into strategies and actions.

In this overview of the paper by Bhopal and Rankin (1996) I have answered the questions in Exercise 7.4. In summary, the strength of the relative risk approach is that it brings to attention potentially rare cancers that might otherwise be overlooked. It is also a means of generating causal hypothesis through reflection on why differences occur. The weakness is that relative measures, alone, are not enough as they give no indication of the actual burden of disease. The absolute (or actual risk) approach has the strength of pointing to the big issues, that are common. If rates can be calculated then their comparison does provide the same information (in different format) as in relative risks but not with the same immediate impact. The danger of over-emphasizing difference is misleading and excessive generalization that could lead to stigma and stereotyping. Yet, if there was no attention to difference, modification and adaptation of priorities could not be achieved.

One of the keys to action in modern health services is evidence of effectiveness, which is becoming an essential ingredient for funding priorities. Yet obtaining such evidence is like searching for gold in a river bed and this applies particularly to minority populations. In Chapter 9, we will discuss what actions are needed to improve on this.

7.5.3 An overview of recent advances relating to prioritization in the field of cancer and the health of minorities

There is, without doubt, a mushrooming of interest in the issue of cancer and cancer services in relation to minority health. Nonetheless, it is still small in relation to the size of the problem and the challenges of delivering equitable preventive and curative services. In the United States, where information systems routinely produce data disaggregated by race and ethnicity and where policies at Federal Government level are strong, the issue is clearly on the agenda, especially in relation to trying to deliver equitable outcomes of treatment.

In Europe, by contrast, progress has been slower, though both increasing amounts of research and modest improvements in routine information systems are leading to an expansion in publication which drives debate. Cancer registries are the major source of information on cancer in Europe. Razum et al. (2011) recently showed that progress was patchy and seriously hindered by a fundamental issue—agreement on how to define and identify the minority groups of interest, and even which concepts to adopt, whether those relating to ethnicity, race, or migration status.

Nonetheless, research is progressing fast on two fronts, the description of the burden and patterns of disease on national or large subnational scales usually using computerized linkage techniques, whereby a source of data on minority status (e.g. censuses in New Zealand and Scotland and hospital records in England) is linked to a source of cancer outcomes, e.g. a death or cancer registry.

A major systematic review has been published by Arnold et al. (2010) summarizing the many interesting findings and bringing together a diverse research literature. Researchers are testing specific hypotheses, e.g. on whether specific dietary components such as spices or food processing methods might explain the huge variations in colon cancer by ethnic group. In Chapter 9 I consider the pursuit of the causes of cancer in more detail.

Yet, cancers have not found their place at the 'top table'. I believe there are two major reasons for this. First, scholars of the field have not yet spent enough time and energy on this. Books are important in portraying the state of the art of a subject. In the first edition of the 701-page US-based multi-author volume *Race, Ethnicity, and Health* (LaVeist 2006), cancer is not dominant in any chapter and the index shows a few small entries, over nine pages. In the two-volume work edited by Ingleby et al. (2012a,b), 14 of the 654 pages are on breast cancer screening. There is a broader account in the book by Rechel et al. (2011), condensed into one and a half pages within the section on non-communicable diseases (other diseases are similarly condensed). The heading of this account, I propose, contains part of the reason why interest in cancer is our field has not risen faster. It reads 'Cancers: higher risks for locally born Europeans'. The perception of relatively low risk endures and is embedded into our thinking by the relative approach. The earlier discussion of Bhopal and Rankin's paper remains of relevance across the whole field of migration-related, racial, and ethnic inequalities.

In Section 7.6 we briefly consider how the case for prioritization is to be made in these difficult circumstances, with particular regard to reducing inequalities.

7.6 Impact of priority decisions on inequalities by migration status, race, and ethnicity

The choice of priorities matters for expenditure decisions on migration-related, racial, or ethnic inequalities in health, as illustrated here in a simplified theoretical example starting with Exercise 7.5.

Exercise 7.5 Effect of priority-setting on ethnic inequalities

◆ Imagine you had £100 000 to spend on only one of five priorities set for health improvement in your minority population, i.e. disease A, B, C, D, or E. Imagine your available interventions will reduce the disease burden by 10% in each of diseases A–E.

◆ Using the data in Table 7.6, consider, before reading beyond the table, the effect on: (1) disease burden for your chosen disease (A–E); (2) inequalities in disease generally i.e. the all-cause death rate.

◆ What do we need to do to reduce inequalities between the minority and majority populations?

◆ What principles are illustrated here?

Table 7.6 shows hypothetical mortality rates for all causes of deaths and for five conditions, which collectively do not account for all the deaths. The minority population here has an overall excess of death of 20%. The death rates for the five conditions show an increasing inequality. The remaining causes of death are not shown here. We assume that these five causes have been selected as priorities for action already and a budget of £100 000 is available to tackle one of them, say, in our population of 250 000 people. Imagine that interventions are available that will reduce mortality by 10%. Again imagine these interventions are specific to one condition. Which condition will you choose? Does it matter? Furthermore, does it matter whether the goal is a reduction in inequalities or a reduction in disease burden irrespective of its effect on inequalities?

Table 7.7 shows the consequences of our decisions. In this table, for simplicity, we make the unlikely assumption that there is no decline in death rates in population X (the majority population). In reality, the majority population will usually be improving even faster than the minority. It is no surprise that an intervention focused on the commonest disorders has the biggest impact on disease burden. In addition, perhaps slightly surprisingly, it also has the biggest impact on health inequalities overall— even though cause A itself shows the least relative excess in the minority population.

It is likely that interventions are already under way to control diseases in the majority population and that the £100 000 budget is designed to help equalize services. Table 7.8 shows that a 10%

Table 7.6 Mortality data for two theoretical populations

	Majority population (X)	Minority population (Y)	Ratio of minority to majority, i.e. inequality
All-cause death rate/100 000/year (at baseline)	1000	1200	1.20*
Death rate from:			
Cause A	300	330	1.1
Cause B	200	240	1.2
Cause C	100	130	1.3
Cause D	50	70	1.4
Cause E	20	30	1.5

* Obviously this is 1200 divided by 1000, i.e. 1.2.

Table 7.7 Effect on inequalities in overall death rate of a 10% decline in death rates in the minority population

	Majority population (X)	Minority population (Y)	Ratio of minority to majority, i.e. inequality
All cause-death rate/100 000/ year (at baseline)	1000	1200	1.20
After an intervention on population Y that reduces the disease by 10% (see Table 7.6 for actual rates) for causes A–E			
Cause A	—	1200 – 33* = 1167	1.167†
Cause B	—	1200 – 24 = 1176	1.176
Cause C	—	1200 – 13 = 1187	1.187
Cause D	—	1200 – 7 = 1193	1.193
Cause E	—	1200 – 3 = 1197	1.197

* The figure is 10% of 330, the rate for cause A in the minority population as shown in Table 7.6.

† 1167/1000.

Table 7.8 Effect of a 10% decline in disease in both majority and minority populations on overall inequalities, and also of a 20% decline in the disease in the minority population

	Majority population (X)	Minority population (Y)	Ratio of minority to majority (Y:X)
All-cause death rate (baseline)	1000	1200	1.2
Overall mortality after intervention on populations X and Y for cause A	1000 – 30 = 970	1200 – 33 = 1167	1.203
After intervention on cause A for majority population and cause E for minority population	1000 – 30 = 970	1200 – 3 = 1197	1.234
After intensive intervention on minority populations (20% effect) and standard intervention on majority population (10% effect) for cause A	1000 – 30 = 970	1200 – 66 = 1134	1.169

reduction in cause A in both populations has no beneficial effect on reducing inequalities. In fact they rise slightly. Imagine that a decision is taken to focus the expenditure on condition E in the minority population (the one showing the highest ratio in Table 7.6) and that, as a result, cause A remains unchanged in that population. Taking into account only the control of cause A in the majority population, with a 10% decline the overall inequality rises substantially.

The message seems to be clear—the reduction of inequalities requires a comparatively more intensive intervention in the disadvantaged population, as shown at the end of Table 7.8 where an intervention that leads to a 20% decline in cause of death A is applied to the minority population.

The principles arising from this simple, theoretical exercise are the following:

1. Making choices on priorities for action to reduce diseases has a differential impact on both on disease burden (obvious) and on inequalities (not so obvious).

2. An equal reduction in absolute terms of disease in two populations that start from an unequal position does not reduce inequalities (which actually widen in relative terms).

3. Choosing to focus on conditions that have the greatest relative excess in minority populations can widen inequalities overall.

4. The reduction of inequalities requires that the disease burden declines faster in the disadvantaged group than in the advantaged one.

These principles require that we have effective interventions that work equally well in all the minority groups, an issue that we consider below.

7.7 Evidence base for interventions in the field of migration, race, and minority ethnic health

The question of what interventions work is always problematic, especially in the case of complex initiatives for complex disorders, e.g. those with social, cultural, and behavioural causes. For many interventions, the evidence is inconclusive (and sometimes non-existent) in any population. The controlled trial, and its strictest variant, the placebo-controlled, randomized, double-blind trial (see Glossary), undeniably provides the most solid evidence for the effectiveness of interventions. These trials are difficult and expensive to conduct, particularly for complex interventions. The critical question is whether we need evidence from such studies to recommend that an initiative is a high priority in minority groups. For example, smoking cessation services are a major priority nationally. Are they a priority for minority groups? On the basis of data on the prevalence of smoking they should be for many minorities, e.g. Bangladeshi men, Pakistani men, and African Caribbean men and women. (There is also the related issue of chewing tobacco, but we will leave that aside for now.) But will the interventions work? We should look for evidence. Unfortunately, we are unlikely to find such evidence, at least not from the UK. The main exception here would be the United States, and even then only for some racial or ethnic groups (e.g. African Americans).

It would be greatly damaging if decision-makers insisted on evidence specific to particular migrant, racial, or minority ethnic groups before providing a budget. We need principles to guide our actions in the absence of concrete, trial-based evidence specific to minority groups.

What do we do when there are no specific relevant studies? Indeed, in the UK setting there are no definitive data (though there are pragmatic evaluations and pilot trials) and internationally they are sparse.

Clearly, it would be excellent to have such trials on minority groups and a research programme needs to be encouraged. As a minimum, studies on general populations ought not to exclude people from minority groups (as some do, often by excluding those who do not speak English, for example). Building up a valid database of this kind for a range of important issues will, however, be a multibillion-pound endeavour which needs to take place internationally, and it will take 10–20 years. In the meantime, surely we cannot permit paralysis in relation to minority health. The solution is appropriate adaptation of effective interventions to ensure their effectiveness across a range of groups.

A substantial body of work on this challenge has been published, most of it very recently. This comprises guidelines based on expert opinion, the description of practice in the field, principles derived from systematic literature reviews, and empirical qualitative research synthesizing the experience of international researchers. In addition to guidelines and principles, decision-making tools have been produced (e.g. RESET; Liu et al. 2012) as well as a 46-item 'Typology of Adaptation'. Even given all this work we remain unsure how much better (if at all) adapted interventions perform than unadapted ones, and we know even less about the cost-effectiveness of adaptation. An open-access report of over 400 pages on this topic was published recently by Liu et al. (2012). The next stage is large-scale international head-to-head comparisons of adapted and unadapted interventions. The principles that could be adopted here are as follows:

1. In planning an initiative for minority groups, start with a systematic review of the evidence in all minority groups, including, of course, the majority group.

2. If an initiative works in one or more populations, it may work in the minority group of interest. If it does not work in other populations it is reasonable to assume it is unlikely to work in minority populations. The essential principle here is this: human populations are more alike than different. No doubt there will be occasional exceptions but the general rule is likely to apply.

3. If the intervention is based on physiology and biology, e.g. folic acid supplementation for pregnant women to prevent congenital abnormalities, one can have a high degree of confidence that it will work across groups because the genome of all human beings is very similar. This is, nonetheless, a matter for evaluation. As a minimum there should be monitoring both of the uptake of the intervention, which may well differ by ethnic group, and the outcome once the intervention is taken up, which is less likely to differ.

4. If the intervention is complex, and likely to be affected by social, economic, cultural, or environmental factors, then we need to take special care. For example, brief advice from the general practitioner helps smokers quit. Most of the evidence comes from White populations. Will this work in Bangladeshi or Chinese men and women? It would be wrong to assume it will. This intervention may be better implemented in the context of a trial or other rigorous research design so it can be evaluated properly. If this is not possible, go ahead with the intervention but in a questioning manner and with a pragmatic evaluation.

5. In most instances, at least for the foreseeable future, health services will need to modify interventions proven to work in one group (very often White populations) to make them cross-culturally effective.

In the first edition of this book I wrote 'This field of study is in its infancy, but needs to be promoted'. It is now a burgeoning field of study and practice.

7.8 **Conclusions**

We can conclude, on the principle that similarities between human populations tend to outweigh the differences, that the general priorities of public health and health-care systems are of great importance to minority groups. These general priorities, alone, are not sufficient. They need adjustment on the basis of careful health needs assessment. For long-settled communities, and minorities born or raised in the country, the adjustments may be modest or even minor. For others—undocumented migrants, asylum seekers and refugees, those who do not speak the local language, or those discriminated against—the adjustments needed may be substantial. Public health and health-care initiatives designed to set priorities must, therefore, consider the majority and minority populations simultaneously, with work of equal validity. The chosen priorities will reflect the pattern of diseases, risk factors, and service utilization of minorities. They will also consider the effectiveness of interventions. Such evidence will be sparse for specific minority populations.

Pending the development of a solid evidence base for the effectiveness of initiatives to improve the health of minorities (a long-term goal), interventions effective in other populations need to be carefully adapted, implemented, and evaluated. In Chapter 9 there will be further discussion of how we achieve more and better research that provides data by ethnic group.

Getting the priorities implemented in practice is difficult, but it requires a continuation of past approaches (education, exhortation, research, taking opportunities to influence management, and influencing policy documents). Increasingly, we need to promote the vigorous mobilization of an increasingly informed community voice. Stories from the community are very powerful in bringing about change, sometimes more so than statistics (which have been described as tragedies without the tears). Nonetheless, better information systems are needed, particularly to foster the evaluation of services and audit of quality of care.

Evidence showing that the quality of care for minority populations is inferior is particularly effective in bringing about change, as it goes against policies and laws promoting equality. Coding of health-care records to include migration status, race, and ethnicity (see Chapters 3 and 8) probably holds the key for setting priorities, audit and new programmes of research, and for monitoring change.

All health-care and public health policies and plans should make explicit what the priorities are, whether they are different for different groups, and how the needs of minority groups are to be met. These needs of minorities should not be relegated to secondary documentation. The health-care system must ensure that its current priorities and policies are evaluated in relation to the changing composition of the population, and especially newly arriving minority groups. Services need to make appropriate modifications to ensure they meet the needs of minority groups. The health-care system must not make the mistake of imagining, assuming, awaiting, or expecting a different set of priorities, though it needs to be alert to the need for modification.

7.9 **Summary**

Whether in research, policy, or health care, the choices for actions to improve the health of minority groups are multiple, especially in complex, multicultural societies. Priority-setting is a process for making rational choices from multiple alternatives. Social values are important to priority-setting and in the context of migration, race, ethnicity, and health the most important of these are equality and equity (discussed in detail in Chapter 10). The public health sciences, particularly epidemiology, can underpin priority-setting, which follows from the process of health needs assessment. Quantitative and qualitative data on health status and service utilization are often available (though they may be crude) but need to be used carefully. In contrast, information on the cost and effectiveness of interventions as applied to specific groups is rarely available, posing a formidable challenge to both priority-setting and future research.

Priority-setting benefits from principles. One principle is that the priorities are those actions that have benefit for the health of a population, and that includes specific minority groups. Another is to prioritize actions that raise the health and health care of the minority group to the level of the population as a whole or, preferably, to the level of the group with the best health. In practice the target standard is usually the health status of the majority population. Integrating these principles will meet the twin goals of maximizing health and tackling health inequalities. Reductions of inequalities, however, can only be achieved if health improvement occurs fastest in the most disadvantaged population. Health improvement requires the use of practical interventions that are cost-effective: evidence of such effectiveness by migration status, race, or ethnic group, is sparse. Pending an international programme of research to rectify this all health policies should use principles to select the priorities relating to minority groups and mandate strategies and actions to achieve them.

Acknowledgments

Text extract reproduced from Bradby H, Genetics and racism in Marteau, T. and Richards, M. (Eds), *The troubled helix: social and psychological implications of the new human genetics*: pp. 295–316, Cambridge University Press, Cambridge, UK, Copyright © 1999 by permission of Cambridge University Press.

References

Arnold M, Razum O, Coebergh JW (2010) Cancer risk diversity in non-western migrants to Europe: an overview of the literature. *European Journal of Cancer* **46**: 2647–59.

Balarajan R, Bulusu L (1990) Mortality among immigrants in England and Wales, 1979–83. In Britton M (ed.) Mortality and Geography: a review in the mid 1980s, pp. 103–21. London: HMSO.

Bhopal RS (1998) Setting priorities for health care. In Rawaf S, Bahl V (eds) Assessing Health Needs of Ethnic Minority Groups, pp. 57–63. London: Department of Health.

Bhopal RS (2006) The public health agenda and minority ethnic health: a reflection on priorities. *Journal of the Royal Society of Medicine* **99**: 58–61.

Bhopal R, Donaldson L (1988) Health promotion for ethnic minorities: current provision and future directions. *Health Education Journal* **47**: 137–40.

Bhopal RS, Rankin J (1996) Cancer in minority ethnic populations: priorities from epidemiological data. *British Journal of Cancer* **74**: S22–S32.

Bradby H (1999) Genetics and racism. In Marteau T, Richards M (eds) *The Troubled Helix: social and psychological implications of the new human genetics*, pp. 295–316. Cambridge: Cambridge University Press.

Donaldson LJ, Clayton DG (1984) Occurrence of cancer in Asians and Non-Asians. *Journal of Epidemiology and Community Health* **38**: 203–7.

Gill PS, Kai J, Bhopal RS, Wild S (2007) Black and minority ethnic groups. In Raftery J (ed.) Health Care Needs Assessment. The Epidemiologically Based Needs Assessment Reviews, pp. 227–389. Abingdon: Radcliffe Medical Press Ltd. Available at: http://www.birmingham.ac.uk/research/activity/mds/projects/HaPS/PHEB/HCNA/chapters/index.aspx

Grulich AE, Swerdlow AJ, Head J, Marmot MG (1992) Cancer mortality in African and Caribbean migrants to England and Wales. *British Journal of Cancer* **66**: 905–11.

Hopkins A, Bahl V (eds) (1993) *Access to Health Care for People from Black and Ethnic Minorities*. London: Royal College of Physicians.

Ingleby D, Krasnik A, Lorant V, Razum, O (eds) (2012a) *COST Series on Health and Diversity Volume 1: Health Inequalities and Risk Factors among Migrants and Ethnic Minorities*. Antwerpen/Apeldoom: Garant.

Ingleby D, Chiarenza A, Devillé W, Kotsioni I (eds) (2012b) *COST Series on Health and Diversity. Volume 2: Inequalities in Health Care for Migrants and Ethnic Minorities*. Antwerpen/Apeldoom: Garant.

Karmi G, McKeigue P (1993) *The Ethnic Health Bibliography*. London: NE and NW Thames RHA.

LaVeist T (ed.) (2006) *Race, Ethnicity, and Health*, 1st edn. San Francisco: Jossey-Bass.

Liu JJ, Davidson E, Bhopal RS, White M, Johnson MRD, Netto G, et al. (2012) Adapting health promotion interventions to meet the needs of ethnic minority groups: mixed-methods evidence synthesis. Health Technology Assessment 16(44): 1–469. doi: 10.3310/hta16440 [open access]

Marmot MG, Adelstein AM, Bulusu L (1984) *Immigrant Mortality in England and Wales 1970–78*. London: HMSO.

Muir KR, Parkes SE, Mann JR, Stevens MCG, Cameron AH (1992) Childhood cancer in the West Midlands: incidence and survival 1980–1984 in a multi-ethnic population. *Clinical Oncology* **4**: 177–82.

Powell JE, Parkes SE, Cameron AH, Mann JR (1994) Is the risk of cancer increased in Asians living in the UK? *Archives of Disease in Childhood* 71: 398–403.

Rankin J, Bhopal R (2001) Understanding of heart disease and diabetes in a South Asian community: cross-sectional study testing the 'snowball' sample method. *Public Health* 115: 253–60.

Razum O, Spallek J, Reeske A, Arnold M (2011) *Migration-sensitive Cancer Registration in Europe. Challenges and Potentials.* Frankfurt: Peter Lang International Academic Publishers.

Rechel B, Mladovsky P, Deville W, Rijks B, Petrova-Benedict R, McKee M (2011) *Migration and Health in the European Union.* Maidenhead: Open University Press.

Smaje C (1995) *Race and Ethnicity: making sense of the evidence.* London: King's Fund.

Stiller CA, McKinney PA (1991) Childhood cancer and ethnic group in Britain: a United Kingdom children's cancer study group (UKCCSG) study. *British Journal of Cancer* 64: 543–8.

Tunstall Pedoe H, Clayton D, Morris JN, Bridge W, McDonald L (1975) Coronary heart-attack in East London. *The Lancet* ii: 833–8.

Other sources and further reading

Balarajan R, Bulusu L, Adelstein AM, Shukla V (1984) Patterns of mortality among migrants to England and Wales from the Indian subcontinent. *British Medical Journal* 289: 1185–7.

Dunnigan MG, McIntosh WB, Sutherland GR, Gordee R, et al. (1981) Policy for prevention of Asian Rickets in Britain: a preliminary assessment of the Glasgow Rickets Campaign. *British Medical Journal* 288: 357–60.

Kilbourne AM, Switzer G, Hyman K, Crowley-Matoka M, Fine MJ (2006) Advancing health disparities research within the health care system: a conceptual framework. *American Journal of Public Health* 96: 2113–21.

Klein R (1993) Dimensions of rationing: who should do what. *Rationing in Action*, pp. 96–104. London: BMJ Publishing Group.

Östlin P, Schrecker T, Sadana R, Bonnefoy J, Gilson L, Hertzman C, et al. (2011) Priorities for research on equity and health: towards an equity-focused health research agenda. *PLoS Medicine* 8: e1001115.

Chapter 8

Policy and strategy to improve health and health care for migrants and minority racial and ethnic groups

Objectives

After reading this chapter you should be able to:

- In outline, appreciate the nature of strategy in relation to policy and tactics.
- Using examples of key strategy documents on migration, race, ethnicity, and health internationally, develop an understanding of the approaches and principles applied.
- In principle, be able to articulate the content of an ideal strategic document, but to accept compromises in the light of constraints of data, expertise, resources, and political circumstances.

8.1 Introduction to policy, strategy, and models of service delivery

Ethnic and racial diversity is increasing in many countries, primarily as a result of increasing migration linked to globalization of trade, education, and markets and to the movement of refugees. This offers formidable challenges in the development of policies and strategies to promote the reduction of inequalities in health and improvements in health care. Challenges in health and health care arising from the increasing diversity of populations include:

- understanding and responding to varying health behaviours, beliefs, and attitudes;
- responding to differences in the pattern of diseases, and in particular reducing inequalities where this is possible;
- maintaining high-quality communications in the face of language and cultural barriers;
- delivering a service that is sensitive to cultural differences, e.g. in relation to modesty among women especially, and the preference for same-sex health carers;
- overcoming both personal biases, stereotyped views, individuals' racism, and institutional inertia and racism;
- ensuring equal opportunities in employment at all stages from recruitment to retirement.

These challenges have, of course, been faced by health policy, medical research, and health-care institutions over many decades, but recent landmark reports and legislation are stimulating change. These challenges require effective policy and strategy that can capture the intent of recommendations and laws and underpin specific plans and local actions.

Before reading on, try Exercise 8.1.

Exercise 8.1 The nature of policy, strategy, and planning

◆ In the health context what is the difference between policy-making, strategy, and health planning?

◆ Why are these three types of activity necessary?

◆ In the field of migration, race, ethnicity, and health how are policies to be reconciled with tactical opportunities?

A policy is a statement, usually issued in writing by a governing body, on its intentions over a relatively long timescale. A policy sets high-level directions and goals. A policy also sets the tone that influences a broader audience, which could be the entire nation, continent, or the world. The importance of tone will be considered later in Section 8.3 on the United States with an example of the controversial effects of editing.

Policies are usually written, but it is common, especially for governments, to announce them in political speeches or political manifestos (or their equivalent). It is generally understood that policy will be backed by political, legislative, managerial, and financial support as appropriate. In practice many policies are never implemented and are either changed, forgotten, or postponed. Good intentions sometimes cannot be implemented for lack of resources. It is not uncommon for new leaders to sweep aside previous policies and start afresh, often merely reinventing what was there before, but with serious loss of time, energy, and expertise. Some policies are quickly seen to be impractical or ineffective. Policies need to be institutionalized and operationalized rapidly if they are not to be forgotten, and this is done through a strategic plan.

A strategy is a general plan to make a course of action promised in a policy actually happen. There is no crystal clear division between a policy and a strategy in practice. Strategies are invariably written. As anyone organizing a party knows, success requires intentions (policy), foresight (vision), general ideas on the type of party and the activities (strategy), detailed planning on menus, music, and other such matters, and meticulous execution including sending out invitations and then being a good host (delivery). On the grander scale of health-care delivery to minorities and whole populations alike, policies and strategies need to be accompanied by detailed plans that outline actions, responsibilities, timetables, and costs. In practice, actions to improve the health and health care of minority populations are not always taken in response to policies and strategies but on a tactical or opportunistic basis. There may be, for instance, some surplus funding that needs to be used for a good purpose before the end of the financial year. Or, alternatively, there may be an urgent perceived need to avert attention from negative publicity or criticism from some important person or media organization. Usually, there are a number of outstanding and well-recognized needs of minority populations that can be attended to in such circumstances. Long-term policies and strategies will make it easier to identify the highest priority needs when such opportunities arrive and to help make the case for using resources in this way.

Health services for minority groups are usually delivered within the scope of policies and strategies for the population as a whole, which in practice means the majority population. Traditionally, such policies and strategies have made no mention of any special needs of minority groups, but this is changing fast. There are a number of approaches to meeting the needs of minority groups, and we should consider the strengths and weaknesses of them.

Before reading on, try Exercise 8.2.

Exercise 8.2 Strengths and weaknesses of various models of service delivery to migrants and minority racial and ethnic groups

What are the strengths and weaknesses of the following policy options for health services for minority groups?

1. One service for the whole population—all individuals and groups are expected to adapt to use it.

2. One service supplemented by special projects to meet special needs.

3. One service adapted to meet needs of all population subgroups.

4. One service purpose-designed to meet diverse needs.

5. Separate services for separate minority groups.

Ideally policies, strategies, and plans for the whole population would address the needs of minority and majority groups simultaneously and in an integrated way. This concept is sometimes known as mainstreaming. In Exercise 8.2 this would mean model 4, but since designing services anew is not usually possible, model 3 is the nearest alternative. In practice, this level of adaptation of services to meet diverse needs has rarely happened, for reasons including one or more of the following: lack of time; lack of understanding of need; the complexity of the task; lack of expertise; or lack of publication space within the key policy and strategy documents. So, the strengths of models 3 and 4 are obvious, but the weakness is that they are hard to achieve.

Mostly, individuals from minority populations are expected to adapt themselves to benefit from the available services, i.e. model 1. Professionals delivering the service may make appropriate adjustments on an ad hoc basic, hopefully with the backing of health service managers. Health professionals, generally, make common sense changes and adaptations. The strength of this approach is that planning and delivering a single model of a service is practical and needs the smallest amount of management input and management cost. Proponents might also argue that it encourages social integration. The weaknesses include that, notwithstanding the efforts of health professionals, the services are likely to be inequitable.

Increasingly, we see two further policy responses—setting up specialist services for minority groups, i.e. model 2, and the development of separate strategies to help reshape existing services, i.e. to move to model 3. The strength of this is its practicality. Altering an entire service, or even a component of it, is very difficult. Adding a component, given resources, is undoubtedly easier (though still not easy). It is also practical, though not ideal, for a generic policy (say on diabetes prevention and control) to be supplemented at a later date by a special policy in relation to minorities. The weaknesses include the observation that such special needs projects are hard to fund sustainably and are not comprehensive. This approach also leads to a delayed response.

Whatever the service model there is a great danger that initiatives to prevent, control, and treat diseases and promote health do not provide their full benefits to minority groups. First, as discussed in Chapter 7, those responsible may wrongly assume that the service under their control is not a priority in one or more minority groups. An example of this, that we discussed in Chapter 7, is a mis-perception that in South Asian populations common cancers, and some of their risk factors including smoking, are not a high priority. The second danger is that any steps that are taken are inadequate, e.g. a media campaign video may be dubbed with the minority group's languages, when it might be more effective to include in the original video some actors from minority groups to convey cross-cultural relevance. The third danger is that the planners are aware of the issues but decide that the strategy for the minority groups should be separate from the main one, and in practice this is the common, perhaps even the usual, response. Such a decision should be carefully justified and implemented. There is a danger that if it is not it could be construed as institutional racism, and counter to the duty to promote racial equality. Such a decision might be undesirable on pragmatic grounds too. Pragmatically, the bulk of the required knowledge, expertise, energy, momentum, and finances will lie with the architects and managers of the main strategy. The strategy for minority groups may, therefore, have a lesser impact, so accentuating existing inequalities. Mostly, it is better for minority groups to be included within the main initiative.

Model 5 is largely deplored in modern, democratic, multi-ethnic societies as both unworkable and undesirable, if not illegal. This model has been the preferred one of openly racist states such as South Africa under the policy of apartheid. In theory, if separate services could be achieved to the same standard, model 5 might be acceptable from a health-care perspective, but it goes counter to the idea of integration. Where integration is not feasible this model has a place. For example, in many countries undocumented migrants have extremely limited access to general services. Special services may be provided by humanitarian organizations or by individuals. Special services have also been designed for indigenous populations, most notably the Indian Health Service in the United States. Special services and strategies are in place for aboriginal populations in Australia. Apart from such exceptional circumstances, where this model has strengths, the approach is out of favour—experience has shown it is not sustainable but it may help meet short-term goals. We will return to these models as we examine some policies and strategies.

This chapter takes an international perspective but also focuses on the UK and particularly on Scotland, and within that the Lothian Health Board. The reasons are that I am most familiar with UK policies and that the UK is advanced in policy-making in the field of ethnicity and health. I have a potential conflict of interest that might have led to an over-optimistic assessment of the situation in the UK. I have served on a number of committees working to improve the health and health care of minority populations, including the NHS (England) Ethnic Health Unit, and chairmanship and/ or membership of committees in the Lothian Health Board, the Scottish Executive, and the National Resource Centre For Ethnic Minority Health (Scotland). These experiences, however, have given me access to, and hence insight into, the decision-making processes. The situation in the UK is compared and contrasted with that in several places, including the United States, to draw more general lessons.

8.2 **Examples of policy and strategy**

Before reading on try Exercises 8.3 and 8.4.

Exercise 8.3 **The importance of political policy and legal background**

- ◆ Why is the political, legal, and policy environment particularly important to the task of meeting the health needs of migrant and racial and ethnic minority populations?
- ◆ Can you think of places where health care for minority groups has been: (1) obstructed by political and legal actions and (2) promoted by political and legal actions?

Exercise 8.4 **Idealized policy and strategy**

- ◆ What might be the principles of an ideal policy and strategy?
- ◆ Given political and resource constraints what compromises might be needed to create an achievable policy/strategy?
- ◆ How will we know that our policy/strategy is being effective?

8.2.1 **General—the international legal and policy context**

All member states of the UN (the vast majority of countries) accept the principle that international law takes precedence over national law. Numerous international laws govern the behaviour of countries in relation to the health and health care of migrants and racial and ethnic minorities. The binding ones are called treaties, conventions, covenants, protocols, or agreements. In addition there are non-binding (soft law) declarations and recommendations that often precede law that must also be taken into account. The requirements of international laws are usually incorporated into national laws, which may go further than international ones. Among the most important rights provided by international laws are the right to non-discrimination and the right to health. The right to non-discrimination permits objective, differentiated treatment to meet needs and rectify imbalances. This right is central to work to promote equality and equity. Non-discrimination on the basis of attributes such as colour, race, and religion is an explicit right, but that is not explicitly so for migration status. In practice, however, the law, as interpreted, does protect migrants.

The right to health applies to migrants and racial and ethnic minorities explicitly, from departure, arrival, and return migration. Poor health of a potential immigrant cannot be an automatic bar to migration.

If health workers are required by national law to report undocumented migrants who seek health care they may deter them from accessing services, so contravening international law. This is a highly controversial area, not least because professional ethics may also be breached.

International laws cover the treatment of asylum seekers and particularly their detention. Arbitrary detention breaches human rights, but limited detention pending decisions on asylum is permitted. If asylum is granted, refugees have the same rights as the general populace.

Other international instruments of importance to the fields of migration, ethnicity and race include the UN Declaration on the Rights of Indigenous Peoples and the Convention on the Rights of the Child.

International law is an important but complex and controversial field. One of the most contentious matters, linked to the rights of undocumented migrants, concerns the rights of those not granted asylum. They do not lose their rights under international law. For example, the return process must not breach their right to health, and they cannot be returned if their death would be hastened. In practice, this happens; and in also practice, those not gaining asylum may not return but become undocumented migrants.

The responsibility for applying international law rests with nation states, though this may occur through regional governments, e.g. the EU. The main international organizations that can support nation states are the International Organization for Migration (IOM), which in January 2013 had 149 member states, and the WHO.

The IOM and the WHO have recently become partners in setting out the issues relating to health in a Global Consultation on Migrant Health in March 2010. The consultation both assessed progress following the 61st World Health Assembly's 2008 Statement on the Health of Migrants, and proposed a way forward. These documents were arguably the most important response from the WHO in this field ever, more so than the 1983 Consultation on Migration and Health by the European Region of the WHO. It placed the subject on the international health agenda for the first time.

The World Health Assembly set the background and made nine calls to Member States (see Box 8.1) and 11 requests to the Director General of the WHO. The 11th recommendation was to report on the implementation of the resolution. The Report of the Global Consultation was presented to the 63rd World Health Assembly. The Report picked four priorities:

1. Monitoring migrant health through standardized and comparable data.

2. Adopting policy and legal frameworks aligned with international standards.

3. Migrant-sensitive health systems delivering comprehensive, coordinated, and financially sustainable services.

4. Addressing the issues through partnerships, networks, and multicountry frameworks.

The idea of a Global Forum on Migration and Development was proposed, amongst other recommendations. Progress at the international agency level has been slow, though the IOM is stimulating new work at the time of writing (January 2013). Progress at national level, however, has both accelerated, and spread to an increasing number of countries even in the face of global economic difficulties since 2008. We will now consider some examples.

8.2.2 The UK and United States in an international context

The UK policy response to ethnicity (and this concept incorporates migration status and race in the UK) and health over the last 50 years, as in many other countries, has been intermittent and

---

Box 8.1 World Health Assembly's Resolution 2008

This calls upon Member States:

(1) to promote migrant-sensitive health policies;

(2) to promote equitable access to health promotion, disease prevention and care for migrants, subject to national laws and practice, without discrimination on the basis of gender, age, religion, nationality or race;

(3) to establish health information systems in order to assess and analyse trends in migrants' health, disaggregating health information by relevant categories;

(4) to devise mechanisms for improving the health of all populations, including migrants, in particular through identifying and filling gaps in health service delivery;

(5) to gather, document and share information and best practices for meeting migrants' health needs in countries of origin or return, transit and destination;

(6) to raise health service providers' and professionals' cultural and gender sensitivity to migrants' health issues;

(7) to train health professionals to deal with the health issues associated with population movements;

(8) to promote bilateral and multilateral cooperation on migrants' health among countries involved in the whole migratory process;

(9) to contribute to the reduction of the global deficit of health professionals and its consequences on the sustainability of health systems and the attainment of the Millennium Development Goals.

Text extracts reproduced from World Health Organization Sixty-First World Health Assembly, 19–24 May 2008, Resolutions And Decisions Annexes, p. 24, World Health Organization, Geneva, Switzerland, Copyright © 2008, with permission from the World Health Organization.

fragmented, with a mixture of both stand-alone projects (model 2) and in more recent years modifications to mainline services (model 3) (separate services—model 5—have not been advocated). This is not surprising as the issue is complex and subject to many external influences, particularly political and financial ones. Progress has been made in the UK on key practical requirements of minority ethnic populations such as equality in employment in health services, interpretation services, and special dietary and spiritual needs in hospital.

The Race Relations (Amendment) Act 2000, which amended the 1976 Act, coupled with explicit or implicit policies from government health departments, drove more widespread changes based on a positive duty to promote racial equality. The requirements of this Act have been absorbed into the single Equality Act 2010 where nine protected characteristics are covered simultaneously. In principle, work on each of the nine characteristics—race being one—should be strengthened by this integrated approach. The concern, however, is that work on each of the characteristics will be diluted, or that one or more of the protected characteristics will be developed to the neglect of others. The clear benefit is that it is much harder to undermine or even sweep away work on the broad equalities agenda than to do this to one single characteristic. In 2010, in the midst of the economic crisis, the governing party changed from the centre-left Labour to the centre-right Conservative and Liberal Democrat coalition. The new government openly declared a crusade against bureaucracy, issuing a red-tape challenge, both as a means of reducing costs and reducing governmental control. Equality laws and policies have been amongst the many undergoing scrutiny in public consultations. The consequences for the long term are unclear. Matters of importance to the field of migration, race, and ethnicity, such as translation and interpretation, are amongst those pinpointed as sources of savings. Aside from financial arguments, there is a view that such services go against social cohesion and integration. Generally, however, there is much support for the principles underpinning the Equality Act 2010, and integration of equality strands has given strength and protection to the components. An equality impact assessment of policies and service changes is an important requirement under the Act that is somewhat under attack. The Prime Minister David Cameron stated on radio words to the effect that such formal approaches are not needed because we have intelligent and skilled civil servants drafting policies. Experience over some 50 years, however, supports the need for a formal approach.

These national initiatives are translated, often with great difficulty, into local action plans and ultimately service changes. Ethnic monitoring in employment and service is an example of a policy that was difficult to achieve until the law came into place, despite excellent intentions and substantial efforts. The combination of a national health-care system, law, and policy has been instrumental in achieving change, albeit slow, in the UK setting.

There has been considerable frustration in the UK among those working to improve the health care of ethnic minority populations. To a large extent this has arisen because of the stop–start nature of policy. I intend to show that the policy infrastructure is in place in the UK, and particularly Scotland, to surmount the formidable challenges (see Section 8.2.3).

Unlike the UK, the United States has had a programme for affirmative action since the 1960s, based on human rights principles, that aims to redress historical wrongs. A racial and ethnic classification of the Office of Management and Budget was explicitly designed to help achieve this goal (see Chapter 2). Despite the country having the most expensive health-care system in the world, more than 40 million people in the United States have no health insurance and many people distrust health services because of their commercially driven ethos. Migrants, especially undocumented ones, and racial and ethnic minorities are most likely to be without insurance, and numerous studies have shown big gaps in the quality of care between the minorities and majority White populations. The United States has been foremost in the world in producing cogent, comprehensive, and clear-cut analyses of the problem. The pluralistic nature of the health care system of the United States, based on private health-care principles even though it is highly reliant on government funding, has made a cohesive national strategy problematic to enact. There are powerful policies in place but their effectiveness seems to be limited. By law and explicit policy based on legislation, minority groups cannot be excluded from research using federal government money without good scientific reason, and this has spurred a substantial research programme. The United States leads the world in the quantity of research on minority racial and ethnic populations, and this is another example of policy and law combining forces to lever change. The Health Care and Education Reconciliation Act of 2010—so-called Obama Care—aims to extend health-care insurance. It has been bitterly contested and challenged in the courts. Over time, it should benefit minority groups, reducing inequalities in access to high-quality care.

8.2.3 Scotland—a late starter, but making rapid progress in the context of a political programme for social justice

8.2.3.1 Background information–demography and politics

I am describing Scotland's approach in detail because I am sufficiently familiar with it to be able to draw generalizable principles and lessons. Moreover, Scotland is recognized as having made rapid progress at a policy and strategy level in recent years. Finally, I believe that those countries that are formulating policy and strategic responses may benefit from examining Scotland's approach, just as Scotland learned from others.

Scotland is one of the four constituent countries of the UK, alongside England, Wales, and Northern Ireland. In 1999 the Scottish Parliament was opened in Edinburgh, with increased devolved powers. Even before that, however, in many respects Scotland had its own systems. Among the devolved powers are the law and health. Given this, it is understandable that Scotland has developed somewhat independently its own policy response.

Scotland has a small population of a little over 5 million, one reason for this being emigration from Scotland on a mass scale over hundreds of years. Scotland has also attracted immigrants mostly from other UK countries and the Republic of Ireland, but also from both western and eastern Europe. Exchange and interchange of populations has been an established part of Scottish life, not least because of the strong, ancient Scottish universities that attracted students from across the world. However, the settlement of non-White people was rare before 1950, a pattern also seen in most of Europe. In Scotland ethnicity is the overarching concept used, inclusive of all migrant, racial, and like groups. The 1991 census recorded about 1% of the population as belonging to non-White ethnic groups, a figure that doubled by 2001 and doubled again by 2011. In the last decade some 60 000 eastern Europeans, mostly Polish people, immigrated.

Data on the social and health context of Scotland's migrant and minority ethnic population was sparse until the 1991 census collected, for the first time, data on ethnic group in addition to country of birth (substantial numbers of elderly White Scottish people were born abroad). Data related to health status have only been available since about 2006, with the exception of special ad hoc studies on specific topics, e.g. vitamin D deficiency. Health-related policy, therefore, was made largely in the absence of health data—a situation that many other countries will find themselves in.

The political parties in power in Scotland in recent decades (Labour and now the Scottish Nationalist Party) have been left of centre, promoting public policy based on social justice with a strong emphasis on reduction of inequality. The key focus of these policies is socio-economic inequality, for Scotland has been and remains an economically unequal society. This social justice perspective embraces the wider inequality strands including gender, disability, sexual orientation, and race.

There is no place for overt racism in Scottish society and all politicians speak against it. There is no power base for ultra-right-wing fascist or racist politics. The biggest problem of this type is sectarianism with hostility between the Protestant and Catholic population, often triggered around football. This is not to claim the situation is perfect—racial and other forms of prejudice clearly exist. The point is that the political milieu has long been favourable for progressing policy in the fields of migration, race, ethnicity, and health.

8.2.3.2 Health inequalities are a priority for the health service in Scotland

Health care in the UK is provided free at the point of delivery to all residents (irrespective of nationality, citizenship, etc.) through the NHS, established in 1948. The Scottish Government is responsible for NHS Scotland and devolves the budget across 14 Health Boards that implement policy, deliver services, and report back to government. Several national-level organizations are also part of the NHS and support the government and the 14 Health Boards.

Tackling health inequalities has long been, and remains, a top priority for the Scottish Government. One reason for this is that Scotland's population is faring comparatively badly in European league tables, and is well behind that of England. The reasons are complex and certainly include the fact that Scotland is socio-economically worse off than some countries, e.g. England, and there are big gaps between the well off and the poor in Scotland. Much of the poorest health is concentrated in the west of Scotland around the city of Glasgow. The critical point from our perspective is that there is already a top-priority policy in place on inequalities that the issues around migration, race, and ethnicity can be aligned with. These issues can then be seen as contributing towards resolving a large problem, and not just as setting out another problem. In Chapter 6 we considered the need to align work on minority health with the agenda on social determinants of health. Indeed, as happened there, the migration, race, ethnicity, and health issue can be squeezed out of national and local policy unless care is taken to avoid this.

The Scottish Executive's (now Government) 1999 White Paper 'Towards a healthier Scotland' identified the reduction of inequalities as a key priority and suggested that research effort 'must focus on the causes of health inequalities and practical means to tackle them'. There had been recognition for some time of ethnic inequalities in health in Scotland, but a lack of quantitative information. There was no information that allowed a description of the level of ethnic inequalities in health or allowed progress to be monitored. The Race Equality Advisory Forum (2001) report, 'Making it real; a race equality strategy for Scotland' highlighted the importance of better information in getting the health of ethnic minorities into the mainstream of service provision, and as the basis for prompt, effective action.

Ethnic coding and other means of getting information were discussed in Chapters 3 and 5. In Scotland, information on ethnic status is not consistently recorded in primary care service settings, although a small financial incentive of about £100 in total was offered (now withdrawn) to practices that record their patients' ethnicity on first registration. Larger payments in some Health Board areas have also failed to achieve comprehensive Board-level coding. Scottish diabetes and CHD registers do not comprehensively and accurately record ethnic status, but there are plans for them to do better and improvements are occurring. Routine hospital discharge data are collated centrally in Scotland. There has been provision for the recording of ethnic status in NHS hospital discharge data for many years, but this is seriously incomplete. A new strategy for collecting these data is being implemented, with earmarked funding to coordinate the process. Rapid progress is being made but data are not yet good enough to be publishable.

Information collated by the General Register Office for Scotland from death certificates includes country of birth but, until 1 January 2012, not ethnic status. For older people, country of birth has been used as a proxy for ethnic status, but it is becoming less useful as the number of people from minority ethnic groups born in the UK increases.

Nonetheless, as part of a larger project to retrospectively accrue data, Fischbacher et al. (2007) analysed mortality for all causes and for circulatory disorders by country of birth. Surprisingly, and overturning decades of generalizations in Scotland, overall mortality was, with few exceptions, highest in the Scotland-born population and substantially lower in some overseas-born populations, e.g. those from India, Pakistan, China, and Hong Kong. This was an example of the healthy migrant effect that is so easily forgotten. On reflection, if these data had been available it would have been harder to argue that minority populations with lower mortality rates require extra attention. This is a general point that applies in many countries. The argument for action should be made on specific points of need rather than general statements which may be shown to be wrong and hence undermine credibility.

The prospective development of ethnically coded information systems was recognized as a high priority for Scotland. Scotland's health information systems provide excellent opportunities, including record linkage schemes that provide information about the outcomes of care. One project in a collaboration between Edinburgh University, the General Register Office for Scotland, and the Information Services Division (ISD) has linked census-derived ethnic codes to health databases (see Chapter 3). This project is now the sole reliable source of data describing the health status of Scotland by ethnic group—papers on cardiovascular health, cancers, mental health, and maternal and child health have been published, and those on a wide range of other matters are under preparation. Table 8.1 summarizes some of the published results. Every major report in the field of migration, race, ethnicity, and health has emphasized the need for data, including the Resolution of the World Health Assembly and the WHO Consultation thereafter (as did the 1983 WHO Consultation). In Scotland there has been rapid progress in the last 10 years, whereas the recognition of need for the 20 years preceding that led to virtually no progress. Why so? The major spur to such action has come from two directions—the law and national policy, as discussed in Section 8.2.3.3. The point is that pleas for data collection by academies and professionals are more likely to be noted when the legal and policy framework is in place.

8.2.3.3 The Race Relations and Amendment Acts and race equality schemes

The 1976 UK Race Relations Act with the 2000 Amendment intended to remove all racial discrimination, direct or indirect, in the UK. Racial grounds are colour, race, nationality, ethnicity, or national origin. Although not explicitly stated, this covers migration status, i.e. it is not permissible to discriminate against a person on the basis he or she is a migrant. These and other such laws are not, by any means, unique to the UK. Rather, they are designed to be the national response to the international laws we considered in Section 8.2.1. They also respond to EU requirements, e.g. the 1997 Treaty of Amsterdam, Article 13 of which gives powers to combat discrimination. While the 1976 Act and 2000 Amendment are now absorbed and superseded by the Equality Act 2010 they were instrumental in the changes described below. (Indirect and direct discrimination were discussed in Chapter 6.)

The Amendment Act came into effect in April 2002 and was a powerful and very ambitious piece of legislation that mandated actions that were open to public scrutiny (Home Office 2001). According to the Amendment Act all public organizations, including the NHS, had a statutory general duty not only to work to eliminate unlawful racial discrimination but also to promote equal opportunities and good race relations. The size of the minority ethnic populations they serve was not deemed relevant.

Table 8.1 Scottish Health and Ethnicity Linkage Study: illustrative overview of some findings with a note of potential policy relevance

Characteristic/topic of study	Key result	Potential policy relevance
Population included	4.65 million people or 95% of Scottish population	The results apply nationally
Ethnic group categories	14 groups, studied with amalgamation for some results. Rare data for mixed ethnic group population	Most groups are included but some important ones, are missing e.g. Gypsy travellers, and data cannot be analysed by migrant status except country of birth.
Cardiovascular diseases	Major variations in incidence of death/hospitalization. Low in Chinese, high in Pakistani populations. Common in all groups. Difference not explained by socio-economic factors or cardiac procedures	Policy priority for all ethnic groups. Potential for setting a new aspirational standard—the disease rate of the Chinese population. No evidence for inequalities in cardio-vascular procedures suggests NHS is meeting such needs equitably
Mental health	Several minority groups have low overall hospitalization but high rates for serious disease (psychoses) and for compulsory admission	Need to examine minority communities' interaction with primary care services and reduce hesitancy to seek medical advice early
Cancers and breast cancer screening	White Scottish population has highest rates of all cancers, and lung, breast, prostate, and bowel cancer. Breast cancer screening rates low in non-White groups	Policies should aim to reduce cancer in White Scottish population and prevent convergence of cancer rates in other ethnic groups. Breast cancer screening service needs to modify itself to reach out more successfully to ethnic minority groups

Source: Data from Bhopal RS, Fischbacher C, Povey C et al, 2011; Bansal N, Fischbacher C, Brown et al, 2012; Bhopal RS, Bansal N, Fischbacher C et al, 2012; Bansal N, Bhopal RS, Steiner MF et al, 2012; Bhopal R, Bansal N, Steiner MF et al, 2012; Bhopal R, Bansal N, Steiner M, Brewster DH, 2012; Bansal N, Fischbacher C, Bhopal RS et al, 2011 and Bhopal RS, Bansal N, Fischbacher CM et al, 2012.

The Commission for Racial Equality (CRE) was the body responsible for overseeing the implementation of this legislation; in June 2002 it published explicit guidance on the nature of the required output to be reported in a public document, known as a race equality scheme, to show that a health organization was meeting its duty. There was, of course, a requirement for a race equality scheme to be published by the Scottish Executive, which implements the will of the Scottish Parliament. So, the political leaders and political institutions were subject to this legislation and were publicly accountable.

The CRE's anticipated outcomes of meeting this duty included the following:

◆ community satisfaction and equal opportunities;

◆ staff satisfaction and equal opportunities;

◆ confidence and respect are increased;

+ leadership is evident;
+ services and policies are better;
+ evidence of meeting the duty is clear;
+ published annual reports;
+ information about services in various languages;
+ a race equality scheme as a 3-year plan, publicly available, in printed and electronic form;
+ race equality objectives for partnership work, and for work carried out under contract;
+ all staff receive training on the Race Relations Act, and on how to prevent discrimination;
+ monitoring of employees by ethnic group.

The Scottish Parliament approved the legislation and noted in its guidance the dangers of adverse consequences, e.g. 'introduction of ethnic monitoring of staff may assist a Board to identify and eliminate unlawful discrimination and promote equality of opportunity, but if staff does not understand its purpose it might actually inhibit good race relations...etc'. Responsibility for success lay with the chief executives of organizations. Shortly before the Amendment Act was implemented, the Health Department of the Scottish Government published its policy for the NHS, 'Fair for All'. This is described in Section 8.2.3.4.

To help organizations to achieve these challenges the Scottish Executive funded a National Resource Centre for Ethnic Minority Health (NRCEMH; see Section 8.2.3.5). Progress with race equality schemes and the Fair for All plans was both supported and monitored by the NRCEMH. The CRE and NRCEMH recognized that integrating the requirements of the Race Relations Amendment Act and Fair for All policy objectives was essential, and a joint monitoring and reporting structure was created.

The key point, widely recognized, was that race equality in Scotland was not an isolated issue. It could not be swept away without dismantling the entire political edifice of social justice and equality, because it was integral to it. Other strategies for equality in NHS Scotland included:

+ The Sex Discrimination Act (1975),
+ The Disability Discrimination Act (1995),
+ The Human Rights Act (1998),
+ The Scottish Executive's Equality Strategy (2000),
+ The Patient Focus/Involving People Strategy (2001),
+ Spiritual Care policy in Health Department letter (2002),
+ The NHS Reform Bill (2004).

Within this challenging context the Fair for All policy, which provided guidance to the NHS, would be welcomed. Nonetheless, given the multiplicity of competing equality challenges, we can see that, in retrospect, greater integration would have been helpful.

8.2.3.4 Health Department letter (HDL) and stock-take: Fair for All

In the 1970s to 1990s sporadic research and consultations took place, often led by community groups or those leading add-on services to meet the needs of minorities. However, I am not aware of an official policy or strategic response at the national level, though undoubtedly there was awareness at the ministerial level. I wrote to the minister responsible in December 1999 requesting ministerial-level support for a vision, policy, and strategy to complement project-level activity, especially given a speech by a minister (see the next paragraph). The official reply in March 2000 indicted that some work was planned, including a stock-take of progress, in the context of national work on inequalities. While no written policy was available, a verbal commitment had been made. It is truly remarkable how much was achieved so quickly by a combination of law, government policy, and professional and academic partnership. In less than 2 years from this official reply in 2000 the detailed policy was in place as now described.

In 1998, the Scottish Minister for Health, Mr Sam Galbraith, gave a speech challenging the NHS in Scotland to meet the health and health-care needs of minority ethnic groups in Scotland and outlined a new vision. Unfortunately, little action was evident as a result. This was, however, one of the events that triggered change, not least because questions were raised about the promises made in the speech. The Scottish Executive supported the effort to reduce inequalities in health by developing several policies with a strong emphasis on social justice. A Scottish Executive policy document called *Our National Health* (Scottish Executive Health Department 2000), for example, made the commitment to ensure that 'NHS staff are professionally and culturally equipped to meet the distinctive needs of people and family groups from ethnic minority communities'. A culturally competent service was defined as a service which recognizes and meets the diverse needs of people of different cultural backgrounds. With this background of enabling policy, the Scottish Executive commissioned an assessment of ethnic health policies of the 15 NHS boards (now 14) that were responsible for the delivery of health care to the Scottish population. The assessment was commonly known as the Fair for All stock-take. The stock-take found positive attitudes, but insufficient actions, expertise, and resources across Scotland. It made many recommendations, as summarized in the quotations in Box 8.2. The recommendations focused on the need for a strategic approach, clear lines of responsibility, assessing needs and planning appropriate actions.

The Scottish Executive Health Department used the stock-take and extensive consultation thereafter to formulate a comprehensive policy, issued in the form of a draft HDL, subsequently finalized in 2002. Box 8.3 summarizes the key points made in the covering letter that accompanied the detailed guidance. Perhaps the most significant elements for its potential success are the importance of the signatories to the policy, the fact it is endorsed by government, and that it was widely disseminated.

The outputs, or elements as they were called, of the HDL were as follows:

1. Element 1: Energizing the organization. Statement of organizational intent; executive leadership; action plan.
2. Element 2: Demographic profile. Surveying the local population; needs assessment; commitment to research.
3. Element 3: Access and service delivery. Access audit; personal care; food; spiritual care; translation and interpretation; advocacy; gender issues; bereavement.
4. Element 4: Human resources. Equal opportunities; improvement policies; bullying and harassment.
5. Element 5: Community development. Collaborative mechanisms; developing the community.

These ideas are not dissimilar to those expressed earlier in Gunaratnam's (1993) checklist (1993), Chandra's (1996) toolkit, and later by the Chief Executive of the NHS in England (Table 8.2). Indeed, the ideas are similar across the world. The commonality seen among these documents is a strength as it shows the principles are lasting, generalizable, and consistent across time and place.

Each NHS health board was required to prepare a detailed, dated, and costed action plan outlining how it intended to respond. The Fair for All policy placed emphasis on population profiling, needs assessment, and research, e.g. upon completing the initial demographic survey and needs assessment, each organization had to actively consider further research on more detailed levels, regarding incidence of disease, service utilization, and other topics as appropriate. Each

Box 8.2 Some quotations illustrating the findings of the Fair for All stock-take

The need for a strategic approach

'A more strategic approach to ethnic minority health issues is a key area for development within NHS Scotland...This will involve securing commitment at executive and non-executive levels, the integration of these issues into Board or Trust strategies and planning processes (including partnership arrangements), and development of implementation plans.'

Managerial responsibility

'Managers and professionals at Board level need to be active in both setting priorities and targets for ethnic minority health improvements and monitoring performance against objectives and standards.'

Assessment of health needs and translating knowledge into action

'[NHS organizations have] little collective knowledge of the ethnic minority populations for whom they are responsible' and 'Even where work has taken place, there is a need for effective processes to translate the knowledge gained into priorities and actions for delivering services that meet the needs of these communities.'

Recruitment/development and retention of minority ethnic staff

'Recruitment and selection processes may need to be reviewed to ensure ethnic minority applicants are not unintentionally discriminated against. More positively managing race equality and equal opportunities issues should be an element of person specification and be tested as part of the recruitment process'.

Dialogue with minority ethnic communities

'More needs to be done to extend consultation beyond those groups and individuals that have traditionally been consulted, in particular to involve young people and women from ethnic minority groups'.

Text extracts reproduced with permission from *Fair for all: Everyone is entitled to fair access to health – This is the founding principle of the NHS*, available from http://www.sehd.scot.nhs.uk/publications/ffar/ffar1.pdf licensed under the Open Government Licence v1.0.

organization was expected to use the results of its assessment to measure how effectively its service provision was in meeting the needs of minority ethnic communities.

One of the structural requirements, seen as essential to the specific tasks, was the development of a forum in partnership with the community to guide the health organization. The guidance included that:

♦ The forum should be jointly chaired by a named member of the executive team and an appropriate member of the local minority ethnic community.

♦ The forum should be used to consult the local minority ethnic community on service delivery issues.

Box 8.3 Fair for All: working together towards culturally competent services (extracts of the letter sent to all key NHS organizations)

Summary

1. This letter accompanies guidance which sets out the responsibilities placed on NHS organizations by legislation, by policy, and by the results of a recent 'stock-take' exercise undertaken on behalf of the Scottish Executive Health Department.

Background

2. The Race Relations (Amendment) Act 2000 develops the responsibilities previously laid down by the Race Relations Act of 1976 and outlaws race discrimination in relation to functions of public authorities not previously covered by the 1976 Act.
3. The Scottish Executive has made equal opportunities for all a key element of all its work, as demonstrated by its Equality Strategy.
4. In addition, the Health Department has underlined its commitment to this agenda by encouraging Chief Executives to follow the example of Mr Trevor Jones [Chief Executive of NHS Scotland] in signing the Commission for Racial Equality's Leadership Challenge.
5. The Health Department has also funded an Ethnic Minorities Resource Centre to provide support to the service.

Action

6. Chief Executives are asked to circulate the attached guidance to executive colleagues and to appoint a senior member of the Executive Team to coordinate and be the point of contact on matters relating to the responsibilities contained within the attached guidance.
7. It is anticipated that local progress in adopting the final guidelines will be assessed on the Scottish Executive Health Department's behalf by the Ethnic Minority Resource Centre after 31 March 2003, as part of the Performance Assessment Framework.

Assessment will be carried out on the basis of relative progress made by organizations.

Yours sincerely

TREVOR JONES Chief Executive Dr E M ARMSTRONG Chief Medical Officer ANNE JARVIE Chief Nursing Officer MARK BUTLER Director of Human Resources

Reproduced with permission from *Fair Enough? Fair For All Progress Report: Analysis of Race Equality Schemes and Fair For All Action Plans*, Appendix B, available from http://www.scotland.gov.uk/Publications/2003/11/18472/28685 licensed under the Open Government Licence v1.0.

◆ This forum must draw sufficient membership from within the NHS organization it is attached to and local external agencies and groups to ensure that it can accurately be described as multidisciplinary.
◆ This forum should be considered to be an informed voice on local service provision.

The Fair for All HDL, therefore, took the previous informal policies into a new, strategic realm. The strategy was seen as needing 10 years to implement. The leadership in relation to the HDL

Table 8.2 The chief executive of the NHS in England's ten-point plan

Action	Responsibility
1. Health services and outcomes	
Strategic direction: Through the forthcoming planning guidance, embed race equality into future local delivery plans to enable more personalized care, reduced chronic disease and health inequalities, increased capacity, and community regeneration	DH [Department of Health] and all NHS leaders with national and local partners
Align incentives: Build race equality into the new standard and target setting regime, into local performance management systems, and into the new inspection model	DH and all NHS leaders with national and local partners
Development: Provide practical support to help NHS organizations make service improvements for people from ethnic minorities	NHS Top Team and NHS Modernization Agency
Communications: Encourage fresh approaches to communications to engage people from ethnic minorities more effectively in improving outcomes	All NHS organizations and DH
Partnerships: Work with other national and local agencies to promote the health and well-being of people from ethnic minority communities	DH and all NHS leaders in concert with national, regional, and local partners
2. Developing people	
Mentoring: Senior leaders to show their commitment by offering personal mentorship to a member of staff from an ethnic minority	All senior leaders in DH and NHS
Leadership action: Senior leaders to include a personal 'stretch' target on race equality in their 2004/5 objectives	NHS Chairs and CEs [chief executives]; DH Board members
Expand training, development, and career opportunities: Enhance training for all staff in race equality issues. Develop more entry points for people from ethnic minorities to join the NHS and take up training. Improve access for black and minority ethnic staff to the full range of development programmes, support networks, and professional training. Encourage appropriately qualified leaders from ethnic minorities in health and other sectors to consider and apply for executive positions	Local WDCs [Workforce Development Confederation] and HR [Human Resources] networks, NHS Leadership Centre, NHSU [NHS University] and other training providers
Systematic tracking: Build systematic processes for tracking the career progression of staff from ethnic minorities including local and national versions of the NHS Leaders scheme	All senior leaders and NHS Leadership Centre
Celebrate achievements: Acknowledge the contributions of all staff in tackling race inequalities and promote opportunities for staff from ethnic minorities to celebrate their contribution to the NHS	DH and all NHS leaders

This action plan has been developed with the help of staff from ethnic minorities within the NHS, building on the advice from leaders in other sectors, and the Commission for Race Equality. It has the full backing of Ministers, the Department of Health's Management Board and the NHS 'Top Team'.

was taken on by the Patient Focus and Public Involvement programme in the Scottish Health Department. A patient-focused service was defined as a service that ensures that the service exists for the patient, and individuals are treated according to their needs and wishes. This Patient Focus programme also funded the NRCEMH.

8.2.3.5 The NRCEMH (Scotland)

The NRCEMH was set up in 2002 to help NHS Scotland deliver a quality service that addresses the needs of minority ethnic communities. The NRCEMH was, intentionally, a small organization. It had a catalytic role, aiming for change through mainstream organizations. It did not deliver any services to patients or the public, but supported those who did. In 2002 its priorities were agreed with the Scottish Executive as: (1) refinement of policy and assistance with its implementation and monitoring; (2) assessing the need for and galvanizing the development of training programmes; and (3) supporting the development of information systems that supply data about and for ethnic minority groups. The demand for these and numerous other challenges was considerable, and the NRCEMH broadened its scope (see Ethnicity and health websites: A selection). It worked by extensive networking, thereby achieving more than its own size would permit. The account of functions in Box 8.4 is taken from the NRCEMH website and is presented with minor editing. There was verbal agreement that work of the NRCEMH would take 10 years, but funding was for 3 years in the first instance. It was extended for another 3 years to 2008. From 2002, following the path of the work on ethnicity and health, Scotland had initiated a range of initiatives on various inequalities strands, mostly under the Fair for All banner. The phrase clearly struck a chord, subsequently being used all over the UK. There were similarities of approach and NHS response across these strands. In addition, there were financial pressures at all levels of the service. It was not possible to fund an organization like the NRCEMH for each equality strand, and then to fund officers for each strand in each health board. The process would have been potentially expensive, unwieldy, and inefficient, especially in duplicating work.

After controversial and difficult discussions the decision was taken to integrate NRCEMH within a new Planning and Equalities Directorate along with five other equality strands. This directorate is in a national NHS health board, i.e. NHS Health Scotland. Prior to this the information-related components of NRCEMH's role were devolved to ISD, part of another national health board (NHS National Services). The education component went to NHS Education Scotland.

This account is important because it is illustrative, perhaps typical, of this area of endeavour. Perhaps the most important of the criticisms of our field are the stop–go nature of initiatives. NRCEMH's work was planned for 10 years but major change took place at 6 years. It is too early to say whether the change was good or bad but it was fortuitous because the work programme, though dispersed, was secured in mainstream large national health boards when the financial storm broke in late 2008. It is unlikely that a small, standalone centre would have survived the ensuing cutbacks. Experience here and elsewhere shows it is important to secure minority health within a larger, more secure base to survive financial and policy storms. The devolution of work has involved large numbers of people, albeit with less concentration of resources.

The 6 years of work of the NRCEMH has been fully described in the final report, and the materials and documents remain available (see Ethnicity and health websites: A selection). The success of a national centre such as NRCEMH depends on the regional and local service response—as discussed in the Section 8.2.3.6.

Box 8.4 The main functions of the National Resource Centre For Ethnic Minority Health (NRCEMH)

The main functions of the NRCEMH are:

- To send explicit and consistent messages about why race equality matters to NHS Scotland.
- To provide specialist guidance, support, and advice to the NHS organizations at local, regional, and national levels.
- To contribute to the development of race equality champions in NHS Boards.
- To develop tools that can assist NHS Boards in their work in race equality and cultural competence.
- To identify and share good practice and encourage learning for staff that will achieve change for patients and carers alike.
- To create a framework of indicators of progress for performance management.
- To contribute to the analysis and interpretation of information about ethnicity of patients in the NHS and about their health needs and health differences (in partnership with ISD Scotland).
- To audit progress by NHS Boards in the development and implementation of Fair for All and Race Equality Scheme action plans.
- To address multiple identity issues by working on specific common areas of interest with other diversity strand teams, for example for disability, lesbian, gay, bisexual, and transgender (LGBT) issues, age, gender, and religion.
- To ensure that NHS Boards respond to population changes and increasing diversity within and between communities—taking account of the inward migration policy of the Scottish Executive.

Source: Data from http://www.healthscotland.com/equalities/index.aspx and National Resource Centre for Ethnic Minority Health, *Final Report–Achievements and Challenges in Ethnicity and Health in NHS Scotland*, pp. 1–38, NHS Scotland, Glasgow, Copyright © NHS Health Scotland, 2009, available from http://www.healthscotland.com/uploads/documents/11260-NRCEMH_FinalReport.pdf

8.2.3.6 Meeting the health needs of minority groups in a locality: Lothian NHS Board

The work of a national centre, indeed the implementation of policy, cannot and should not be a simple top-down process. If it were so it would fail for lack of resources, lack of support, and lack of sensitivity to local needs and local innovations and advances. Rather, it should be based on a relationship of mutual learning and development where local work is supported by national policy and perspectives, and vice versa. The NHS in Scotland funds 14 health boards that are responsible for all health services to their geographically defined populations. NHS Lothian Board is responsible for health care for about 675 000 people in and around the city of Edinburgh in the east of Scotland. In the NHS Lothian area, as in the remainder of the UK, numerous attempts have been made to improve health care for migrants and minority racial and ethnic groups over several decades.

Community organizations concerned with the health and welfare of minority groups in Lothian have worked with service providers, including the NHS and local government councils, to raise awareness of the issues, and to improve services and access, e.g. in interpretation and translation services. Consultations have been done on several occasions, and reports have been produced identifying areas where action is needed. These reports cover a wide variety of issues including the needs of particular groups such as children, carers for the sick and disabled, older people, men and women; appropriate acute health services; particular diseases (such as CHD, diabetes, mental ill-health); and many other issues like housing and domestic abuse.

Initiatives funded and established within the NHS in Lothian in the 1990s designed to improve services included a Minority Ethnic Mental Health Project, with a worker based in the Royal Edinburgh Hospital, and the Minority Ethnic Health Inclusion Project (MEHIP) which was an advocacy service. Other projects included action to improve services for refugees and asylum seekers and Gypsy travellers. In the north-east locality of NHS Lothian an innovative project to prevent heart disease called Khush Dil was set up with short-term funding (Mathews et al. 2007). All these activities were achieved largely in the absence of a policy or strategic framework, and by widespread testimony were very difficult to set up and sustain.

Collective experience of these projects testifies to the need for enormous energy, commitment, and effort to set up limited initiatives. These initiatives have struggled around one or more of the issues of resource constraints, multiple demands exceeding available resources, short-term funding, insufficient managerial or peer support, insufficient cross-coordination, and difficulties in moving from project to mainstream service status even when success was demonstrable. The outstanding, impressive feature of these services is the gratitude and support of the minority groups served and the dedication of the staff. I think that this situation is commonplace, i.e. hard and often excellent work is done by community workers and health professionals but often with little managerial support because managers are busy with explicit policy goals.

In the mid-1990s a strategic document on ethnicity and health was prepared by a senior public health practitioner in the NHS Lothian Health Board's Public Health Department. For reasons that are unclear, this document was not published or progressed, even though many of its recommendations were later to be echoed in the board's strategy developed independently only a few years later. We can only assume that the issue was not perceived to be a sufficiently high priority at that time, but national policy very shortly changed that.

In the late 1990s and early 2000s the NHS Lothian Board noted that the need to tackle ethnic health inequalities was, or was going to be, recognized in the Scottish Executive's public health policy, Towards a Healthier Scotland (Scottish Executive 1999), the UK's Acheson Report on Inequalities in Health (Acheson 1998), the Scottish Executive's Equality Strategy, a Management Executive letter in 1999 asking Scottish health boards to improve health services for minority ethnic communities, in the stock-take of action in Scottish health boards, in the Race Relations (Amendment) Act 2000, and in the HDL of 2002 (Fair for All). The new chief executive of NHS Lothian, later chief executive of the whole of the NHS in Scotland and signatory to the HDL 2002, had experience of the challenges of serving multi-ethnic populations in England and a proactive approach to this agenda. He convened and chaired an informal interdepartmental group to galvanize action across the board. I was appointed in 1999 to Lothian Health Board as an honorary consultant. For this informal group I prepared a brief ten-point plan (see Chapter 6) to guide action. It was clear that there was national support for local actions.

The next stage was to move from specific local projects and initiatives to integrating the needs of minority ethnic groups across the services (mainstreaming). The definition of mainstreaming by the Scottish Executive Equality Unit was the guiding one, i.e. making sure that concern for equality is built in from the start in the development of policy, the design of services, and the monitoring and evaluation frameworks.

Lothian NHS Board, and specifically its chief executive, was a signatory to a pan-Lothian declaration to root out racism. This document signified a public commitment to work to promote equal access to all citizens, regardless of skin colour, race, culture, or religion, and to make this part of Scotland a safer place for people from minority communities.

Within such a supportive context at national and board level the task of preparing an ethnicity and health strategy for Lothian NHS health-care delivery services was made much easier. Lothian Health developed a strategy that slightly preceded the 2002 HDL (developed by a committee chaired by me) on the health needs of minority ethnic groups (Lothian NHS Minority Health Group 2003), which was summarized and embedded in the board's health improvement plan for 2000–5. The challenge of the strategy was to get all NHS Lothian's health policies, particularly those on inequalities, to take into account the ethnic dimension. We foresaw that the implementation of this recommendation alone would be a huge step forward, particularly for mainstreaming. We also emphasized that the health of people from minority groups in Lothian is affected by their relative levels of disadvantage due to socio-economic factors including poverty, poor housing, and unemployment, and by their experience of racism reducing their employment prospects and career success.

Such broad issues could only be addressed in partnership with minority ethnic communities and other service providers, including local government councils. Monitoring and evaluation needed to be set up, including ethnic monitoring of primary care and hospital services.

The process of agreeing and producing the strategy was a collaborative exercise involving staff from health services, representatives of local communities, local government, and the voluntary sector. The draft strategy was focused around four principles and a 10-point plan shown in Box 8.5. The draft was widely disseminated for consultation with minority ethnic individuals, institutions, and community organizations. The draft plan was widely endorsed with only minor changes suggested.

The plan, in turn, linked to hospital- and primary care-based equivalent documents that provided more detail. For example, extracts from the primary care document include these on refugees and Gypsy travellers:

◆ Services should improve links between Lothian NHS Trusts and other agencies including the Scottish Refugee Council.

◆ Refugee issues should be included in training for staff.

◆ Scottish gypsy travellers who have a nomadic lifestyle should have patient-held health records.

After 6 years of strategic activity lead by inequalities managers and backed by NHS Lothian Board, NHS Lothian had an integrated race equality scheme (required by law) and Fair for All action plan (required by NHS policy), overseen by the Lothian Ethnic Health Forum. Projects were contributing to policy. It would be dishonest to pretend that everything that had been agreed was achieved, but coordinated progress was made, including the appointment of a full-time member of the management team dedicated to coordinating and managing the performance of the ethnicity and health agenda. The equalities managers gave regular reports to NHS Lothian's Ethnic Health Forum and reported to the NHS Lothian Board itself. Most of the 10 action areas were reportedly fully or largely tackled satisfactorily. However, in the absence of quantitative data it is not possible to objectively record progress, and ethnic monitoring of staff and patients was not well achieved. That is a vital ingredient and is discussed separately in Section 8.2.3.7. Other obvious problems were non-attendance by

Box 8.5 Core principles of the Strategic Action Plan on Minority Ethnic Health

The work was based on four principles.

1. Mainstreaming of minority ethnic health so that it becomes an automatic part of all NHS activities.

2. Tackling racism. The NHS must be an advocate against racism, and work to ensure that racism does not occur in any part of its activities.

3. Providing accessible, equitable, high-quality, and appropriate services to all members of minority ethnic groups.

4. Partnership working with organizations, community groups, and individuals so that the experience and knowledge of people from minority ethnic groups contributes to developing services.

The ten action areas

Ten action areas and aims were listed in the draft plan for the NHS in Lothian:

1. Mainstreaming minority ethnic health needs into the planning and delivery of all health services.

2. Advocacy and action against racism; to take action against racism in any form, and to reduce racist attacks, harassment, and discrimination.

3. Appropriate, culturally sensitive, high-quality, and accessible healthcare, available to all people from every ethnic group.

4. Involving people and communities so that people from minority ethnic groups are involved in consultation over health services.

5. Interpretation and translation services; to ensure that interpreting and translating are available.

6. Health and health-care information for minority ethnic groups; to ensure that appropriate information is available.

7. Provision of advocacy and facilitation services; so that health advocates are available, and to respond to the specific needs of particular groups, such as refugees and asylum seekers, and Gypsy travellers.

8. Training for NHS staff; to raise awareness of racism, ethnicity, and health, and to enable staff to provide appropriate and accessible services.

9. Employment; to ensure non-discriminatory employment practice and to work towards a workforce which reflects the diversity of local communities.

10. Patient profiling; monitoring of ethnicity; to obtain and use information about the ethnicity and health of people from minority ethnic groups.

Reproduced from Bhopal R, and Donnelly P (eds), Lothian NHS minority health group. *Strategic Action plan on minority ethnic health: being fair for all in the NHS in Lothian*, pp. 1–64, 2003, with permission from the editors.

staff at pre-arranged training sessions, leading to a switch to on-site training at the workplace which was increasingly integrated with other training requirements. Staff turnover, pressures on budgets, the economic crisis from 2008 onwards, and the increasing pressures created by the need to accommodate the other equality strands have meant that the 10-year vision in NHS Lothian is still a work in progress. The Equality Act 2010 is changing the direction, while the 2002 Fair for All strategy and NHS Lothian action plans are, effectively, out of date. The race and ethnicity officer resigned, the ethnicity and mental health officer moved positions and was not replaced, and the Lothian Ethnic Health Forum ceased to meet in 2012. Overall, with the exception of ethnic monitoring, this is a period of relative strategic inactivity and reassessment. However, service development has continued, particularly to address the needs of the large, young Polish community that immigrated into the area, with much augmentation of translation and interpretation services, staff and patient education, and a health and lifestyle survey. While this new area of activity undoubtedly benefited from the strategic and policy drivers, it was not done under the umbrella of the Lothian Ethnic Health Strategy. The potential reasons for this are worth speculating on. Firstly, the timing was out with most of the Polish migration after the plan was completed and largely implemented. Second, the team who developed an interest in the health and health care of Polish people was largely uninvolved in the Ethnic Health Forum. Thirdly, there is a tendency to equate 'ethnic' and 'race' with non-White, and the Polish people are White Europeans. There is a tendency to wall-off areas of work, and so it is also possible that Polish health was seen as a migrant health rather than an ethnic health issue.

There are general lessons from this relatively full account of action in this locality. Local activity will take place, but proponents will find it hard to articulate their case and get the ear of budget holders and managers. Once policy and strategy are in place the case for service development is easier to make, and the support of managers and colleagues is easier to gain. Scarcity of funding and competing priorities will remain an obstacle, so progress will still be slow. External factors, including new policies and laws, will bring about new changes. Interestingly, in the UK some of the strongest pressures have come from the desire to extend the race equality principles to many other domains of potential inequality, and the resulting need to integrate the work. Race equality no longer stands alone. Policy is not fixed forever, even though it is neither annulled nor updated. For example, the Scottish HDL Fair for All 2002 still stands, though it is out of date. The local application of policy is greatly dependent on local champions, and these change. Champions for one aspect of minority health (Polish health in NHS Lothian) may be independent of champions for other aspects. This is a fast-changing scene, but the pace of change is not the same at national, local managerial, and local practitioner level. Finally, progress is heavily dependent on scarce resources. Staff working on these issues are thin on the ground and not easy to recruit or train. In times of financial restraint maintaining staffing is a massive challenge. One of the toughest and most important actions has been race or ethnic monitoring, a challenge that has needed national and local action simultaneously.

8.2.3.7 Monitoring migration status, race, or ethnicity—experience in one locality

Try Exercise 8.5 before reading on.

Exercise 8.5 Coding by migration status, race, or ethnicity

◆ What is migration status, race, or ethnic coding? Why is it centrally important to implementation of policy?

◆ Why is it so difficult to achieve?

Coding by migration status, race, or ethnicity was discussed in detail in Chapter 3. In essence, it is the incorporation into routine records simple information on the service users' migration status, race, or ethnic group. It is mostly known as racial or ethnic monitoring or coding.

Following a very long period of debate, and numerous failed attempts to have ethnic monitoring—subsuming migration status and race—implemented comprehensively (see Chapters 3 and 5), we now have a virtual consensus in the UK at policy and strategic levels that it is essential (this is also the view in the United States and several other countries). In 1995 the NHS in England, through its NHS Executive, published comprehensive guidance in a volume called *Collection of Ethnic Group Data for Admitted Patients* (Shaw 1994). This itself arose from an Executive letter issued in 1994 declaring that ethnic group is to be recorded for all hospital inpatients. The policy failed because the data collected thereafter were incomplete.

The difference, now, is that policy is backed by legislation (even though the law, at least in the UK, does not explicitly require it) and at the highest levels in management. *Ethnic Monitoring—A Guide for Public Authorities in Scotland* (Commission for Racial Equality 2002) was published to help public authorities to comply with the requirements of the Race Relations (Amendment) Act 2000 (Home Office 2001). Ethnic monitoring was seen as the process by which an authority maintains an informed view of the extent to which its race equality policy is working.

The strongest impetus towards ethnic monitoring, according to the 2005 guidance from the Department of Health, is the business case, i.e. meeting needs cost-effectively. Other influences, e.g. the Race Relations (Amendment) Act 2000, are acknowledged.

The fundamental principle for ethnic coding in the UK is self-classification from the ethnic group codes on offer. Consent and confidentiality are to be respected with no-one being forced into giving their ethnic group against their will. Collection of such data is expected to be routine. Service providers are also expected to collect data on service users' religion, language, and diet, where appropriate. There are arguments to have coding relevant to a wider range equality (diversity) strands and on what are called additional needs. The arguments are solid. The problem is of implementation. The experience of attempting to collect one data item—ethnicity—is salutary as services move towards collecting a multiplicity of patient profile details.

Staff, patients, and the public should, obviously, receive training, relevant to their needs, on the collection and use of ethnic group and related data. In Scotland, with earmarked funding, senior staff have been appointed to lead the initiative, and a national-level committee was formed to coordinate action within the broader diversity agenda, which started with demonstration projects working with primary and secondary care staff. It rapidly became clear that even with law, policy, guidance, and steering groups the challenge remained formidable The progress in Scotland can be described as slow, geographically variable, reliant on local enthusiasm and technical capacity, and subject in some places to indifference and even hostility. These problems apply both to ethnic coding by centrally managed hospital services and to the decentralized, independent primary care sector. Experience across the world has shown that ethnic coding is difficult to achieve, and this was anticipated in several of the guidelines, e.g. see Table 8.3 which summarizes some of the anticipated issues. The points in Table 8.3 are insightful. The critical questions, however, are how to rapidly achieve high levels of ethnic coding and how best to use the data once this is achieved.

In late 2008 the particularly low level of ethnic coding of hospital records (about 7%) for NHS Lothian Board was criticized by both central NHS management and the CRE. An Ethnic Coding Task Force was convened in April 2009 to help resolve the problem (I was the chairperson). A seemingly impossible target of 90% valid coding in hospitals and general practice was agreed by the task force—to be achieved in 3 years. This target was selected by me, as chairperson of

Table 8.3 Communications guidelines for the introduction of ethnic monitoring in health boards in Scotland

Audience group	Objection/barrier
White majority	No need for them to reply as their ethnic identity is obvious
	The end result will be preferential treatment for black and minority ethnic groups
	Nothing in it for me
Black and minority ethnic groups	Fear of being identified and suffering harassment or discrimination as a result
	Scepticism about the ability of NHS organizations to deliver real change of benefit to them
	If status is known, the patients may not be eligible for NHS treatment (would only apply when following the Overseas Regulations)
NHS managers	Additional burden on managers to no clear result
	No connection to assessment of their performance
	Technical difficulties in launching monitoring and managing data
NHS front-line staff	Another burden that will interfere with clinical duties
	Will involve confrontation if patients refuse to complete the forms
	Procedural difficulties with the introduction of the monitoring
Media	More bureaucracy in health service
	More political correctness
	NHS services being geared to needs of minorities rather than majority
All audiences	Data protection issues
	Raising expectations of service change well ahead of this happening in practice

Reproduced from *Communications Guidelines for the Introduction of Ethnic Monitoring in Health Boards in Scotland*, p. 4, produced by NHS Health Scotland in collaboration with Information Services Division of NHS National Services Scotland, Copyright © NHS Health Scotland, 2005 with permission from NHS Health Scotland. Available from http://www.equalitiesinhealth.org/public_html/publications/COMMUNICATIONSGUIDELINES.pdf

the task force, as being sufficiently high to command external attention and allow valid analyses of data. The target was said to be impossible for accident and emergency services, so these were exempted.

The task force worked by visiting hospital and general practice premises and holding discussions with key staff; by offering information, materials, and education on the topic; by working alongside information system staff to resolve technical issues including codes for ethnic group categories; and holding dialogue with senior managers, clinicians, and medical records staff. The end result was 90% coding in hospital systems, including near 100% in the exempted accident and emergency services. This target was not achieved in general practice. Indeed, in the latter context it was not possible even to have an accurate assessment of the level of coding at the beginning and end of the 3 years. The lesson from the work was that ethnic coding is a tough challenge that needs policy and legal backing, active management, and focused resources (albeit modest). Above all it needs management agreement, technical support, and public education. The critical turning point was an agreement by senior managers at NHS Lothian that ethnic group should be a mandatory field in the hospital information system. Once this decision was taken the target was rapidly achieved. By contrast, in general practice no such managerial control was available.

The next and existing challenge is to show that these data are useful. NHS Lothian Board dissolved the Ethnic Coding Task Force (as planned) but started an even more ambitious data collection project named the 'Additional Needs and Diversity Information Task Force'. This is looking at how a wide range of patient profile data relating to the full span of equality issues will be collected routinely. The experience of the Ethnic Coding Task Force will be applied on a comparatively grand scale. As with ethnic coding, this work is also in response to national Scottish Government initiatives on equality, in this case a ministerial report (*Equally Well*; Scottish Government 2008). A review of equality health data needs was published in 2012 which outlined what had been achieved and what was to be done in relation to age, disability, ethnicity, gender, religion and belief, sexual orientation, and transgender identity. It colour-coded progress in relation to initiation, collection, and use of data with green, amber, and red indicating, respectively, good progress, some progress, and poor progress. For Scotland as a whole the judgement for ethnicity was amber for initiation and collection and red for use. With the exception of age and gender, the colour code for the other equality strands was red. It is likely that in other countries there will be the same kind of pressures to integrate the migration, race, and ethnicity agenda into the broader equality challenge. There are obviously benefits—the topic gets attention at the highest policy level. The problem, as here, is one of dilution. At the local level, e.g. NHS Lothian Board, instead of focusing on making use of the collected ethnicity data this major task has become one of many of the new task force which is primarily considering the challenge of collecting new data. This said, the ministerial interest in data has also led to a new analysis of Scottish Health Survey data by a range of equality variables including ethnicity. While the substantive results are of modest interest because of small sample sizes, the mere production of the analysis has brought to the fore the importance of such data.

Readers from most countries, with the partial exemption of the United States (where, at least nationally, data by race and ethnicity are relatively plentiful) will recognize commonalities with their own circumstances. This is a particularly good example of how policy alone is not enough—its enactment depends on strategy, plans, resources, monitoring, and above all tight management.

In this second edition I have sought to show how the topics of migration, race, and ethnicity are best integrated in the health arena. Just as we considered here, however, integration can have the unwanted effect of dilution. In Scotland, ethnicity is the dominant concept and migration status and race are subsumed within it. There is no separate consideration in ethnic coding schemes for different kinds of migrants, whether asylum seekers, refugees, etc. There is merit in considering the needs of different kinds of migrant groups, within the broader concept of ethnicity, but more thoughtfully and explicitly so than in Scotland hitherto.

8.2.3.8 Delivery and evaluation of policy—*Checking for Change*

Try Exercise 8.6 before reading on.

Exercise 8.6 Evaluation of policy in the field of migration, race, and ethnicity

- Why is evaluation of policy important?
- How would you evaluate policies of the kind we have discussed?
- What difficulties can you foresee?

Monitoring is a means of describing what is happening and is a vital ingredient for planning, delivery, and evaluation of services. (As well as assessing health status.) Evaluation is obviously important for finding out whether something works. The prospect of evaluation helps policy implementation, and for ensuring it happens to the expected standard. Without evaluation, or the expectation of evaluation, tough jobs would not be done, or would be done poorly. We have just examined this in relation to ethnic coding, which failed for so many years due to a lack of evaluation. It is in recognition of this basic aspect of human nature—so well known by teachers and their students in relation to examinations—that the migration, race, ethnicity, and health field has expended considerable energy on evaluation tools.

Legislation, policy, and strategy in the ethnicity and health arena is not generally amenable to evaluation using the gold standard of the randomized controlled trial. This is not because of any scientific principle but the need for pragmatism. Mostly, the intervention would need to be randomized at the level of country or large law- or policy-making region. Even for global programmes such as polio eradication or tobacco control such trials have not been done. The possibility, however, should not be discarded. It is for a future era when evaluation of policy by trials becomes acceptable, just as it now is for medical treatments and procedures (after decades of resistance).

Basic evaluation designs, such as before-and-after studies, which are about the best that we can currently strive for, are very difficult to interpret, because change is slow and the effect of one policy cannot be isolated from that of others and from the relatively rapid demographic and other changes. Nonetheless, before-and-after designs should be routine. Currently they are not. Making them feasible requires good-quality monitoring data so that such evaluations do not require new, expensive research-based information systems to be set up.

Policies on minority health are highly complex interventions in complex political and social environments. These policy interventions are not without risks or side-effects, and they come with financial and other costs, though these are seldom made explicit. Their implementation invariably demands an act of courage and faith that they are beneficial. Is it not irresponsible to implement such important policies without assessing them? Mostly, however, evaluations are based on whether the actions have been taken (and sometimes not even at this level) rather than on the effects of the actions, especially on health status and health-care outcomes. This lack of evaluation of effectiveness, and even cost-effectiveness, is a weakness—and possibly one that cannot be easily remedied—though this requires fuller debate. The approach is illustrated in the following quotation from the English Department of Health's ten-point plan lead by the then Chief Executive Sir Nigel Crisp and published in 2004 (table 8.2):

> As well as my oversight, Ministers will take a keen interest in progress. Staff in black and minority ethnic networks from the service will be encouraged to express views and keep this plan under review. And, to make sure we benchmark ourselves against the best, I have invited an independent expert panel to review our progress and report back to the September Chief Executive's conference this year.
>
> Reproduced from the Department of Health, *Race Equality Action Plan, Ten Point Plan of the Chief Executive, Nigel Crisp*, Copyright © 2004. Reproduced under the Open Government Licence v1.0.

This kind of assessment presumes that checking the structures and processes, mainly through testimony and observation, is sufficient: while not enough it is a good start.

Tools for both deciding on a set of actions and assessment of progress have been developed, and an old but excellent example is *Facing up to Difference* (Chandra 1996), designed to help in the creation of culturally competent health services for black and minority ethnic communities and which still remains remarkably modern and relevant. There are benefits to examining older materials such as Chandra's toolkit, e.g. we are encouraged not to re-invent what has already been invented, and are reassured that our current thinking chimes with that of others. We might even learn why past work was not widely implemented. In addition to comprehensive guidance on what needs to be done, it gives a set of core standards and targets. This kind of work sets the stage for quantitative and qualitative evaluation. Remarkably, the organization that published Chandra's work, the King's Fund, had published a *Checklist: Health and Race* (Gunaratnam 1993) with the subtitle 'A starting point for managers on improving services for black populations'. It starts with a set of core race equality standards on patients' rights and needs, service provision, and employment. The main part of this document is a comprehensive set of questions. Other than the language on outdated service organizational structures the questions are to the point and comprehensive. Gunaratnam's *Checklist* points out that it concerns what needs to be in place to achieve better health outcomes and is not designed to measure the health outcomes themselves. A more recent checklist is given in Box 8.6.

The Scottish NRCEMH published the toolkit *Checking for Change: a building blocks approach to race quality in health* in 2005 (http://www.healthscotland.com/resources/publications/search-result.aspx). It is structured around the five key Fair for All elements, i.e. energizing the organization (Chandra used this identical phrase in 1996), demographics, access and service delivery, human resources, and community development. The main novelty and additional strength of this toolkit, other than the fact it is tailored to Scottish policy and legislation, is that it assesses the stage (or level) that the organization has currently achieved and what its next challenges are.

Box 8.6 A checklist for evaluation

Best practice checklist for planning services for Black and minority ethnic groups (BMEGs)

1. Services for BMEGs should be part of 'mainstream' health-care provision.

2. The amended Race Relations Act should be considered in all policies.

3. Facilitate access to appropriate services by: providing appropriate bilingual services for effective communication, education and training for health professionals and other staff, appropriate and acceptable service provision of religious and dietary choice within meals offered in hospitals.

4. Promote ethnic workforce issues, including addressing racial discrimination and harassment within the workplace, and promoting race equality and valuing diversity in the workforce.

5. Promote community engagement and participation.

6. Systematize structures and processes for capture and use of appropriate data.

7. Ask questions such as:

   ◆ with what population or patients (how many and how severely ill) are we concerned?

   ◆ what services on average are currently provided?

   ◆ what is the evidence of the effectiveness and cost-effectiveness of these services?

   ◆ what is the optimum configuration of services?

Source: Data from Gill et al, Health Care Needs Assessment: Black and Minority Ethnic Groups, in Abingdon (ed.) *Health Care Needs Assessment: The epidemiologically based needs assessment*, Third Series, pp. 227–389, Radcliffe Medical Press Ltd, Oxford, UK, Copyright © 2007.

There are four levels for each key area. It also clarifies the source of the evidence. For example, under energizing the organization, Level 1 (the lowest) is indicated by the organization having a race equality scheme that is more than 3 years old (or none at all) while Level 4 (the highest) is feedback from ethnic minority communities and other partner agencies that the organization's activities are successful.

Checking for Change was widely tested and found to be useful. However, in the current integration of equality strands a new multi-equality-strand tool is required, though the basic ideas are clearly transferable. (This kind of approach is echoed in the recently issued guidance by the Robert Wood Johnson Foundation in the United States; see Section 8.3.)

One indirect way of evaluating outcome is to get feedback from service users, e.g. in satisfaction surveys. This approach is periodically in fashion. Gauging satisfaction is not easy. Respondents may be reluctant to admit dissatisfaction (and they may not have the facts on which to base their view) and an overall rating of 'satisfactory' may hide dissatisfaction with specific aspects of services. There may also be cross-cultural differences both in what gives satisfaction and how it is reported back. Satisfaction studies in the field of migration, ethnicity, and health are unusual, though in the UK, incorporation of an ethnic group question in large national surveys is producing data. The reliability can be questionable, not least because of variable response rates. Studies by Madhok and colleagues (Madhok et al. 1992, 1998) in a Pakistani population in the north-east of England were, however, detailed and focused. They used home interview, by a person of the same sex and ethnic group as the respondent, and in the language of the respondents' choice, to safeguard partially against such problems. Questioning on a range of services together with probing on a few, lessened the danger of finding overall satisfaction and yet missing specific criticisms. In these studies satisfaction was generally high. This kind of result is surprising. One interpretation of such findings was that the expectations of the minority communities were low. This kind of interpretation may hold some truth but questions the quality of the perceptions of the respondents, and the good work of health services in meeting most needs. Given the relatively small number of data it would be wrong to generalize except to say that the common perception that services do not meet minorities' needs is not always upheld by this kind of work, and this is also shown in service utilization data.

Another route to evaluation is to gauge utilization and quality of services. Again, the research base in most countries with the exception of the United States is small. Recent systematic reviews of the European situation have confirmed the picture emerging from individual studies, i.e. migrants and racial and ethnic minorities are mostly users of services. Most studies show that compared with the majority or entire population they use more accident and emergency and primary care services, about the same level of hospital services, and less of 'fee-for-service' facilities such as dentistry. These generalizations will not hold for every group, and certainly not for undocumented migrants, but they are reasonably consistent. Fears that minorities do not engage with services have been shown to be unfounded. Rather, migrants and their descendants may be particularly supportive of health services—perhaps because they have experience of more basic or costlier services in their countries of origin.

Policies and strategies may have to engage with specific issues and not just matters of access. Quality of care is one such specific issue and it is not an easy one to study. The literature mostly supports the view that minority groups have a lower quality of care than the majority population. This has been shown to be reversible, at least in relation to structured cardiovascular and diabetes care, as shown in a series of papers from the UK examining data in general practice.

Examining trends over time gauges change, and is an indirect indicator of whether policies are working and the way they may need adjustment. Again, routine monitoring data are required to make this feasible. The production, uptake, and effects of health education and health promotion materials and services can be assessed. The acceptability of these can also be examined, as well as levels of health knowledge and changes in attitudes, beliefs, and behaviours. These kind of evaluations (and consultations) lead to service adjustments that can benefit minorities and the majority alike. For example, in many countries medicine is practised in an asexual way, i.e. it is not supposed to be important whether the doctor is a man or a woman. In other countries, modesty is greatly prized. People from minority groups often express a preference to see a doctor of the same gender as themselves. Such preferences are greater when physical, and especially gynaecological, examination may be involved. These kinds of specific preferences can lead to adaptation of services. The preference for health professionals of the same sex is also expressed in majority White ethnic groups, though less strongly and usually only for intimate examinations and care procedures (e.g. cervical smears). When a choice is made available the entire population may advantage from the new opportunity. This is one of many potential examples of how attending to the needs of minorities can potentially benefit the entire population—others include more choice in hospital food, careful consultation with the community, and more use of symbols in signage in buildings rather than text. This insight is not novel or particularly profound but it is often overlooked.

An issue that is prominent in relation to minority health is the utilization of alternative (or complementary) systems of healing or health care. Sometimes, their use is interpreted as a criticism of the main health-care system. Certainly, migrants are likely to be familiar with health-care practices in their country of origin, and may continue to use such practices either in visits to their country of origin or while in their new country of residence. The use of complementary or alternative therapies (e.g. including use of hakims and Ayurvedic remedies) in minority ethnic communities tends to be additional to rather than an alternative to the mainstream service—as with the population generally. Alternative or complementary medicine is flourishing within the general population. These are not good indicators of the extent to which mainstream services are, or are not, meeting needs.

These forms of evaluation are focused on the effects of health policies, but many other kinds of policies have an impact on the welfare of minority groups, e.g. transport, education, employment, housing, and enterprise. Unless these also meet the needs of minority populations we will not narrow the socio-economic status gap. A simple idea has been implemented in Scotland and England—race equality impact assessment, whereby all policies are to be screened to ensure equality.

The impact assessment process is a set of questions that assesses whether the policy/strategy/programme is having or might have differential or even adverse effects on different migrant, racial, or ethnic groups. The aim is to ensure and demonstrate that we are promoting equality of opportunity and good race relations. Impact assessment of this kind is now an integral part of the policy-making/development process with guidance provided by the Scottish Executive's Equality Unit.

The challenge that we have barely confronted is to evaluate the outcomes of change in relation to health status, costs, cost-effectiveness, and cost–benefit ratios. It is probably true to say, certainly in Europe but probably across the world, that the fields of migration, race, and ethnicity policy, and health outcomes research have overlapped too little. Researchers have focused on health status to a great extent but not in relation to testing the effectiveness of policy actions. This would require much better data systems and, in particular, high-quality monitoring and research on migration status, race, and ethnicity. Policies would also need to be reframed in terms of expected health status and health-care outcomes; this is a difficult task, not least because setting the standard is difficult both conceptually and technically. This theme will be picked up in

Chapter 9. A guiding policy on research and an ethical code to ensure its benefits are, however, discussed in Section 8.2.3.9 as a prelude to examining policy in other countries and then research in Chapter 9.

8.2.3.9 Research policy and an ethical code for researching migration status, race, ethnicity and health

Try Exercise 8.7 before reading on.

Exercise 8.7 Research

♦ Why is research important to policy, and vice versa?

♦ Do you see any evidence of personal or institutional racism in research?

♦ What principles would you emphasize for ethical research with migrant or minority racial or ethnic groups?

Most modern health policy documents recognize the need for data, whether from the census, routine vital statistics, or research. Although policy-making is at core a political process, there is increasing emphasis on using evidence to inform policy (evidence-based policy). Evidence underpinning policy is usually quantitative but it may be that qualitative research (or a case study, anecdote, or a newspaper article) was the original spur to policy development. This is a hazard for minorities because relevant evidence is usually very sparse and is rarely available by migrant status, or racial or ethnic group. Health policies, nonetheless, are increasingly noting the need to consider the diversity of the population in their guidance. This is usually general and not backed by either evidence or practical recommendations. This was demonstrated in a recent review of guidelines on diet, physical activity, and smoking by Liu et al. (2012) This is at least partly due to a lack of data, with the one major exception of the United States (see Section 8.3 and Chapter 9).

However, even available research on the health and health care of minorities tends to be neglected in policy and in its implementation. The reasons are not difficult to understand. Expertise is limited, experience and examples are hard to find, funds are always tight, and the immediate tasks such as policy implementation for the population generally are urgent and demanding. Both specific studies and policies often recommend that research on minorities should be done to fill evidence gaps. These recommendations are difficult to act upon because funding for research is usually routed separately and is granted on a highly competitive basis whereby committees and peer reviewers choose from a range of projects on the basis of scientific quality and promise. There is no automatic match between the needs of health policy and the priorities of research. Indeed, there is a clash, because policy requires basic information for a region or nation while research is concerned with original and novel (leading-edge) questions that produce internationally generalizable results.

Minority groups have been shown to have been largely bypassed in large-scale and expensive kinds of research such as trials and cohort studies (see Chapter 9). The United States is now leading the world in addressing this imbalance, as discussed in Section 8.3.

Researchers interested in, and able to work in, this field are few; timescales for research are usually much longer than for policy and service change and the different funding streams are an obstacle. As an example the NRCEMH in Scotland though chaired by an academic (me) did not prioritize research at its inception although its later efforts to raise funds for research were largely successful.

Qualms are sometimes expressed by practitioners, especially by leaders of community organizations, about spending money on research. One common viewpoint is that they cannot see the benefits of the research to the minority communities (except for researchers' careers, which is arguably a gain, although it might not be seen that way). There is sometimes a view that minority groups are over-researched, which is contrary to the reported experience of people recruited into studies—empirical evidence from several extensive studies shows that few trials and cohort studies report results by migration status or racial or ethnic group (see Chapter 9). There is also a fear that researchers are drawing away scarce funding from more pressing and obvious needs. It is usually true that community organizations have little access to funding, while academics working in universities may, apparently, have a great deal. Research grant applications sometimes dwarf the annual budgets of partner community organizations, yet there may be little or no funding for such partners.

Even more important than these pragmatic matters is the anxiety that research may do harm rather than good. The answers to these understandable fears is good research governance. The history of racism in research has been referred to throughout this book and will be considered again in Chapter 9. Currently, however, in the realms of health and research policy it is the lack of inclusion of minority groups in large-scale research that is causing most concern, with a gathering fear that this might reflect institutional racism in the research world. Indeed, the United States has enacted legislation and policies to counteract this problem and the debate about following this path has lately been opened in the UK. Research on migration, race, ethnicity, and health is growing rapidly, in response to both research and health policy, and it behoves us to agree a governing code of conduct that reduces the possibility of harm and maximizes benefits. The Scottish Executive Central Research Unit (2001) published *Researching Ethnic Minorities in Scotland* summarizing a consultation in 2000 where the criticism was made that researchers and funders had failed to acknowledge the existence of institutional racism in research. This was seen, at least in part, to be a result of the absence of an ethical code for researching race. Subsequently, *An Ethical Code for Researching 'Race', Racism and Anti-racism in Scotland* was published by a group of researchers called the Scottish Association of Black Researchers (SABRE). SABRE was a network of 'Black' researchers within universities, local authorities, and the 'Black' voluntary sector in Scotland. The principles of the code state that ethical research on race should:

- be embedded in social justice and human rights concerns and legal obligations;
- be explicit in its commitment to antiracism and to promoting social inclusion;
- empower and be actively inclusive of the perspectives of Black and minority ethnic people;
- address the complex and problematic nature of concepts of 'race', racism, and ethnicity;
- ensure that it does not pathologize, stereotype, or be exploitative, particularly of Black and minority ethnic people;
- value and address the diversity within the Black and minority ethnic population and recognize the interconnections with colour, age, gender, disability, sexuality, culture, class, language, belief, context, and other socially defined characteristics;
- acknowledge the power relations inherent in social research processes, e.g. between 'White' and 'Black', 'researchers' and 'researched', and families and communities;
- ensure that the whole research exercise is underpinned by a commitment to confidentiality.

The code also gives some attributes of sound researchers, including that they:

- make explicit their respective racial and ethnic origins, principles, ethics, and authority and acknowledge the potential impact that this has had;

- provide a full description of the scope, constraints, and procedures for gaining access to Black minority ethnic communities, the ethnic categories used, and their effects on the results in terms of plausibility, validity, reliability, and generalizabilty.

(These lists comprise edited extracts reproduced from *An Ethical Code for Researching 'Race', Racism and Anti-racism in Scotland*, SABRE, Copyright © 2001, with permission from the authors.)

Even many years later these principles seem radical. The challenges to values, perspectives, attitudes, and behaviours inherent in these principles are still present and difficult to deal with. In 2009 NHS Health Scotland published, on behalf Scotland and following wide discussion, an official strategy for health research in relation to its multi-ethnic society—*Health in Our Multi-Ethnic Scotland: Future Research Priorities*. Some of the specific content will be considered in Chapter 9, but the relevant point here is that the strategy included ethical principles for research into ethnicity and health, organized in a more traditional way than the SABRE statement but incorporating many of its key points.

Several codes of this kind are now available, not just for research on minorities generally but on specific topics such as genetics in relation to race. The Leeds Consensus Statement providing 10 principles supported by leading UK researchers and verified as consensual through a Delphi exercise is a recent example (Mir et al. 2013), and one that goes beyond the more common expression of guidelines by individuals or small groups of researchers. These and other guidelines will be examined in Chapter 9.

Although policy and research have not been fully integrated this does not mean a lack of mutual influence. The power of research in influencing policy and then practice is diffuse and is discussed in Section 8.2.3.10. I will use the example of CHD to consider how research can do good, not harm, albeit in ways that are hard to pinpoint.

8.2.3.10 Interaction of health and research policies: the example of CHD in South Asians in Britain

I have chosen this disease outcome because it is one of my specialist interests. However, the points made here are not unique to CHD—the same would apply to mental health, cancer, and a wide range of other problems, albeit with different kinds of responses at different stages. CHD is a dominant cause of death and disability in all ethnic groups in the UK (and increasingly globally) and as a result there have been well-documented efforts in policy, research, and practice. The White UK population is internationally notorious for its high CHD mortality, so much higher than in comparable European countries, especially France. It is remarkable, therefore, that Indian-, Pakistani-, and Bangladeshi-born residents of England and Wales, coming from countries where the disease is comparatively rare (especially so in the 1950s to 1970s when most migrated), have mortality rates 40–50% above those of the population in England and Wales as a whole. The disease risk does not fit clearly with a lower prevalence of causal factors such as smoking. Similar conclusions have arisen from work in Scotland, and in many other countries too. There is virtually a consensus that emigrant South Asians, and possibly even those still living in the Indian subcontinent, are highly susceptible to cardiovascular diseases. By contrast those residents of England and Wales who were born in Africa, the Caribbean, or China/Hong Kong have comparatively low CHD mortality. Again, such patterns have been corroborated elsewhere. Such stark ethnic inequalities in a top-ranking health problem, together with the comparatively high absolute rates of disease in all ethnic groups, compel policy attention.

Any policy or strategy needs to grapple with the question—why is CHD so common in South Asians? There is no simple, unequivocal answer. Assuming that the high rates are not an artefact of data collection or differentials in diagnostic activity, and it seems they are not, there several kinds of explanation (e.g. see Chapter 1 in Patel and Bhopal 2004):

1. South Asians are more exposed to the established CHD risk factors. (This explanation has usually been dismissed.)

2. South Asians are more susceptible to established CHD risk factors. Mechanisms proposed include genetic differences (as yet unidentified) or a mismatch between fetal/early life metabolism and that in middle age with rapid change in some risk factors.

3. There are risk factors that are not yet established (or discovered) that could specifically explain the high risk.

4. There are fewer competing causes of death in middle-aged South Asians, particularly as cancer rates are comparatively low so CHD deaths are higher because people don't die of other causes.

The high rates of CHD in South Asians are likely to arise from a complex mix of these and other explanations. While causal understanding helps direct policy, it is not as vital as having appropriate effective responses.

The control of the CHD epidemic in South Asians requires coordinated and vigorous responses based on evidence on effectiveness, and the required standards of care. The *National Service Framework for Coronary Heart Disease* (NSF) published by the Department of Health in 2000, setting 12 standards, is the key governing policy for NHS England, particularly as it gives attention to ethnic variations. The NSF requires NHS organizations to ensure that the services they provide are accessible and acceptable to the people they serve, regardless of their ethnicity. This includes accessing and meeting people's needs in ways that are culturally, religiously, and linguistically appropriate. It also states that staff will need to have or to acquire the relevant skills, knowledge, and experience to enable them to be sensitive to the cultural and religious needs of the individuals and communities that they serve. These kinds of policy directions were unusual in national policy documents of that time (and still are in many countries). The equivalent Scottish document (*Coronary Heart Disease/Stroke Task Force Report*, Scottish Executive Health Department 2001) made no mention of ethnic variations.

It is worth reflecting on why the English policy did, and the equivalent Scottish policy did not, explicitly consider the minority health dimension. The obvious answer is population size. The minority population in England was much bigger in actual numbers and as a percentage of the whole. That is not a satisfying explanation; this remains the case, but at present Scotland is producing more and stronger policy than England. I think the answer lies in the volume of research and scholarship (and interested researchers and scholars). England was a world leader in researching this issue, whereas Scotland had no published work on mortality for CHD by country of birth, race, or ethnicity. Not only did the researchers' voices reach the committee that developed the policy, but interested and active researchers (me included) served on it. In recent years Scotland has produced and published extensive data on CHD by ethnic group—it is not conceivable that future policy documents will fail to mention these. Although it cannot be proven, research has raised the subject of variations by migration status, race, and ethnicity in CHD to a central place in policy and practice in England (as in the United States) and is now doing the same in several European countries. The policies in turn spur the development of information systems and change in practice and in turn further higher-order research (e.g. interventions), creating a virtuous cycle. As one of the leaders of the Newcastle Heart Project focusing on Chinese, Indian, Pakistani, Bangladeshi, and White populations I recall in about 1990 a close academic colleague being resistant to the idea of doing that research on the basis that action, not research, was needed. The synergy between policy, research, and action (not linear) requires full recognition in the field of migration, race, and ethnicity.

Specific evidence from clinical trials of the effectiveness of interventions on South Asian populations is virtually non-existent. The actions required of health services, therefore, need to be based on first principles and include those in Box 8.7.

The Director of Equality and Human Rights for the NHS in England, Surinder Sharma, reminded those managing the NSF and working on CHD control that the NHS was founded on the unachieved principle of equal access for all (DH, BHF/NHS 2004, p. 3). Sharma asks for an explicit commitment to equality, diversity and respect in everything we do. These issues are discussed in a joint Department of Health and British Heart Foundation (2004) publication, *Heart Disease and South Asians: Delivering the National Service Framework for Coronary Heart Disease*.

Two vital principles are illustrated in this example. First, it is important that migrant health, race, and ethnicity are incorporated into primary policy documents, as secondary documentation (detailed planning) will turn to these. Research and scholarship do influence policy, albeit slowly, indirectly, and even opportunistically. A very specific example concerns heterogeneity of populations. Until the publication of papers in the 1990s on heterogeneity of CHD risk factors, nearly all discussions, including those of highly informed researchers, treated South Asians as a homogeneous group. The following extract from *Heart Disease and South Asians. Delivering the National Service Framework for Coronary Heart Disease* illustrates how this scholarship had a great influence on policy:

> It is generally agreed, however, that certain risk factors are more common among South Asians. These vary between communities, but include high levels of smoking, particularly among Bangladeshi men, low rates of exercise across all South Asian communities and a diet high in fat and low in fruit and vegetables in certain groups.
>
> Department of Health/British Heart Foundation (2004, p. 6), licensed under the Open Government Licence v.2.0.

This emphasis on differentiating South Asian subgroups (still in its infancy in the United States) is, without question, a result of research and publications that are easily accessible and impactful. Subsequent to these policy publications an enormous amount of work has taken place including in the voluntary sector, the NHS, and research funders.

Box 8.7 Some action required of health services to control CHD in South Asians

1. Adopt broadly based strategies focusing on the major risk factors, and taking account of language and cultural needs, relative poverty (especially Bangladeshis), and the heterogeneity of South Asians populations. Disease registers and practice lists may need to have a valid ethnic code so services can be targeted. An example of such a strategy is available with information on how it was developed and is on the internet [Elliot 1997].

2. Ensure that South Asian patients are well informed about CHD (their knowledge is low).

3. Ensure that standards of care for secondary and tertiary prevention follow national guidelines with equity in the quantity and quality of care.

4. Be particularly vigilant in controlling risk factors in South Asians. Thresholds for action may need to be set lower for South Asians than in the population as a whole (a topic for new research). [In Chapter 9 there is a discussion of how BMI has underestimated the proportion of Asians that are carrying too much adipose tissue (fat).]

8.3 **The United States: leading in policy and practice**

Try Exercise 8.8 before reading on.

Exercise 8.8 United States' policy relating to race, ethnicity, and migration status

♦ What factors might make the United States particularly conscious of health in relation to migration, race, and ethnicity?

♦ What might be the barriers to improving the health of minorities in the United States?

♦ What might be the strengths of the United States in the field of migration, race, and ethnicity?

The United States is one of the most race-conscious countries in the world. As a country where immigrants or their recent descendants have comprised the majority of the population for some hundreds of years, it is multiracial almost everywhere. This multiracial society, paradoxically, also has a great deal of segregation, both in location of residence and the employment sector. It has a multiplicity of highly advanced policies. The UK, like many European countries, even taking into account recent attempts at decentralization, is organized in a relatively unified way with legislation and political power underpinning extensive statutory services paid from general taxation. By contrast the United States' preferred stance (though not always practice) favours privatization of services and slicing up of political powers at federal, state, and county levels. Funding, likewise, tends to be from diverse sources. Policy analysis, policy-making, and policy implementation may well be in separate domains. It is a characteristic of US federal policy that it does not outline who is to do what and when, the practicalities usually being the responsibility of states or federal agencies. This contrasts with the UK system where a government policy is rapidly followed by both plans and instructions led by government civil servants, usually developed after consultation, but nonetheless moving from the top to the bottom of the hierarchy. Of course, such plans and instructions are often not followed—UK services do not run on a military basis. In the United States the creation of such plans is devolved. The US approach can create local energy, and local achievement, as it is not so reliant on top-down leadership. Equally, the federal policy may be ignored. Federal funding power is enormous, however, and may drive and effectively mandate change.

Race and health is incredibly controversial in the United States. Words matter greatly, and considerable controversy can occur when the language of reports is changed. The fear, of course, is that downplaying the magnitude of the problem of minority health will reduce funding for research and policy initiatives.

The following account gives a synopsis of policy in the United States. The work on race and ethnicity is done within the civil rights framework (Title VI), with legislation that protects against discrimination on race, colour, or national origin. There are many documents, but I have not found an overarching government policy that applies to the entire US health-care system, such as the Scottish HDL or English ten-point plan (Table 8.2). The recent history of policy activity in this field can be traced to the landmark *Report of the Secretary's Task Force on Black and Minority Health* (US Department of Health and Human Services 1985). This was rapidly followed by inclusion of relevant health targets in the 10-year public health plan Healthy People 2000 (US Department of Health and Human Services 1990), and in the same year the Disadvantaged Minority Health Improvement Act. This Act provided wide ranging provision of powers to tackle the disadvantages of racial and ethnic minorities in health care, data collection, research, and socio-economic, cultural, and linguistic barriers in services. It is this context, of increasing activity that the report *Unequal Treatment* was published.

8.3.1 Institute of Medicine report on unequal treatment

The Institute of Medicine is one of the most influential and respected health-related institutions in the United States, and perhaps the world. In March 2002 it published a report, *Unequal Treatment: what health care system administrators need to know about racial and ethnic disparities in healthcare* (Institute of Medicine 2002). The report recognized that health system managers worked hard to provide high-quality health-care services to an increasingly diverse population. The report acknowledged that, nonetheless, minorities and non-English speakers have comparatively greater difficulty accessing health care, and are over-represented in publicly funded health systems. Even when they are insured, racial and ethnic minorities tend to receive a lower quality of health care than White people. This report concluded that 'the sources of these disparities are complex, are rooted in historic and contemporary inequities, and involve many participants at several levels, including health systems, their administrative and bureaucratic processes, utilization managers, health care professionals, and patients' (Institute of Medicine 2002, abstract, p. 2).

The committee that wrote the report reviewed over 100 studies on the quality of health care for racial and minority ethnic groups, while taking into account explanatory factors such as income, which did not wholly account for differences.

The report considered whether minority patients could receive a lower quality of health care as a result of differences in health-care-seeking behaviours, e.g. refusing recommended services and delaying seeking health care. Such issues were judged unlikely to be major sources of health-care disparities. (Most likely such delay results from lack of insurance, lack of money, and fear of taking time off work.) Uncertainty was also considered important, e.g. when faced with patients from different racial or ethnic backgrounds, doctors' uncertainty about the patient's condition and best course of treatment is increased. Another potential explanation was that the diagnostic and treatment decisions of health-care providers, as well as their feelings about patients, were influenced by patients' race or ethnicity and stereotypes associated with them. The ways in which systems are organized and financed, changes in funding, language barriers, and time pressures on physicians in the face of cultural or linguistic barriers were all considered.

The report argued for a comprehensive, multilevel strategy to eliminate health-care disparities. Among the suggested contents of such a strategy were: base decisions about resource allocation on published clinical guidelines; take steps to improve access to care—including the provision of interpretation and translation services where community need exists; ensure that incentives for physicians do not disproportionately burden or restrict minority patients' access to care; and collect and monitor data on patients' access to and utilization of health-care services by race, ethnicity, and primary language.

The report recommended that federal, state, and private stakeholders should continue efforts to increase the proportion of under-represented US racial and ethnic minorities among health professionals, to improve access to care among minority patients, and to reduce cultural and linguistic barriers to care. Cross-cultural curricula should be part of the training of these professionals. The report proposed that such strategies were likely to reduce health-care disparities and improve the efficiency and equity of care for all patients.

In many respects, the issues were similar to those in other countries, as were the broad policy recommendations. In contrast to UK documents, it was less clear who was going to see these recommendations through. One of the most important of the US health agencies for implementing policy is the Centers for Disease Control and Prevention (CDC), and its role is considered next.

8.3.2 The CDC REACH programme

Healthy People 2010 (US Department of Health and Human Services 2000), which succeeded the 1990 publication *Healthy People 2000*, was the overarching document that describes the United States' health objectives, including goals to eliminate racial and ethnic disparities in health. The CDC's leadership role in this initiative includes a programme called Racial and Ethnic Approaches to Community Health (REACH) 2010 which was designed to eliminate disparities in cardiovascular disease, immunizations, breast and cervical cancer screening and management, diabetes, HIV/AIDS, and infant mortality. The groups targeted by REACH 2010 were African Americans, Native Americans, Alaska Natives, Asian Americans, Hispanics, and Pacific Islanders. In 2005 $34.5 million was available for this programme. REACH 2010 supported community coalitions comprising a community-based organization and three types of other organizations, at least one being a health department or a university or research organization.

In a report on the REACH programme, the Acting Director of the CDC, G. A. Mensah, gave several examples to illustrate the extent of health disparities in the United States. Mensah advocated culturally appropriate, community-driven programmes based on sound prevention research and supported by new and innovative partnerships among governments, businesses, faith-based organizations, and communities.

One REACH project is targeting the Cambodian community and its leaders, health-care providers, and public health researchers. Community health educators teach people how to decrease risks and enhance protective behaviours associated with diabetes and cardiovascular disease. The number of Cambodians accessing health care at a local health centre increased from 1070 in 2000 to 3080 in 2004. Of those who had attended educational workshops and peer support groups, 50% reported favourable behavioural changes such as limiting salt intake.

The REACH programme developed a dissemination plan to help others develop and implement culturally appropriate prevention and intervention strategies. REACH also expanded policy initiatives that target environmental change, document the impact of cultural competency in collaborative partnerships, and build capacity to include research on social determinants of health.

Although REACH clearly is linked to national policy, it was a project-orientated initiative and did not aim to shift the entire health-care system to meet the needs of minorities. This is not surprising, as the system in the United States is pluralistic, and the CDC (and federal government) has no direct jurisdiction over health care. By contrast in our third example, on research, a federal agency has extensive powers to enforce its policies.

8.3.3 The National Institutes of Health: legal, policy, and financial drives to promote equity in research

The importance of research in improving, the health of minorities has long been recognized in the United States, and key laws and policies encourage expanded efforts, particularly to narrow disparities (the preferred term in the United States for inequalities that are unjust—or inequities). It is obvious that for this to succeed high-quality research would need to be focused on these disadvantaged groups. The research record clearly showed that this was not happening. The route to change was through the federal government's health research agency—the National Institutes for Health (NIH), the largest health research funding agency in the world (its 2012 budget exceeded $30 billion).

The too common failure of researchers to include minority racial and ethnic populations (and women) in research led to legislation (the NIH Revitalisation Act of 1993) and NIH policy in the mid-1990s (amended 2001) that required researchers funded by the NIH to either ensure inclusion of minority racial and ethnic populations or to justify their exclusion on scientific grounds. (The same applied to women.) The consequence has been a great expansion of research focusing on minorities (and women). In this regard the United States easily leads and influences the world. Several studies have examined how inclusion of minorities in research compares in the United States and other parts of the world. Invariably, the United States does better, and NIH-funded studies do better than other US studies. For example, Ranganathan and Bhopal (2006) showed that of 31 North American cardiovascular cohort studies 15 provided some data by ethnic group, while none of 41 European ones did. Bartlett et al. (2003) reported that all eight of 47 trials that were specific on the matter of ethnicity were US based. These are only two of many such observations, and I have chosen them because this is the position with cardiovascular disease, which has been long recognized as a matter of priority for minority ethnic groups. The situation is likely to be worse for other outcomes.

The NIH policy has been controversial but it has withstood criticisms and is still in place. Research underpins US strategies to reduce racial and ethnic disparities. These strategies have far-reaching consequences and need evaluation. In 2000 the US Congress created within the NIH the National Center on Minority Health and Health Disparities (NCMHD), which is backed by legislation and serves to coordinate research. This legislation mandated the *Strategic Research Plan to Reduce and Ultimately Eliminate Health Disparities* (National Institutes of Health 2000).

The NIH's strategic plan identified goals for research, research infrastructure, and public information and community outreach. The strategic plan was developed with input from the public, professional and patient advocacy groups, health-care organizations, academic institutions, and the scientific community. The NCMHD asked the Institute of Medicine to assess the plan in achieving the NIH's goals and objectives. As targets for health outcomes have been set, the United States is ahead of the UK. The plan and budget were updated twice following publication, showing the intent of this strategy. Nonetheless, it seems improbable that disparities in health status will narrow without a broader, integrated, and government-led approach to simultaneously tackle income and wealth and environmental inequalities. In terms of legislative backing, policy, funded strategy, sheer volume of activity, state of the art methods, and flow of academic and service-related publications the United States has a global lead and is an exemplar in the field of research on minority health.

8.3.4 From policy generally to policy on a key service component: the National Standards on Culturally and Linguistically Appropriate Services (CLAS)

In virtually every policy document ever written on the subject of the health of migrant, racial, ethnic, or indigenous minorities, one dominant and perennial theme is better communication that transcends language barriers, with a recognized need for cultural competence at level of both the organization and individual practitioners. Yet experience shows that a simple and obvious policy is exceedingly difficult to implement effectively—at least partly because this measure creates heated resistance especially amongst politicians and every few years progress is set back.

Given this context, and in recognition of political resistance in many parts of the United States, including attempts to ban health and other professionals from speaking in languages other than English, the National Standards on Culturally and Linguistically Appropriate Services (CLAS) are remarkable. These were first launched in 2000, with the third revision being published in 2013 (see Box 8.8). The content is comprehensive but not in itself remarkable—similar statements have been made in many places. The remarkable factor is the vigour with which they have been disseminated and the widespread impact they have had.

Box 8.8 National Standards on Culturally and Linguistically Appropriate Services (CLAS)

The CLAS standards are intended to advance health equity, improve quality, and help eliminate health-care disparities by establishing a blueprint for health and health-care organizations to:

Principal standard:

1. Provide effective, equitable, understandable, and respectful quality care and services that are responsive to diverse cultural health beliefs and practices, preferred languages, health literacy, and other communication needs.

Governance, leadership, and workforce:

2. Advance and sustain organizational governance and leadership that promotes CLAS and health equity through policy, practices, and allocated resources.
3. Recruit, promote, and support a culturally and linguistically diverse governance, leadership, and workforce that are responsive to the population in the service area.
4. Educate and train governance, leadership, and workforce in culturally and linguistically appropriate policies and practices on an ongoing basis.

Communication and language assistance:

5. Offer language assistance to individuals who have limited English proficiency and/or other communication needs, at no cost to them, to facilitate timely access to all health care and services.
6. Inform all individuals of the availability of language assistance services clearly and in their preferred language, verbally and in writing.
7. Ensure the competence of individuals providing language assistance, recognizing that the use of untrained individuals and/or minors as interpreters should be avoided.
8. Provide easy-to-understand print and multimedia materials and signage in the languages commonly used by the populations in the service area.

Engagement, continuous improvement, and accountability:

9. Establish culturally and linguistically appropriate goals, policies, and management accountability, and infuse them throughout the organization's planning and operations.
10. Conduct ongoing assessments of the organization's CLAS-related activities and integrate CLAS-related measures into measurement and continuous quality improvement activities.
11. Collect and maintain accurate and reliable demographic data to monitor and evaluate the impact of CLAS on health equity and outcomes and to inform service delivery.
12. Conduct regular assessments of community health assets and needs and use the results to plan and implement services that respond to the cultural and linguistic diversity of populations in the service area.

(Continued)

Box 8.8 (Continued)

13. Partner with the community to design, implement, and evaluate policies, practices, and services to ensure cultural and linguistic appropriateness.

14. Create conflict and grievance resolution processes that are culturally and linguistically appropriate to identify, prevent, and resolve conflicts or complaints.

15. Communicate the organization's progress in implementing and sustaining CLAS to all stakeholders, constituents, and the general public.

Reproduced from The Office of Minority Health, *The National CLAS Standards*, US Department of Health and Human Services, Copyright © 2013, available from http://minorityhealth.hhs.gov/templates/browse. aspx?lvl=2&lvlID=15.

Their success is attributable to some factors that are generalizable and some that are particular to the United States. The generalizable factors include their preparation via an inclusive dialogue, leadership from a major government agency (the Department of Health and Human Services, Office of Minority Health), their focused nature, and that they capitalized on a wave of previous policies that we discussed above. Other generalizable factors include the formation of a wide network of participants, cemented and broadened through a very active web listserve (CLAS-talk, http://www.diversityrx.org/activities/clastalk-listserv), and the timelines, given the ever-increasing diversity of the US population. I see at least three factors that have led to success that are not easily reproducible in other places. First, there is considerable vigour in the private and entrepreneurial sectors in the United States. Implementing CLAS standards is an industry, and the private sector, both small and large operations, is busy with it. In other countries, certainly the UK, the primary means of implementing such policies is through the civil service, managers, and professionals. While the community sector and private sector are present, it is not easy for them to lead. By contrast, numerous individuals and companies are taking leading roles in the United States. (To get a taste of this I recommend readers attend the annual DiversityRx Conferences on Quality Health Care for Culturally Diverse Populations.) The second factor is the strong system of quality evaluation of US health organizations, with re-licensing of individual professionals and institutions at stake. The CLAS standards have become integral to this in many places. The third factor is the emphasis on the business case, with evidence that these standards save money. The world's most expensive health-care system (and possibly one of the most inefficient too) is rightly looking to save money. This may well work because good interpretation services are associated with shortened hospital stay and reduced readmission.

8.4 Policies relating to migrants, Roma/Gypsy travellers, and indigenous populations and their relation to those on race and ethnicity

In international laws and policies—and hence reflected in national laws and policies—the primary concept is race. This is not at all surprising, because these laws are designed to prevent the barbarism and exploitation implemented so wrongly in the past as a result of racism, partly underpinned by misguided race science. These laws and policies recognize fully the various facets of the race concept—well beyond biology—so apply to discrimination on the basis of ethnicity, religion, language, colour etc. The 'etc.' is deliberate and very important because the law has the discretion to include discrimination on unspecified matters. It is already clear that these laws apply to migrants. They also apply to indigenous minorities in so far as they are an ethnic group. So all migrants and all indigenous minorities recognized as an ethnic, religious, or linguistic minority are protected. In the United States and the UK the concepts of race and ethnicity have long been accepted and are part of day-to-day discourse. This is also true in countries such as New Zealand, Australia, and Canada. In South Africa, an established but unjust discourse using a politically driven race classification is under reconsideration. In other countries, especially in continental, north-west Europe, the race and ethnicity concepts are awkward for the same reason as in South Africa—sensitivities stretching back to the Nazi atrocities based on both these concepts. In such countries the concentration of activities is on migrants and their descendants. It is, obvious, however, that the issues are much the same. European guidelines (http://www.euro.who.int/__data/assets/pdf_file/0005/127526/e94497.pdf) show much overlap with and similarity to those in the United States (see Box 8.8).

There are policy advantages and disadvantages to using both the race and ethnicity concepts and the migration concept. The problem with race and ethnicity (aside from acceptability) is that it is too easily and too often equated with applying to just non-White (or even more crudely non-Western) people. This is an error that needs correction. The problem with migration status is that it does not cover the indigenous minorities and long-established populations such as the Roma (Europe's largest minority group) or the children of migrants (who become ethnic minorities and are not migrants). Very quickly, migration status also starts to focus on non-White (non-'Western') populations and becomes a proxy for ethnicity or race.

The viewpoint in the second edition of this book is that the common ground is so large that we should unify the field—not splinter with different groups working on migrant health, indigenous health, race, and ethnicity.

There are, however, at least three major groups where a specialist policy, and possibly legislative outlook, is needed. One group is undocumented migrants, also widely known as illegal migrants. Although in international law their right to health and freedom from discrimination and fairness is relatively clear, the practice at national level is both variable and mostly unacceptable, particularly from the perspective of health professionals who are caught between their duties under medical ethics and their duties under often unclear government policy. New policies are needed, preferably at international, supra-regional, and national levels, working contemporaneously. Ideally, these new policies would dovetail with the general ones dealing with disadvantage, migration, race, and ethnicity.

The second group is indigenous minorities. (These people are also sometimes known as aboriginal peoples—the original inhabitants of the land.) Their exceptionally poor health and socio-economic circumstances are well known. Despite the existence of a UN Permanent Forum on Indigenous Issues and documentation of needs of indigenous groups (including objectives) the situation is somewhat dire. The rights of indigenous peoples are often ignored, and progress is extremely slow. While most attention is devoted to indigenous people in North America (American Indians, First Nations people, Inuit, etc.), and Australia (Aborigines and Torres Strait Islanders) and New Zealand (Maoris), the vast majority live elsewhere. In China there are an estimated 91 million indigenous people, compared with 2.7 million in the United States and 120 000 in the Arctic.

Some vigorous policy and service responses have been mounted, e.g. the Indian Health Service in the United States and work with Australian Aborigines and Torres Strait Islanders, and especially progressive work with Maoris. Some responses have taken a largely separatist approach, e.g. the US Government Indian Health Service for 566 federally recognized tribes provides a wide range of services to American Indians and Alaska Natives. The Australian Government has also done similar policy and service work. The approach of the New Zealand Government is less separatist and more one of mainstreaming and inclusion (though it is separate from the more general efforts on the health of ethnic minorities).These approaches—with the partial exception of the Maori—have not been successful in moving rapidly to equitable health outcomes. Reappraisal and reconsideration of mainstreaming policies—as in New Zealand—is warranted.

The third group that clearly needs fresh policy implementation is the long-established minorities such as indigenous travellers, Gypsy travellers, and Romani populations. Their health status is extremely poor, and their health services are usually comparatively poor. In Europe, there are an estimated 10 million people of Roma origin. They migrated over a period of 1000 years from India. National policies—though they may be good in content—have not been effective. A Europe-wide policy effort is currently under way but it is too early to judge its effectiveness.

These three groups are clearly living at the margins of mainstream society—sometimes out of choice in the case of indigenous people and the Roma, but not so for undocumented migrants. In times past, and even now in some places, the same applied to legally settled minority ethnic and racial groups.

I propose that work that integrates across these strands—race, ethnicity, migration, indigenous health, and long-established minorities—will provide mutual strength, learning, and power. The European Public Health Association's Migrant and Ethnic Health Section is currently following this path. In turn this work needs to be embedded within the strategic and policy framework of the Social Determinants of Health Programme led by the WHO.

8.5 **Conclusion**

While there are many policies, strategies, and action projects in existence, health services internationally have struggled with the challenge of equitable health care in multicultural societies. While I have focused on the UK and the United States, I am on reasonably safe ground in stating that matters are not better, and are sometimes much worse, elsewhere. New Zealand has long-standing and superb policies but the health of Maoris is poor; Australian Aborigines living in one of the world's richest economies have appalling health despite targeted efforts; and many European countries have yet to properly confront the challenges, including those relating to long-settled populations such as the Roma.

To date the challenge has been tackled mostly at the level of structure and process—which systems might work and what should we do? Equity in service delivery is increasingly the central focus, with outcomes in terms of health-care delivery and its quality as the benchmark. The achievement of outcomes measured in terms of health status is seldom the centrepiece of discussion, although the United States has recently moved to this. Intuitively, this is currently too great a challenge for most countries, not least because the causes of differences in health status are often not clear. Even conceptually, it is difficult to set a benchmark. What would be the goal? Racial and ethnic inequalities in health are far more complex than socio-economic inequalities, not least because socio-economic factors are part of them. Racial and ethnic inequalities are very hard to predict, vary by cause of ill-health and by risk factor, and are rapidly changing; social class inequalities, by contrast, are mostly predictable—on the great majority of indictors the poor are worse off than the wealthy. As considered in Chapters 6 and 9, a different conceptual approach will be needed for tackling inequalities in health status in minorities—and logically it would be based on the benchmark being the group with most desirable state of health for each indicator.

Current opinion favours mainstreaming, i.e. adaptation of general existing services, and incorporation of the needs of minorities into the design stage of new services. The importance for minority groups of the wider determinants of health, such as wealth, housing, employment, and education, is clear. Policies and strategies to achieve better health for minorities are strengthened and sustained by their incorporation within a broader agenda for social justice and civil rights, and within wider policies to reduce inequalities. Methods for race equality impact assessment are being developed. These are being applied to a wide range of policies, e.g. transport, health and safety, and employment practices. In this way there is an interconnection, and synergy, across the different sectors of social life. When everyone is speaking with the one voice, action is more likely, as we saw with the example of CHD services in England where research, policy, strategy, and service delivery came together with a commonality of perspective that itself was in harmony with other national policies. These increasingly accepted ideals are constrained by lack of funds, expertise, data (particularly on what works and why), and the ongoing political controversies (usually negative in tone) around immigration, asylum, racial equality, and human rights. These constraints mean that progress is slower than ideal.

While policy, strategy, and action are highly dependent on local context, many of the principles, experience, and lessons are transferable internationally. Perhaps the most important of all the principles is that policies are most powerful and effective when they are supported by a legal and ethical framework. As illustrated well in relation to undocumented migrants, they are weakest when laws and ethics clash. These frameworks, of necessity, reflect the values of the society and particularly those of the politicians and other holders of power. Policies to improve the health and health care of minority groups depend crucially on the value that all humans and human groups are equal and all have the same rights to health and health care.

8.6 **Summary**

A policy is a statement of intent that sets high-level directions and goals; a strategy is a general plan to make an intended action happen; and these policies and strategies need to be supported by detailed plans that specify tasks, responsibilities, timetables, and costs. In practice, actions are not always taken according to policies and strategies but on a tactical or opportunistic basis. However, a pre-existing policy increases the likelihood of grasping such opportunities.

Health services for minority groups are usually set within policies and strategies for the population as a whole, in practice the majority (or most powerful) population. Ideally, policies for the whole population would address the needs of minority groups in an integrated way. This concept is known as mainstreaming. In practice this may not happen for reasons including absence of understanding or agreement that this is important, the complexity of the issues raised, and lack of expertise, time, and publication space within policy and strategy documents.

Mostly, minority populations are expected to adapt themselves to benefit from the available services. Professionals delivering the service tend to make some adjustments on an ad hoc basis. Increasingly, we see two further policy responses—setting up specialist services for minority groups but within the main service; and the development of strategies to help reshape existing services to meet needs. The complete separation of services for minorities, as under apartheid, is currently not in favour. However, this approach may be needed when minorities are unwilling or unable to access main services, e.g. undocumented migrants, and indigenous populations living apart, e.g. on reservations.

The UK policy response until about 1990 was intermittent and fragmented, with a mixture of stand-alone projects and modifications to mainstream services. Progress has been made on key requirements such as interpretation services and dietary needs in hospital. The Race Relations (Amendment) Act 2000 building on the 1976 Act, coupled with explicit or implicit policies from government health departments, drove more widespread changes based on a positive duty to promote racial equality. These national initiatives affect everyone and are being translated, often with great difficulty, into local action plans and ultimately service changes. Ethnic monitoring is an example of a policy that is difficult to achieve despite evident need and good intentions. The work on race and ethnicity was incorporated within the wider equality agenda, and formalized in the 2010 Equality Act.

The United States has had a long-standing programme for affirmative action based on human rights principles that aims to redress historical wrongs. Its racial and ethnic classification is explicitly designed to help achieve this goal. The pluralistic nature of the health-care system of the United States, based on private health-care principles, makes a cohesive strategy impossible to enact nationally to serve the whole population but huge progress is being made with global leadership, especially in research. By law, minority groups cannot be excluded from research using federal government funds without good reason, and this has spurred a substantial research programme in the United States.

While many policies, strategies, and action projects exist, health services internationally have struggled with the challenge of equitable health care in multicultural societies. These struggles are especially seen in relation to undocumented migrants, indigenous populations, and long-established populations such as Roma. Current opinion favours mainstreaming with adaptation of general existing services, and incorporation of the needs of minorities into the design of new services. These ideals are constrained by lack of funds, expertise, data, and the ongoing political controversies around immigration, asylum, race equality, and human rights. While policy, strategy, and action are highly dependent on local context, many of the principles, experience, and lessons are transferable internationally.

References

Acheson D (1998) *Independent Report into Inequalities in Health*. London: HMSO.

Bansal N, Bhopal R, Fischbacher C, Povey C, Chalmers J, Brewster D, et al. (2011a) Linkage of data in the study of ethnic inequalities and inequities in health outcomes in Scotland: the Scottish Health and Ethnicity Linkage Study (SHELS). *Journal of Epidemiology and Community Health* 65(Suppl. 1): A33.

Bansal N, Fischbacher C, Bhopal R, Brown H, Steiner M, Capewell S (2013b) Myocardial infarction incidence and survival in Scotland: the Scottish Health and Ethnicity Linkage retrospective cohort Study (SHELS). BMJ Open; 3:e003415.

Bansal N, Bhopal RS, Steiner MF, Brewster DH (2012) Major ethnic group differences in breast cancer screening uptake in Scotland are not extinguished by adjustment for indices of geographical residence, area deprivation, long-term illness and education. *British Journal of Cancer* 106: 1361–6.

Bartlett C, Davey P, Dieppe P, Doyal L, Ebrahim S, et al. (2003) Women, older persons, and ethnic minorities: factors associated with their inclusion in randomised trials of statins 1990 to 2001. *Heart* 89: 327–8.

Bhopal RS, Fischbacher C, Povey C, Chalmers J, Mueller G, Steiner M,et al. (2011) Cohort profile: Scottish Health and Ethnicity Linkage Study of 4.65 million people exploring ethnic variations in disease in Scotland. *International Journal of Epidemiology* 40: 1168–75.

Bhopal RS, Bansal N, Fischbacher C, Brown H, Capewell S (2012a) Ethnic variations in chest pain and angina in men and women: Scottish Ethnicity and Health Linkage Study of 4.65 million people. *European Journal of Preventive Cardiology* 19: 1250–7.

Bhopal RS, Bansal N, Fischbacher CM, Brown H, Capewell S (2012b) Ethnic variations in the incidence and mortality of stroke in the Scottish Health and Ethnicity Linkage Study of 4.65 million people. *European Journal of Preventive Cardiology* 19: 1503–8.

Bhopal RS, Bansal N, Fischbacher CM, Brown H, Capewell S (2012c) Ethnic variations in heart failure: Scottish Health and Ethnicity Linkage Study (SHELS). *Heart* **98**: 468–73.

Bhopal R, Bansal N, Steiner M, Brewster DH,on behalf of the Scottish Health and Ethnicity Linkage Study (2012d) Does the 'Scottish effect' apply to all ethnic groups? All cancer, lung, colorectal, breast and prostate cancer in the Scottish Health and Ethnicity Linkage Cohort Study. *BMJ Open* **2**: e001957.

Chandra J (1996) *Facing up to Difference: a toolkit for creating culturally competent health services for black and minority ethnic communities.* London: King's Fund.

Commission for Racial Equality (2002) *Ethnic Monitoring—a Guide for Public Authorities in Scotland.* London: CRE (http://www.equalityhumanrights.com/uploaded_files/PSD/13_ethnic_monitoring_scotland.pdf).

Department of Health (2000) *National Service Framework for Coronary Heart Disease: modern standards and service models.* London: Department of Health.

Department of Health/British Heart Foundation (2004) *Heart Disease and South Asians: Delivering the National Service Framework for Coronary Heart Disease.* London: Department of Health.

Elliott B for the Newcastle Strategy Group (1997) *Taking Heart. Reducing Diabetes and Cardiovascular Disease Among Newcastle's South Asian and Chinese Communities.* Newcastle upon Tyne: University of Newcastle upon Tyne.

Fischbacher CM, Steiner M, Bhopal R, Chalmers J, Jamieson J, Knowles D,et al. (2007) Variations in all cause and cardiovascular mortality by country of birth in Scotland 1997–2003. *Scottish Medical Journal* **52**(4): 5–10.

Gunaratnam Y (2003) *Researching Race and Ethnicity: methods, knowledge and power.* London: Sage Publications.

Home Office (2001) *Race Relations (Amendment) Act 2000.* London: Home Office.

Institute of Medicine—Committee on Understanding and Eliminating Racial and Ethnic Disparities in Health Care (2002) *Unequal treatment: confronting racial and ethnic disparities in health care* (ed. Smedley BD, Stith AY, Nelson AR). Washington, DC: National Academies Press.

Liu JJ, Davidson E, Bhopal RS, White M, Johnson MRD, Netto G,et al. (2012) Adapting health promotion interventions to meet the needs of ethnic minority groups: mixed-methods evidence synthesis. Health Technology Assessment **16**(44): 1–469. doi: 10.3310/hta16440

Lothian NHS Minority Health Group (2003) *Strategic Action Plan on Minority Ethnic Health: being fair for all in the NHS in Lothian.* Edinburgh: NHS Lothian.

Madhok R, Bhopal RS, Ramaiah RS (1992) Quality of hospital service: an 'Asian' perspective. *Journal of Public Health Medicine* **14**: 271–9.

Madhok R, Hameed A, Bhopal RS (1998) Satisfaction with health services among the Pakistani population in Middlesbrough, England. *Journal of Public Health Medicine* **20**: 295–301.

Mathews G, Alexander J, Rahemtulla T, Bhopal R (2007) Impact of a cardiovascular risk control project for South Asians (Khush Dil) on motivation, behaviour, obesity, blood pressure and lipids. *Journal of Public Health* **29**: 388–97.

Mir G, Salway S, Kai J, Karlsen S, Bhopal R, Ellison GTH, Sheikh A (2013) Principles for research on ethnicity and health: the Leeds Consensus Statement. *European Journal of Public Health* **23**: 504–10.

National Institutes of Health (2000) *Strategic Research Plan to Reduce and Ultimately Eliminate Health Disparities.* Bethesda, MD: National Institutes of Health.

Patel KC, Bhopal RS (eds) (2004) *The Epidemic of Coronary Heart Disease in South Asian Populations: causes and consequences.* Birmingham: South Asian Health Foundation.

Race Equality Advisory Forum (2001) *Making it Real. A Race Equality Strategy for Scotland.* Edinburgh: Scottish Executive.

Ranganathan M and Bhopal R (2006) Exclusion and inclusion of nonwhite ethnic minority groups in 72 North American and European cardiovascular cohort studies. *PLoS Medicine* **3**: 1–8.

Scottish Executive (1999) *White Paper, Towards a Healthier Scotland*, Cm 4269. Edinburgh: The Stationery Office.

Scottish Executive Central Research Unit (2001) *Researching Ethnic Minorities in Scotland.* Edinburgh: Scottish Executive (http://www.bemis.org.uk/source/Researching%20BEM%C9otland%20 2001.pdf)

Scottish Executive Health Department (2000) *Our National Health. A plan for action, a plan for change.* Edinburgh: Scottish Executive (http://www.scotland.gov.uk/Resource/Doc/158734/0043082.pdf).

Scottish Executive Health Department (2001) *Coronary Heart Disease/Stroke Task Force Report.* Edinburgh: Scottish Executive (http://www.sehd.scot.nhs.uk/publications/cdtf/cdtf-01.htm).

Scottish Executive Health Department (2002) *Fair for All: working together towards culturally competent services*, HDL 51. Edinburgh: Scottish Executive.

Scottish Government (2008) *Equally Well: Report of the Ministerial Task Force on Health Inequalities.* Edinburgh: The Scottish Government (http://www.scotland.gov.uk/Publications/2008/06/25104032/0).

Shaw J (1994) *Collection of Ethnic Group data for Admitted Patients* (EL(94)77). Leeds: NHS Executive.

US Department of Health and Human Services (1985) *Report of the Secretary's Task Force on Black and Minority Health*. Washington, DC: US Government Printing Office.

US Department of Health and Human Services (1990) *Healthy People 2000*. Washington, DC: US Government Printing Office (http://www.cdc.gov/nchs/healthy_people/hp2000.htmx).

US Department of Health and Human Services (2000) *Healthy People 2010*. Washington, DC: US Government Printing Office (http://www.cdc.gov/nchs/healthy_people/hp2010.htm).

Other sources and further reading

Adelstein AM (1963) Some aspects of cardiovascular mortality in South Africa. *British Journal of Preventive and Social Medicine* 17: 29–40.

Anonymous (2001) American Indian health: insights and reservations. *The Lancet* 357: 1810.

Arnold M, Razum O, Coebergh JW (2010) Cancer risk diversity in non-western migrants to Europe: an overview of the literature. *European Journal of Cancer* 46: 2647–59.

Bhopal R, Unwin N, White M, Yallop J, Walker L, Alberti KG, et al. (1999) Heterogeneity of coronary heart disease risk factors in Indian, Pakistani, Bangladeshi, and European origin populations: cross sectional study. *British Medical Journal* 319: 215–20.

Chambers JC, Obeid OA, Refsum H, Ueland P, Hackett D, Hooper J,et al. (2000) Plasma homocysteine concentrations and risk of coronary heart disease in UK Indian Asian and European men. *The Lancet* 355: 523–7.

Chaturvedi N, Bathula R, Shore AC, Panerai R, Potter J, Kooner J,et al. (2012) South Asians have elevated postexercise blood pressure and myocardial oxygen consumption compared to Europeans despite equivalent resting pressure. *Journal of the American Heart Association* 1: e000281.

Clyne MB (1964) Indian patients. *Practitioner* 793: 195–9.

Ineson A and Bhopal R (2000) *Meeting the Health Needs of Minority Ethnic Groups in Lothian*. Report of the Director of Public Health. Edinburgh: Lothian Health Board.

Lothian Health Board (2002) *Strategic Action Plan on Minority Ethnic Health: Being Fair for All in the NHS in Lothian* [draft for consultation]. Edinburgh, Lothian Health Board.

Rocheron Y and Dickinson R (1990) The Asian mother and baby campaign: a way forward in health promotion for Asian women? *Health Education Journal* 49: 128–33.

Steinbrook R (2004) Disparities in health care—from politics to policy. *New England Journal of Medicine* 350: 1486–8.

Taylor AL, Ziesche S, Yancy C, Carson P, D'Agostino R Jr, Ferdinand K, et al. (2004) Combination of isosorbide dinitrate and hydralazine in blacks with heart failure. *New England Journal of Medicine* 351: 2049–57.

Tunstall Pedoe H, Clayton D, Morris JN, Bridge W, McDonald L (1975) Coronary heart-attack in East London. *The Lancet* 2: 833–8.

Woolhandler S, Himmelstein DU, Silber R, Bader M, Harnly M, Jones AA (1985) Medical care and mortality: racial differences in preventable deaths. *International Journal of Health Services* 15: 1–22.

Chapter 9

Research on and with minority migrant, racial, and ethnic groups: Past, present, and future

Objectives

After reading this chapter you should:

+ Be familiar with a history of research that has done harm to minority migrant, racial, and ethnic groups, and hence be forewarned about the potential pitfalls.

+ In outline, be familiar with the range of research methods that can yield understanding of both variations in health and disease in, and the health and health-care needs of, minority groups.

+ Be able to apply existing terminology, classifications, and measurement methods as appropriate to the research questions and study design (or develop new concepts).

+ Be able to discuss the key issues of: recruitment of study populations, consent and participant information, response rates, validity of research methods and measurements, interpretation of data, application of research for improving the health of minority groups, and publication.

+ Be able to articulate an ideal approach to research with minority groups but adapt it in practice in the light of financial and other constraints.

9.1 Introduction: potential, limitations, and pitfalls of migration, race, ethnicity, and health research

The theme of research has permeated this book because there is so much overlap between the practice and science of medicine, epidemiology, public health, and health-care delivery (and perhaps also because the writer is a both researcher and a practitioner). The contents of Chapters 1, 2, 3, 5, and 6 are particularly relevant to research. In Chapter 8, I discussed research in the context of policies and strategies. Overlap between this chapter and earlier ones is, therefore, inevitable. This chapter will draw together the challenges we face and the principles and methods that will help us overcome them. Among the challenges is the question of whether we need more or less research showing variations in health status and health in minorities.

A discussion of specific methods and how they can be used in the context of minority health requires a book, indeed a series of books, of its own. However, many of the points incorporated in this book can be integrated with the methodological and conceptual ones in general research textbooks (though the challenges are not insubstantial). (See the Bibliography for some specialist books.) Above all, this chapter aims to demonstrate the potential pitfalls and problems (so as to avoid them) in counterbalance to the benefits of minority health research.

There are many motivations underlying research, and not all are altruistic. Health scientists aspire to discover the causes and processes of disease and related problems, while health policy-makers and planners need to meet the health and health-care needs of minority groups. Additional motives for research include a wish to reverse the health and social disadvantages of minority groups, curiosity and interest, especially about more exotic matters, and an unfortunate interest in ranking migrant, racial, and ethnic groups. This latter work can be abused to justify inequalities in resources and social status. The opportunities for causal research and hypothesis generation are huge, though often missed, as illustrated by the classical migration study discussed in Section 9.1.1.

9.1.1 The classical migration study: a route to disentangling the effects on health of nature and nurture

Even though it is somewhat obvious that nearly all diseases (and other health status outcomes) arise from the interplay (or biological interaction to be more technical) of genetic and environmental factors, one of the most lasting paradigms of health research is the attempt to dissect out their separate effects. (To what extent this paradigm has proven its worth is beyond the scope of this book.) The potential contribution of migrants and different racial and ethnic groups to this scientific enterprise has long been recognized and extolled.

The classical migration study, whereby migrants are tracked as they move from one place to another, undoubtedly helps separate the effects of environmental and genetic influences. These studies can be of local migrants, e.g. as people move from a rural village to an urban slum. Unsurprisingly, their health-related behaviours and risk factors change quickly and subsequently so does their pattern of disease. Leaving aside problems of bias, and the difficulties of making comparable measurements across long distances and times, migration studies offer rich opportunities for generating and testing hypotheses. One problem, however, is the multiplicity of changes that arise. This makes it difficult to be sure of causes and effects, e.g. salt intake tends to rise rapidly and blood pressure follows. It is tempting to ascribe cause and effect—but perhaps the real cause was the stress of migration or indeed the gain in weight in the new environment. Although migration studies are sometimes thought of as 'natural experiments', they are not able to control variables as would be the case in a true experiment. These difficulties in interpretation are compounded by international migration. Migrants are a selected group—usually, the health of migrants is not the same as that of the people left behind. Most often migrants are healthier, and perhaps more ambitious, skilled, educated, and energetic than their non-migrant counterparts. Sometimes, this is not true, especially for those facing enforced migration, e.g. people who are trafficked—enticed, tricked, and even kidnapped and forced to migrate (usually to be exploited as servants, labourers, or sex workers).

Adding to this the racial or ethnic dimension, where both the migrants and their offspring are compared with other racial or ethnic groups within one territory, enriches the possibilities and potential. Obviously, this enrichment comes at the cost of even greater complexity. The ideal migration study might comprise people in the country and place of origin, their migrating counterparts in the country of destination (perhaps several countries), and other populations in the country of destination. This kind of study is extremely rare because it is difficult to set up. Changing social and environmental circumstances within and between generations in different migrant, racial, and ethnic groups in such ideal studies can be linked to changing health states.

The message from many publications on race, ethnicity, and health is that this wonderful opportunity must not be missed. One of the chapters in the book by Rothschild (1981) was entitled 'Ethnic groups: a paradigm' and offered ethnicity as a paradigm for understanding diseases of complex aetiology. Marmot et al.'s (1984) report *Immigrant Mortality in England and Wales* opens with the words 'Studies of mortality of immigrants are useful for pointing to particular disease problems of immigrants, investigating aetiology and validating international differences in disease'. Before we turn to the methods for achieving these goals, let us consider the pitfalls and limitations.

9.1.2 **Research, values, harm, and good**

Research of any kind, whether in the human population at large, the laboratory, or on animals, is not a value-free activity. Values in research are particularly important when that research is on living human beings, and arguably even more important when it compares and contrasts different human populations. Migration status, race, and ethnicity, as variables that distinguish human populations, are extremely important to the structure and function of human societies, and it is inevitable that research using these concepts is of interest to, and has influence upon, social organization and will be interpreted to serve social goals. In the UK, as in most countries, this is openly recognized: the Data Protection Act classifies information on race and ethnicity as sensitive personal data requiring particularly stringent control. Interestingly, data protection laws on fair processing of data may allow the release of a variable, e.g. a name, but that does not mean investigators can use it to derive other personal information from it, e.g. ethnic group by name analysis. Permission should be sought for such secondary use. Even where such Acts do not specify immigration status specifically, it can be assumed that variables such as country of birth, language spoken, or asylum status are personal data and hence protected by the Data Protection Act. Researchers and practitioners who wish to access such data may find it irritating to find them closely controlled. A historical understanding is helpful for understanding the reasons.

Before reading on try Exercise 9.1.

Exercise 9.1 Harm from research

◆ What kind of harm can you envisage from health research demonstrating
   (1) similarities and (2) differences between migrant, ethnic, and racial groups.

◆ Can you recall any examples of such harms, whether historical or current?

◆ Why do you think such harm may occur? Is it inherent to the field of research or
   dependent on social context?

◆ Why do migration, race, and ethnicity variables still remain popular in population
   health research?

Modern-day work showing differences by migrant, racial, and ethnic group in the health status and health care of populations is mostly used to further current social goals of equality and justice. Equally, much research in the same field in the past was used to further previous social goals such as the continuation of slavery, the justification of Empire, the maintenance of social and material inequality including apartheid in South Africa, anti-immigration policies, eugenics, and the Nazi final solution that included the total extermination of Jews, the disabled, the mentally handicapped, and Gypsies. These events are recent and currently affect the circumstances of people around us. We have in our midst descendants of slaves and slave-owners, and people who themselves lived under Empire, apartheid, and the Nazi terror and are currently struggling because of immigration laws. The memories of these and similar horrors are still fresh—and they should remain so forever.

The most important lesson from this history is that research on migration status, race, ethnicity, and health needs to be done within an ethical framework emphasizing the potential benefit, primarily to the population studied. Benefits to society at large are secondary benefits but not trivially so, as I will discuss in Chapter 10. Some issues on ethics in research were discussed in Chapter 8, and a more general consideration of ethics in relation to ethnicity and health is given in Chapter 10.

Harm from minority health research is not inherent or inevitable, but is dependent on social and political context. Just as differences can be misused to bolster arguments justifying and promoting inequality, similarities can be used to ignore the needs of minorities. Researchers and practitioners will find themselves in a quandary as emphasizing differences can lead to action and interest (and money) but can be harmful, while emphasizing similarities can lead to their work being ignored as uninteresting. The argument that past research has done harm can impede new proposals that aim to undo such harms. This argument of past harms has value in cautioning us on potential dangers, but it must not be allowed to block ethical research.

Migration status, race, and ethnicity are controversial and difficult epidemiological variables, as discussed in Chapter 1. They are, however, effective in contributing to a crucial aspect of medical and public health strategy: demonstrating differences and similarities in the health, disease, and health-care experience between subgroups of the population, as discussed in Chapters 3, 5, and 6. Much research on ethnicity and health is epidemiological or sociological. Such research has two prime purposes: to describe the health status of ethnic minorities in the context of their life and environmental circumstances, and to use the information to redefine scientific understanding, health policy, and practice.

As illustrated in Chapter 8, by learning that CHD is common in migrant South Asian populations (and in other studies discussed in chapter 6 that the relationship between the rate of heart disease and social class is both complex and shifting over time), we can develop appropriate policies. Simultaneously, we can use these observations to seek understanding of the causal mechanisms of CHD. We might ask why heart disease is so high in a population originally from countries where heart disease was uncommon at the time of migration, and why it does not display the same social class gradient as in the general population. In the answers to such simple questions lie fundamental truths about the nature of disease. Clearly, the analysis and interpretation of such data may lead to hypotheses that in turn lead to an understanding of aetiology (cause)—and such understanding in turn should lead to better policy-making and practice.

Research which cannot, on its own, lead to causal understanding, such as the estimation of disease prevalence and incidence (and the derived rates and ratios), must not be over-interpreted to make hasty causal inferences. Its true value in generating testable hypotheses, shaping health policy, and improving practice can be overlooked in the excitement of premature causal analysis. The emphasis of researchers has been on comparing the health experience of the minority with that of the majority population (relative approach), and not on the numbers of cases of disease or the derived rates (absolute approach). As discussed in Chapters 5 and 7, by combining both approaches the power of the data to shape priorities and health strategies can be enhanced.

Characteristically, descriptive studies of minority health have concluded by emphasizing both enthusiastically and over-optimistically the great potential of their findings for understanding the fundamental causes of disease. Causal knowledge usually follows a spark of inspiration, which is pursued with detailed, painstaking, and carefully planned research designed to test hypotheses. No amount of enthusiasm about minority health research can overcome this basic requirement, and over-interpretation of data will, in the long term, impede progress, as discussed below.

9.1.3 Association and causation—black box epidemiology

An association is the scientific term for a statistical relationship between one factor and another. In the population health sciences associations are a vitally important starting point for the discovery of causes of illness, disease, and death. The analysis of associations is a complex aspect of epidemiology, and comprises both statistical and conceptual matters. Because understanding the cause of a disease can transform medicine and public health, the uncovering of new associations with the potential for understanding causes is exciting. As association implies there is an inequality. For example, one of the most important associations ever discovered is the one between smoking and cancer. Smokers have more cancer than non-smokers, i.e. there is an inequality. We have already discussed in detail the extent of inequality in disease outcome by migration status, race, and ethnicity (e.g. in Chapter 6). These inequalities are simply associations between minority status and health outcomes. For reasons already discussed, such inequalities are almost inevitable and unsurprising; and also, therefore, the discovery of associations is also unsurprising.

Indeed, thousands of associations between migration status, racial or ethnic group, and both disease and other health outcomes have been published with the expectation and proclamation that they will help in elucidating disease causation. However, few such associations have been explained in a way which gives new insight into causation. Most research on migration, race, ethnicity and health is black box epidemiology, described by Skrabanek (1994) as epidemiology where the causal mechanism behind an association remains unknown and hidden (black) but the inference is that the causal mechanism is within the association (the box). The metaphor is derived from the modern electronics industry where the circuitry and components are packaged in a closed box. Users make no attempt to examine or understand the contents (indeed there may be a warning not to open the box) and even a mechanic is not expected to open the box and diagnose the problem. When problems occur the entire component is replaced. Skrabanek argued that science must open and understand the black box. He likened black box epidemiology to repetitively punching a soft pillow (i.e. doing the same kind of research), and when the dimple refills (the association is perhaps forgotten) taking another blow, perhaps in a different place, but with the end result being the same (the association is rediscovered).

This black box metaphor and Skrabanek's general warning is of the utmost importance in the field of minority health research. If the field is expected to deliver causal advances then it will lose its credibility, funding, and researchers if it does not do so. One of the longest-standing forms of epidemiology that generates associations is international comparison. For example, many studies have looked at patterns of cancer in immigrant populations internationally. These studies have typically found huge variations in most cancers, effectively clarifying that, given the homogeneity of the human genome across countries, cancers are primarily caused by non-genetic causal factors. These international studies spurred migration studies that showed, generally, that cancer patterns in the migrating populations converge towards those of the recipient (or host) population. It is within this context that we need to ask the critical question of what the additional research value of studying the health of minorities within a country or region actually is. Cancers are poorly understood from a causal perspective, so it is pertinent to trace the history of the contribution of minority health research.

I will briefly examine this history in the UK. Marmot et al.'s (1984) analysis of cancers in immigrants in England and Wales around the 1971 census period found many differences. Overall, immigrants had lower cancer rates, although for specific cancers the picture was very varied—sometimes higher, often lower. The authors' approach is illustrated by their emphasis on causal hypotheses. For example, they note high correlations in international data for cancers of the large intestine and female breast with both heart disease and fat consumption. This raises the possibility that fat consumption is an underlying common causal factor. Their observation of low rates for these two cancers in Indian immigrants, but high rates for heart disease, leads them to question the assumption that dietary fat is the common factor in cancer of the large bowel and breast. They query whether the high fibre content of the Indian diet modifies the effect of fat on large bowel cancer. This is a very interesting observation, and is one of many that could, potentially, have led to detailed causal research and novel understanding. The next large scale contribution was the study of immigrant populations by region of origin by Balarajan and Bulusu (1990) around the 1981 census. This study also found many differences from which causal hypotheses were drawn.

On a more local scale Donaldson and Clayton (1984) found numerous ethnic differences in cancer registration patterns in the Leicestershire health district. The authors rightly concluded that 'The results indicate the need for formal epidemiological study to test specific aetiological hypotheses which may account for these apparent differences'. Examples of this type of local work have been reported by Barker and Baker (1990) in Bradford and by Matheson et al. (1985) in Scotland. Similar work has been done on children. The conclusion is almost predictable: differences exist and need detailed study. Wild et al. (2006) published on the cancer data by country of birth around the 2001 census. Again, marked variations were shown. Unfortunately, our level of causal understanding shows little advance (if any) from the analysis of 1971 data by Marmot et al. (1984). The main difference, however, is that the work of Wild et al. (2006) puts more emphasis on the value of such data for policy, planning, and health needs assessment. Using the SHELS, Bhopal et al. (2012) analysed rates of all cancers, lung, breast, colorectal, and prostate cancer by ethnic group in the period 2001–8. As in previous such work, the findings showed very interesting associations by ethnic group. Unfortunately, the explanations for these associations were, with one exception, of the kind already advanced in several previous papers. The one exception was a new idea on why South Asian populations have low rates of colorectal cancer. The main hypothesis under scrutiny is the potential protective effects of spices in Indian cuisine and high levels of fruit, vegetables, and fibre in the diet. By contrast, Bhopal and colleagues proposed that it was a result of low exposure to processed meats. In this paper, and in a major review by Arnold et al. (2010) of European work on migrant groups, a few, small-scale research projects testing hypotheses are cited but most projects describe variations and come up with similar observations. Skrabenek's repeatedly punched pillow comes to mind. In the Scottish study Bhopal et al. (2012) called for a research unit to be set up specifically to study ethnic variations in cancer from a causal perspective, based on testing hypotheses. Bhopal et al. also emphasized the separate importance of such work in public health policy and strategy and in spurring the improvement of cancer-related health for the entire population, especially the White Scottish population that had the highest rates of disease.

There has been too little progression in causal thinking, in my view, because few studies have explored the often ingenious and potentially invaluable ideas generated by observational epidemiology over the very long timescales required. In any place, population health research starts with description. As we have considered, given the state-of-the-art in relation to data collection systems, description is a difficult task in itself. Given the small research workforce working on minority health it is not surprising that capitalizing on causal potential has been hard. One illustrative exception, where a hypothesis has been doggedly pursued, is the study of diabetes and insulin resistance as the potential basis of the surprisingly high rates of CHD in South Asian communities. The observation of Marmot et al. (1984) places this in context:

> This high rate of diabetes could contribute to the high rate of ischaemic heart disease in Indians. This explanation would then pose the problem of why immigrants from the Caribbean, with their high rate of diabetes do not also have a high rate of ischaemic heart disease.
>
> Marmot et al. (1984, p. 51).

The answer to this question has been pursued tenaciously from studies of South Asian groups and African Caribbean groups, and sometimes both together. It turns out that the role of diabetes and insulin resistance is probably a partial but important explanation, and new avenues still need to be explored.

The research effort around this question has been UK-led but has also been international, and it has been ongoing for some 30 years. In pursuit of this and related questions we have seen the development of new prospective cohort studies and the redesign of cross-sectional studies. It will probably be another 10–20 years before we get more definitive answers. The lesson is that for causal advances we need to move on from the repetitious demonstration of disease variations which have previously been shown either in migration, race, ethnicity, and health research, or in work on international variations, or in social and gender variations. Minority health studies are able to provide models and contexts for advancing causal knowledge if research questions are clearly articulated and pursued using sound methods. However, they do not provide an easy route to causal understanding. It is wiser for our field to emphasize the importance of data for policy, strategy, and planning, especially in relation to public health improvement, than to make scientific promises that are seldom fulfilled.

Of the medical sciences, with the possible exceptions of medical sociology and medical anthropology, the one that has grappled with minority health issues most seriously is epidemiology. As with other sciences, epidemiology has been beguiled by migration, race, and ethnicity and has sometimes become racialized. Racialization is the idea that race is a primary, natural, and neutral means of grouping humans, and that racial groups are distinct in other ways, e.g. in their behaviours (see Chapter 10). (The equivalent for migrant health would be migrantization and for ethnicity would be ethnicization, but racialization will do to cover these variations.) There are modern lessons to be learned here, especially from the racialized research of the 19th century.

9.2 **Race and related research, history and harm: some lessons**

This book has provided examples of research that has done harm, e.g. in Chapters 1 and 6, but this topic deserves a more detailed discussion, even at the risk of repetition.

Racialized research of the kind now referred to by the phrases 'race science' and 'scientific racism' has an inglorious history, and many books have recorded in detail the extent of the work that has been done (see, e.g., Gould 1984, Kiple and King 1981). Some important scientists of the 19th century, in particular, were focused on race, and their fascination was encouraged by influential and powerful politicians and social commentators. The power behind scientific racism is illustrated by the prowess of some of the researchers involved, including Louis Agassiz, Francis Galton, Paul Broca, and John Down. (The details of their contributions are given in Gould (1984) and other volumes listed in the Bibliography.). All four are men of huge scientific stature, often listed in even small recently published encyclopaedias. The lesson for the present is that scientists work within the framework of thought of their times. Scientists also shape this framework—they are not merely passive onlookers. Currently, we are under similar influences that in future may be obviously flawed even though they seem sensible to us now. I am conscious, for example, that the Glossary in this book may be seen as a product of the times.

In the 19th century, northern European scientists were influential and busy ranking races on their biological and social worth, in particular using measurements of the size and shape of the head and the volume of the brain as an indirect means to measure intelligence (is it surprising that the northern European groups ranked highly?). Such research was undoubtedly interesting, at least to those doing it. It was also useful to politicians and others as a partial argument to justify slavery, imperialism, anti-immigration policy, and the social status quo. After all, if this viewpoint on intelligence was true, and at that time both common sense and science seemed to coincide on it, and northern Europeans were indeed the most intelligent of humans, their world dominance was inevitable and possibly even desirable, if not essential, for the well-being of humanity. In 1899 the Imperialist poet Rudyard Kipling published 'The White Man's Burden' which captures the idea that the superiority of the White man imposes a duty to colonize and rule even against the will of those so dominated, for their good. Reading the poem now one wonders whether it was political satire, but apparently it was not. Similar arguments and data were used to analyse the role of men and women in society and justify the subordinate role of women. One underlying value of this 19th-century research was that biology, i.e. genetics, determined social position—biological determinism. If this were true, there was nothing to be done about the social hierarchy—it was an act of nature and an act that was most attractive to the advantaged groups.

As we noted earlier, doctors were important contributors to racialized medical science. Disease labels such as drapetomania (the irrational and pathological desire of slaves to run away) and dysaethesia Aethiopica (rascality) were invented to describe the behaviours of slaves. Cartwright (1851), who invented the label drapetomania, said 'It is unknown to our medical authorities, although its diagnostic symptom, the absconding from service, is well known to our planters'. Again, this kind of writing comes over now as zany humour but it was a serious matter then.

To quote a textbook of obstetrics and gynaecology 'the pelves becomes increasingly lower and broader the more civilized the race from which it is obtained' and 'coloured children weigh considerably less than white, a fact which, in large cities at least, is indicative of the physical degeneration which characterizes the race' (Whitridge Williams 1926). The words and tone (civilized, degeneration) display very clearly the writer's stance and the arrogance of the society he represented. At the time this language would have been seen as justifying the self-evident truth. These phenomena of differences in skull size and shape, pelvic dimensions, and birth weight (still there and causing great controversy in relation to cause) are still noted and discussed but in different language and different interpretation. The great debate at present on birth weight differentials by race or ethnicity revolves around socio-economic circumstances or biology, not physical degeneration. It seems a sensible dialogue to us but it may be judged naïve or harmful by future generations.

John Down's theory of 'mongolism' (trisomy 21 or Down syndrome) (Down 1867) was that such infants were from an inferior, Mongoloid, race. Down interpreted this in a positive and humanitarian way and proposed that this demonstrated the unity of the human species, i.e. Europeans could give birth to children like those of another race. The problem here is that Down syndrome is characterized by mental handicap. It is insulting to Mongoloid peoples to offer this analogy. The example is an apt one because it shows the deeply ingrained thinking around race and inequality at that time.

Dr James McCune Smith, an African American who graduated from the University of Glasgow, Scotland in 1837 and worked in the United States, argued that the environment, not innate biology, was responsible for health differences, showing that poor White families had similar patterns of diseases to Black ones. Such challenges to biologically driven explanations for health inequalities are still needed. Remarkably, some very recent research papers in the United States are showing exactly what McCune Smith said. As then, so it is now—very often it is people from minorities who have the insights and knowledge to provide the more valid accounts of the causes of differences.

Gamble (1993) has argued that the Tuskegee syphilis study, discussed in Chapter 1, has left a legacy of mistrust that has continued to undermine good medical practice up to recent times. Gamble also recounts Thomas Hamilton's experiments testing remedies for heat stroke and those of Dr J. Marion Sims on surgery for vesico-vaginal fistula, done on slaves. While the Tuskegee study cast a long shadow, recent work shows African Americans are both trusting of their health services and active users of them—their main problem being lack of easy access to high-quality services. It is undoubtedly true that race science died out following the Second World War—killed off by the Nazi horrors. This does not necessarily mean that research, even when meant to be beneficial, cannot be harmful.

Osborne and Feit's (1992) review of modern American health research on race and ethnicity concluded that much of it is racist in its effect, if not in intention, because many projects focus on Black/White differences in diseases associated with promiscuity, under-achievement, and anti-social behaviour and imply that the underlying explanation lies in internal factors such as race rather than external factors such as class, lifestyle, or socio-economic status. This is a very important point—it's not just the intent of the research that matter but its interpretation. There is also the closely related issue of what is studied by researchers. Osborne and Feit noted that the research topics given special significance to public health policy makers were those where the minority is perceived to be doing worse than the majority. Giving attention to such matters makes some sense, but the negative effects of the resultant publications are predictable. Disease and health problems become associated with minorities to the detriment of their social standing.

The concept of a package of specific 'ethnic' diseases which are associated with minority ethnic groups, and therefore worthy of special study and exploration, has echoes in the history of medicine and racism. The susceptibility of Negroes to particular diseases, such as leprosy, tetanus, pneumonia, scurvy, and sore eyes was, as Kiple and King (1981) argue, misinterpreted, and the differences, on which scientists' attention was riveted, led to nonsensical race-related hypotheses on causation.

It may well be that in the future our hypotheses will also be seen as nonsensical. In this historical sketch I have mostly referred to African Americans—the current terminology that reflects an increasing population preference. However, for most of their history they were called Negroes (see Glossary), reflecting their lack of power in self-determining their own description. Since those times our field has de-emphasized biology and shifted to culture and socio-economic status. With the partial exception of the United States, the subject of racism has not achieved prominence.

Indeed, Krieger et al.'s (1993) review of racism, sexism, and class concluded that science was unable to explain a myriad of racial/ethnic differences in health. They criticized current models of ethnicity and health research which focus on racial differences but usually do not study racism. (Since then, a modest increase in the research effort on racism and health has occurred.)

Before the end of the Second World War few scientists questioned whether their work in this field was ethical. They could not be aware, of course, that such work would inspire Hitler, the Nazis, and the Final Solution, but they would have been well aware of the contemporary effects and uses of their work. Given the circumstances of the time, their 'racist-in-effect' work was probably welcomed as important. With hindsight, much of the race-oriented science of the past was unethical, invalid, racist, and inhumane, even though it was perceived at the time to be of great importance. Nevertheless, there is absolutely no doubt that many medical practitioners and researchers were openly racist. In Chapter 6 I discussed how strongly the medical profession supported Hitler. The South African Medical Association colluded with the policies of apartheid in South Africa, not least through its *South African Medical Journal*, as discussed by Ellison and De Wet (1997). In April 2006 *The Lancet* published articles reopening the debate on whether racists who have achieved distinction through eponyms should have their names stripped from the disease or disorder they helped to define, e.g. Reiter was a Nazi doctor known to have committed war crimes but his name is hallowed through its association with Reiter's syndrome (Woywodt et al. 2006).

In the last 60 or so years, the concept of race as a valid and important way of defining human subspecies biologically has been eroded under the impact of scientific and social scrutiny. The idea of biological race, however, is far from extinct. The application of the concept of ethnicity is often indistinguishable from that of race, with a heavy and unwarranted emphasis on genetics, which means that the same criticisms apply. *The Bell Curve*, by Hernstern and Murray (1994), is a reminder that research which purports to demonstrate the innate inferiority, particularly in intelligence, of some racial groups continues and that race science is alive. This book was a best-seller and re-ignited long-standing controversies. This is not to deny the possibility that some contemporary authors have benevolent motives, which seems less likely for 19th-century writers. In April 2006, *The Sunday Times*, one of the UK's most influential newspapers, published a letter from a number of distinguished scientists stating that racial differences in IQ are a matter of fact, and claiming that it is likely that the lower IQ of some races is genetic (Lynn et al. 2006). The controversy around race and IQ simmers, but shows no signs of dying. I see no end to this debate because there is no way of moving from association to causation (or no causation). In complex situations such as this the normal way to resolve the controversy is to run a controlled trial or experiment. In the case of IQ and race one cannot envisage any practical or ethical trial that will lead to a definitive answer. The interpretation of the available non-trial, observational data is open to bias by the values of observers. Unlike the past, the contemporary dominant values are that all human groups are equal and the undeniable group differences in IQ mostly, if not wholly, reflect social, economic, and cultural variations between populations. It is important to note that this is also only one possible interpretation of the data, just as the biological one is, but one that better chimes with the mores of the 21st century.

In taking their stance on modern-day controversies, researchers can benefit from an understanding of how race and health research was abused in the past. Epidemiologists who think that racial prejudice could not influence science in the modern era might read about the Tuskegee syphilis study which examined the natural history of syphilis in 600 poor 'Negroes' in Alabama between 1932 and 1972, actively denying them effective treatments and hastening many deaths (see Jones 1993). I introduced this study in Chapter 1. It is not that these researchers, working under the noble auspices of the US Public Health Service, wanted to do harm or be racist. Rather, they were influenced by the racist ethos of the society they were part of.

Similarly, I believe that few modern-day researchers in the field of migration, ethnicity, and health research are racist, and I know that most hold humanitarian views. However, many researchers are working to a racialized research agenda (my own work is no exception—I have, after all, been using British census type ethnic group categories on the presumption they delineate meaningful population groups). If most of the current work under way is in a future era judged as racist as well as racialized, future historians should remember that it was unwittingly so. It may be, however, that this defence also applies to much historical work, and it looks very weak now.

Our current work may be seen in the future as being done within a framework of institutional racism in research, and as bolstering such racism. (See Chapter 6 for a discussion of various forms of racism.) Simply switching from race to ethnicity or migration status does not solve the problem. Applying these arguments to ethnicity, might our work be seen as 'ethnicized' research, and the fuel of 'ethnicism'? (A similar perspective can be applied to migration research and work on indigenous groups.) In a wide-ranging review of UK research through to the early 1990s, Donovan (1984) warned that we were heading this way:

> A great deal of the published research in this area has come from the medical profession, published in journals such as The Lancet, *the* British Medical Journal, *the* Proceedings of the Royal Society of Medicine, *with* very little contribution from the black population. Consequently, there has been a bias in the work, characterized by a concentration on illnesses and diseases that interest doctors, central Government and the health service administrators; rickets, tuberculosis and sickle-cell anaemia being examples. This concentration on 'interesting' or 'unusual' ailments has meant that the opinions of black people about their own health have been largely ignored, as have the obvious links between health and the large and growing literature on 'race relations', including levels of deprivation and racial discrimination experienced by black people in Britain.
>
> Donovan (1984, p. 663), reproduced with permission from Elsevier.

Certainly the focus in the UK in the 1970s and 1980s on 'ethnic problems' such as the high birth rate, 'Asian rickets', the haemoglobinopathies, congenital defects, and consanguinity, was at the expense of common problems such as CHD (now being tackled), smoking, alcohol, and cancer. Health education materials for minority ethnic groups in the 1980s were available on birth control, lice, child care, and even spitting but there was nothing on heart disease, and little on smoking and alcohol. In the 1990s through to the present day a better balance has been achieved. Looking at the research agendas of other countries we also often see a similar pattern, e.g. in recent years female genital mutilation has been a prominent topic. It would be interesting to assess whether the relevant minority populations would also perceive it as a prominent priority.

In the 19th century millions had their skulls measured by craniologists to no discernible lasting benefit either to themselves, their racial or ethnic group, or society at large. As we have seen, there are many such examples of abuse and harm. Yet health research based on migration status, race, and ethnicity remains popular. As sizeable and potentially important differences by migration status, race, and ethnicity have been easy to describe, the literature on minority health is growing rapidly. This trend will accelerate as more societies become multicultural. We must work to ensure that this accelerating research endeavour does not suffer the fate of 19th-century work.

It is already clear that much race, ethnicity, and migration research is unsound because the questions posed are not relevant or answerable or because the underlying theories, concepts, principles, and methods are not adequate. We must do better. The remainder of this chapter will focus on good practice in research.

9.3 Research: application of the migration status, race, and ethnicity measures in a variety of research designs

Try Exercise 9.2 before reading on (readers unfamiliar with research methods in epidemiology may want to read a little on that first; see Bhopal 2008). The Glossary provides brief definitions, and the text following the exercise also introduces these methods.

Exercise 9.2 Strengths and weaknesses of study designs in relation to minority health

Choose a topic that interests you, and is relevant to minority health. What are the strengths and weaknesses of the following research methods in advancing minority health research in your chosen topic:

- (traditional) literature review, systematic review, and meta-analysis,
- case reports,
- clinical case series,
- population register studies (also known as population case series),
- case–control studies,
- cross-sectional studies,
- cohort studies,
- trials,
- studies of genetic structure, family pedigrees, and genetic associations?

There are many forms of research with distinct purposes, processes, and outcomes. Neither the claims that minority health research is of great value, nor the criticisms, are likely to apply uniformly to all forms of research. My answers to Exercise 9.2 are summarized in Table 9.1. In addition, we will consider qualitative methods later in this chapter.

Table 9.1 Strengths and weaknesses of a number of methods of research in the context of migration status, race, ethnicity, and health

Method	Strengths	Weaknesses
Literature review	Quick, brings experience from all over the world, cheap	Often there is no good literature by minority group for many topics; much work is unpublished or difficult to obtain; work may be published in local reports; may be in languages other than English so adding translation difficulties and costs; hard to generalize between studies because of different contexts and terminology; and the review may lead to biased conclusions and recommendations
Systematic review	As above, except that it is much more time-consuming, but in return this ensures work is more comprehensive and minimizes biases	As above, and synthesis may be impossible for lack of comparable work, e.g. lack of clarity in concepts and terminology and heterogeneity of populations or study methods
Meta-analysis	Permits quantitative synthesis of key outcomes and relations between risk factors and outcomes	As above, and may not be reported in a way that permits synthesis of questionnaire data; getting hold of original data may prove too difficult because researchers are scattered and not organized into cooperative groups
Case reports	Rapid highlighting of issues for fuller investigation	Likely to be on rare and obscure or exotic issues, e.g. a case report is not going to be on lung cancer but may be on lead poisoning. This will skew understanding of minority health priorities
Clinical series	As above, but brings together experience of a clinician or group of clinicians. Rapid publication of admittedly selective statistics on large populations; gives overview of a clinical problem	As above, but more likely than a single report to be on matters common enough to be of importance at a population level
Population registers or case series	As above but the series is of all the known experience in a defined area and population so is less biased	The statistical summary is often not stratified by minority group (for lack of ethnic coding); the information is limited; errors such as numerator/denominator mismatch arise
Case–control studies	Feasible at reasonable cost and timescales, particularly when based in places where minority populations are large	The number of cases (outcomes) of interest may be too small, particularly for studies of incident as opposed to prevalent cases; problem of identifying cases and controls by minority group in the absence of minority status coding in population health databases; recall bias may be great and medical records may be incomplete for recent migrants in particular

(Continued)

Table 9.1 (Continued)

Method	Strengths	Weaknesses
Cross-sectional studies	The most feasible design for new research and best for burden of risk factors and common diseases	Needs a sampling frame so representative samples can be identified—these lists are not usually coded by minority group status; response rates may not be consistent across study subgroups
Cohort studies	Excellent for measuring incidence rates, survival, and risk-factor outcome relationships	Need to be large, long-term, and so are very expensive. Hard to set up and maintain. Experience in such work is limited but growing worldwide
Trials	The definitive method for evaluation of drugs, services, and public health interventions, especially if it is the placebo-controlled, randomized design	For legal and ethical reasons trials are even harder to set up than cohort studies but otherwise have similar weaknesses. Trials deliberately designed to compare effects by ethnic group are few and usually from the United States. The theoretical basis and need for such studies is under intense debate
Genetic studies	These are necessary to quantify what we already know—that health states arise mostly from gene–environment interactions. The large family size and close family links (including consanguinity in some populations) makes some minority populations attractive for such work	The techniques are evolving and the ideas are unfamiliar to all populations but particularly minority groups. There is the danger that these studies will focus on specific issues and stigmatize minority groups. There are fears of the return of race science

   Researchers must clarify the purpose for which the research is being done and carefully choose the research design, analysis, and presentation to meet it. Sometimes there will need to be a mix of methods and designs. Excepting the migration study, which applies the above designs in a specific way (considered in Section 9.1.1), there is no form of research that is unique to the field of minority health.

   Literature review is a starting point for all work, whatever the purpose, and preferably it should be a systematic one whenever possible. Literature review is simply a written summary of published work on the question of interest. Traditionally, the researcher would make a personal selection of publications to summarize. The problem is that this process is potentially biased. At worst the researcher might choose the articles that provide the answer wanted either by the scholar or the authorities, e.g. minorities have higher rates of schizophrenia. At best, the selection might be random but not pointing to the depth of knowledge available, especially from sources that are not easily accessed. The logical response to this problem is to have an objective procedure for finding, accessing, retrieving, and summarizing available data. This is the systematic review—but this also poses problems, e.g. what kind of databases will be searched? In the field of minority health it is common for work to be published either in reports (perhaps nowadays only on websites but previously only in limited circulation) or in the less readily available specialist journals. Yet most systematic reviews concentrate on the best established scientific journals, where peer review systems are designed to maximize quality. For example, a search of MEDLINE would be considered essential—and for some purposes sufficient. MEDLINE, however, only covers a fraction of all journals. Notwithstanding this criticism, systematic reviews should be done wherever possible, though they are far more difficult and expensive than traditional ones. A meta-analysis is simply the quantitative joint summary of the work included in a systematic review. This requires comparable quantitative data, which are scarce in the field of migration, race, and ethnicity research. Such reviews serve a vital function in exposing gaps in the research record and pointing to what needs to be done. There is a strong argument that this kind of work should be a prior requirement for all new empirical research. The problem is time and money—systematic reviews typically take 3–6 months of full-time work and sometimes much longer.

Is your purpose to improve the quality of care? Remarkably, even a single case report of poor care can help spur improvement. It would be even better to look at quality of care in a series of patients, and even better still if all people attending a service were included (population register/population case-series). Then one could design a study around one of the priority issues, such as communication between minority patients and professionals. Such a study is likely to include evaluation of the outcomes and an audit of whether expected standards of care are being met and improved. Perhaps, ultimately, you will conduct a trial as a definitive test of the effectiveness and/or cost-effectiveness of any intervention you recommend.

Is your purpose to measure how common risk factors or diseases are and to set public health priorities? Then measure their incidence or prevalence, or both. The study is likely to be one based on routine statistics on death, or diagnosis of diseases held in population health registers, or will use cross-sectional or cohort designs to collect new data.

Do you wish to generate hypotheses about the causes of specific diseases? Then you will need to read the scientific literature in great depth (not in the way of a systematic review), and examine published statistics and cross-sectional and cohort data for group variations. That occasionally might be enough to develop some brilliant insight into causation. If not, you may undertake a hypothesis-generating case–control study. Typically, in a case–control study people with the health outcome we want to understand are compared with a control or reference population, ideally one that is representative of the population that gave rise to the cases. In the field of minority health we have the interesting added option of having two or more case groups and two or more control groups, i.e. one for each ethnic group under study. Such refinements in the design are rare but feasible (see, e.g., Chambers et al. 2000). Case–control studies can test prior well-defined hypotheses and generate new ones, e.g. through the analysis of stored research materials or data linkage.

You may, however, develop ideas from first principles and publish a data-free hypothesis paper. As we have already discussed in relation to cancer, the observation of variations by migration status, race, and ethnicity does trigger many interesting ideas that are too seldom taken forward. Hypothesis or, even better, theory papers are a prelude to new research for they force a detailed consideration of the question, including consideration of how the hypothesis is to be tested.

Typically, to test hypotheses in epidemiology you need cohort study data. Alternatively, you test your hypotheses one by one using the experimental approach. Investigators should expect to spend years or more probably decades before their hypotheses are accepted or rejected, though the latter result is usually quicker.

Differences in disease patterns do not always yield testable hypotheses, but even testable hypotheses have too often remained untested or been superficially examined. There are numerous disease patterns in the literature on migration, race, and ethnicity which have been little studied beyond the initial observation of difference, even though they could be. Explaining them is just too difficult within the short time periods that most researchers devote to a project. One reason is the lack of long-term funding, as most projects are funded for up to 3 years and researchers' contracts may be much shorter.

Different forms of research may need, generate, and apply different facets of the concepts of race and ethnicity and of migration status. The population subgroup classifications required are also likely to vary according to the type of research. For illustration of these points, three forms of research are considered here: surveillance, health services research, and causal epidemiological research (introduced in Chapter 3 in less detail).

Before reading on try Exercise 9.3.

Exercise 9.3 Applying concepts of migration status, race, and ethnicity in research

In what ways might the concepts be applied differently for:

+ monitoring/surveillance research?
+ research on the quantity and quality of care?
+ research trying to understand disease causation?

9.3.1 Surveillance and its relationship to coding of routine health data systems

Surveillance is the analysis, interpretation, and feedback of systematically collected data with methods distinguished by their practicality, uniformity, and rapidity, particularly to detect change in the pattern of disease or death. In the context of minority health, the main objective of surveillance is to detect and track variations in the health of populations grouped by migration status, race, or ethnicity. Of course, the data should be used to monitor the impact of interventions to improve health and reduce variations.

In practice, surveillance systems usually use simple indicators such as colour (black/white), nationality or ancestral origins (Indian/Pakistani), or country of birth as the foundations of their classification. Surveillance systems almost always use routinely collected health and health-care data, often needed for administrative or other non-health reasons. These data systems need to have space for appropriate codes for migration status, race, or ethnicity. (We have discussed the challenges in Chapter 3.) In respect to self-reported race and ethnicity, current classifications in the United States and the UK are primarily based on the concepts underlying race, i.e. colour and region of the world (continental grouping). The same is true for indicators of migration status, such as country of birth of self, parents, or grandparents. We have already discussed the limitations of definition of race as a reflection of biology. These kinds of categories are actually used more as indictors of social and political context and not primarily as sources of biological information. Exactly the same applies to the US ethnic group category 'Hispanic'. It is purportedly based on language (Spanish), but in effect it is a mix of region of origin and history of ancestors living in a place under Spanish colonial rule. Generally, surveillance indicators, with the exception of Hispanic, are closely tied to the race concept or migration status. Other markers of population characteristics such as language or religious origin, more closely tied to the ethnicity concept, may also be used, but are rare in surveillance systems that are focused on health status. These other characteristics are increasingly recognized as important for surveillance systems for health-care access, utilization, and quality and are likely to be increasingly prominent in the future.

Mostly, surveillance systems have adopted and incorporated migration status, racial, and ethnic classifications that were developed for political or health policy purposes. The OMB classification, first published in 1977, still dominates in the United States (see Chapter 2). Occasionally some databases report data using the classification of White and non-White. It is important to reflect on the nature of categories required for surveillance.

Hahn and Stroup (1994) recommend that a surveillance category should be conceptually valid, accurately measurable, exclusive and exhaustive, meaningful to respondents, reliable, consistent, and flexible. Those recommendations are ambitious, and are rarely if ever achieved in practice. They and others have questioned the conceptual validity of categories such as Hispanic, Latino, and Asian but, interestingly, they (and a few others) have not criticized the category White. Given its importance, both in terms of population size and the role of this category as a point of comparison of other groups, it also deserves scrutiny. Bhopal and Donaldson (1998) pointed out the severe limitations of White as a valid category. While the US census has 10 subcategories for Asian or Pacific Islanders, it has none for White, which accounts for most of the population. The focus of surveillance is therefore necessarily on non-White minority groups. This is not justifiable rationally, even for the purposes of anti-discrimination policy (the OMB categories are for this), because some White populations may be disadvantaged, e.g. those arriving as refugees, particularly from non-English-speaking countries, but also economically disadvantaged sub-populations, e.g. eastern Europeans migrating to western Europe. In recognition of this the SHELS has taken care to examine data for White Scottish, White Other British, White Irish, and Other White populations separately. The case for doing so becomes clear once this is done. The 2011 Scottish census increased the White subgroup categories to specifically count disadvantaged groups such as White Gypsy Travellers and people of Polish origin. There were five specific categories and one write in category for White in the 2011 census.

Surveillance has been constrained by the need to use the census classifications to obtain the population size (denominator for the calculation of a rate) data so essential for constructing the rates and summaries of rates (such as SMRs) which are the basis of surveillance. If changes are to be made to surveillance systems, the migration status, race, and ethnicity categories used need to be comparable with census or population registry codes.

For reasons of historical practice, perceived need, cost, simplicity, and stability over time, the classifications used in surveillance systems divide populations in a fairly crude way. It would be unfortunate if the pragmatic uses of these categories in surveillance systems imply that they were in any sense fixed, natural, or scientifically validated. Future surveillance systems are likely to change to the use of more specific variables reflecting not just the needs of disease surveillance but also health-care surveillance.

9.3.2 Health services research

Unlike surveillance, health services research is not easily defined and it takes many forms, although in its essence it is broadly about evaluation of services. It is about the organization, costs, effectiveness, quantity, and quality of health services, particularly in relation to processes and health outcomes. Where health services research is examining issues of access to and utilization of care, the migration status, race, and ethnicity concepts to be used and classifications needed are likely to be similar to those for surveillance (it is health-care surveillance) and subject to the same limitations and criticisms. However, more so than for surveillance, heterogeneity within each category is a major limitation.

Consider the uptake of breast cancer screening by mammography. The health services research question—'Is the programme being accessed by all racial or ethnic groups?'—is akin to surveillance. (The equivalent disease surveillance question might be what is the rate of breast cancer across racial and/or ethnic group categories and how is it changing over time?) There is an important difference, however, and that is one of heterogeneity. Categories used in surveillance—perhaps sufficient to detect variation and change—such as South Asian, Hispanic, Black, etc. are unreliably crude in this health-care context. The programme may be accessed well by South Asians, overall, but not well by an important subgroup such as, say, Bangladeshi Muslims. Nonetheless, in terms of answering this question and tracing progress, a relatively simple classification by migrant group, race, or ethnicity would suffice. The South Asian group might be subdivided into Indian, Pakistani, and Bangladeshi and perhaps also (or alternatively) by religion (say Hindu, Muslim, Other) and language (Hindi, Urdu, Punjabi, Gujarati, Other). A mix of relevant group categories could be derived, the relevant data could be collected quickly, and this research question could be answered.

However, when the issue is research for the development of new policy or to effect change, or the evaluation of the quality or effectiveness of care, a deeper understanding of the populations under consideration is necessary. The question here might be 'Why is mammography less well taken up by some minority groups?'. To understand why, say, the uptake of mammography was low in the South Asian community, is a question which focuses on causes. Here issues such as the group's religious views, language of communication, and beliefs about the importance of disease prevention, screening, cancer, and the nature of the service available become important. The socio-economic standing and educational attainment is likely to be influential. This is also the case, of course, for all populations, including majority White ones.

In addition, the attitudes and behaviours of service providers are crucial. In so far as racial discrimination may play a role, the migration status, ethnicity, or race of a group will be important. Service providers, and the system they work within, may not treat populations equitably, for reason we considered in Chapter 6. They may perceive some populations to be unentitled (say undocumented migrants) and others uninterested for cultural reasons (say women from populations with low rates of disease or high levels of personal modesty). The service may not have made provision to inform some populations, e.g. those who do not read the main language of the nation. In exploring this question, then, crude indicators such as religion, race, ethnic group, or place of birth are no more than a means of describing the situation and a way of deriving a sample for more detailed work which will include measuring directly those population characteristics thought to be causally relevant. Here, migration status, race, and ethnicity are variables which, in themselves, generate little or no understanding of the underlying problem and hence do not serve the purpose of health services research on their own. The 'black box' of causality needs to be opened to answer the causal question. We shall now develop this theme further.

9.3.3 **Causes of disease**

For research on disease causation the principles are the same as in the kind of health services research which seeks to understand why something happens. Here the question is 'Why is there variation in disease pattern by migration status, race, and/or ethnic group?'. The explanation is, conceptually, that either the variation is a chance result, an artefact of study bias, or it is real. If it is real either exposure to the risk (causal) factors varies by migration status, race, and/or ethnic group or the effects of the risk (causal factors) differ. If it is the latter then we can say there is effect modification (or interaction), i.e. the association between risk factor and disease outcome varies across categories of migration status, race, or ethnicity. This conceptual framework, simple as it is, is a great challenge in medical and population health research generally. The field of migration, race, and ethnicity is only now acquiring databases that are detailed and large enough to make serious progress.

Migration status, ethnicity, and race are, without question, good markers (or indicators) that can help us to discover and measure variations which merit investigation, and are also excellent for identifying relevant populations for the detailed studies that are required. They are also appropriate for sparking hypotheses, but are rarely in themselves, for reasons already discussed, the source of causal knowledge. The same also applies to other epidemiological variables such as age group or social class. Indeed, difficulty in causal interpretation is intrinsic to population health sciences. The contribution of population sciences to scientific understanding of causation is too complex to do justice to here, but it has been discussed in my book *Concepts of Epidemiology* (Bhopal 2008). The process of establishing causality is a long and difficult one, starting with associations—links between risk factors and the diseases (or other health outcomes)—of interest. Mostly, the associations arise by chance or from errors and biases in the research methods. Confounding is a huge problem in population sciences where experiments are not possible. Confounding arises when there are differences between the populations being compared that have not been fully controlled for. Confounding is especially important to the migration, race, and ethnicity field and is worth reflecting on with an example.

One classic example of confounding is the observation that those who drink alcohol are more likely to develop lung cancer. There is an association between alcohol consumption and the disease, but is it causal? Assume that we have assembled a group of 50-year-old male alcohol drinkers and compared them with men of the same age who do not drink alcohol, and that there are no errors in study measurement and the results are unlikely to have arisen by chance. What explanation is there that you can think of except that alcohol causes lung cancer?

Is it possible that alcohol drinkers are either more likely to be smokers or to be exposed to tobacco smoke? Perhaps, if so, alcohol is not itself a cause of lung cancer but tobacco use is? This phenomenon is known as confounding. Here the variable under study is alcohol consumption, but imagine it was migration status (foreign born compared with locally born), race (African Americans compared with White Americans), or ethnicity (Punjabis compared with Bengali Indians). The issues of confounding would be even more difficult to think out and resolve.

The best way of controlling for confounding is experimentation. We can do animal experiments where the effects of alcohol on lung cancer are studied. In the migration, race, and ethnicity fields there are no possible equivalent animal experiments. We can with more difficulty imagine experiments on humans too, either where people are given alcohol, or perhaps more likely stopped from drinking alcohol, to see the effects on disease outcome (here lung cancer or its precursors, e.g. malignant change in cells). With a few exceptions on very specific issues it is not possible to alter the indicators relating to migration, race, and ethnicity in this way. The comparison in the population sciences such as epidemiology is, ideally, between the population with the risk factor and exactly the *same* (so-called counterfactual) population without the risk factor. This is obviously impossible in practice but it clarifies what we are trying to do. Changing the exposure of one randomly chosen subgroup of the population in an experiment and comparing with a similarly chosen control group, where exposure has not been altered, comes close to this ideal. In population sciences, experimentation with randomization of populations is usually problematic and mostly we make do with a similar population (not randomly chosen) without the risk factor. The similar population is called the control, reference, or comparison population. This thinking in epidemiology is based on the idea of counterfactuals and has been discussed in the context of ethnicity and health by Kaufman et al. (1997).

In causal epidemiology indicators of migration status, race, and ethnicity are treated as risk factors which are potential causal factors. These risk factors are, as discussed in Chapter 1, also known as exposure variables, as opposed to outcome variables. The focus here is on differences between migrant, racial, and/or ethnic groups. The ideal (counterfactual) population does not exist, i.e. the same population but with a different migrant status, or racial or ethnic identity! The risk factor (or exposure) of migrant status, race, or ethnicity cannot be manipulated or changed by the investigator, so no experimentation is possible. This is similar to age, sex, and adult height, to take some examples, but different from drug use, exercise habits, and alcohol use. It follows that establishing causation is going to be difficult, and some people have argued it is impossible (others, including myself, disagree here).

The specific underlying, potentially causal components of migration status, race, and ethnicity are, however, more amenable to change, e.g. the diet (rapidly), religion (rarely), language (between generations and slowly within one). The children and grandchildren of migrants also allow opportunities for observing change in facets of ethnicity. The closest model I can think of in terms of a natural experiment in race is studying mixed race or ethnic group populations (admixture studies). Admixture studies tend to be associated with genetics and put an emphasis on the genetic underpinning of racial and ethnic variations in disease. It is hard to predict where this kind of research will lead us, but hopefully it will not return us to the days of race as, primarily, biology. (The health of admixed groups is an important topic but not primarily from a genetic perspective—rather from a societal one. The limited data we have are pointing to some concerns, notwithstanding the general principle of hybrid vigour.) One of the influential ethnicity and health researchers in the UK, Paul McKeigue, is developing this field from both a conceptual perspective and from a methodological one (1997).

McKeigue (1997) has argued that (a) when migrant groups living in the same environment have different disease rates that are not accounted for by adjusting for known environmental determinants of disease risk, genetic explanations should be considered and (b) genetic explanations are most likely where differences in disease rates persist even in migrants who have been settled outside the home country for several generations and where such differences are consistently found in all countries where the migrant group has settled. Most ethnicity and health research is non-experimental, and does not use admixture-type approaches but relies on comparison, i.e. a control or reference group. So, what is to be the control group? In practice, the pragmatic control is another racial or ethnic group, but we already know that this does not come close to an ideal control, i.e. the counterfactual population. The pragmatic control group will have a multiplicity of differences in comparison with the group under study. It is not possible to control confounding completely in these circumstances. This does not mean that migration status, race, and ethnicity have no role at all to play in the endeavour of medical and population sciences to find causes, but it does mean that there are theoretical limitations.

Since all disease arises from the interaction of the genome, the host (phenotype), and the external environment, in causal research the process of migration and the concepts of both race (as biology) and ethnicity are of interest. Historically, the role of biology has been invoked too readily as the prime explanation for racial differences. For example, in the 19th century inherited biological susceptibility was wrongly assumed to be a prime explanation for the high rates of syphilis, tuberculosis, conjunctivitis, and nutritional disorders in African Americans. Unfortunately, current research also gives prominence to genetic explanations and downplays environmental (and especially economic) ones. To take one modern example, the high rates of hypertension in populations of African origin are widely attributed by medical scientists and clinicians to genetic and related biological factors with comparatively little attempt to test other explanations. The role of genetics in explaining hypertension in populations of African origin is slowly being clarified, but nonetheless needs to be studied along with environmental and social factors, including the experience of racism. Studies across the globe, led by Richard Cooper (e.g. Cooper et al. 1997), are contradicting the emphasis on genetics by showing that there is a tremendous variation in blood pressure in populations of African origin across the world, and that their blood pressure is by no means uniquely high, being lower than in some European populations.

A useful contribution to hypothesis generation and testing requires direct measurement of the components of the concepts which define the race and ethnicity of a population group. The black box needs to be opened. This, unlike in most health services research, will include genetic studies. The approach to genetics that needs to be taken is exemplified in the quotation below, which is one of a number of recommendations made by the authors:

> Race/ethnicity should not be used as a proxy for genetic variation. Statements about genetic differences should be supported by evidence from gene studies. Genetic hypotheses should be firmly grounded in existing evidence, clearly stated, and rigorously tested.
>
> Kaplan and Bennett (2003, p. 2712)

The first step in bioscience may indeed be work using migration status, racial, and ethnic categories but it needs to move to the next step rapidly. The study of heart failure in African American populations and its treatment by a drug licensed to be used in this population specifically (BiDil) has caused huge controversy, and this will need genetic studies to resolve.

Table 9.2 illustrates the approach I am recommending using the example of variations in stroke.

Overall mortality rates and life expectancy differ among migrant, racial, and ethnic groups living in the United States and Europe. Populations of Far Eastern origin, such as the Chinese, do particularly well. Are these differences attributable to genetic or environmental factors? We don't know, but it would be unwise to attribute this to genes. Until genetic studies of ageing demonstrate

Table 9.2 Categorizing and analysing the factors which may underlie an epidemiological variable: the example of stroke

Category of potential explanatory underlying difference	Example of possible specific differences by migration status, race, or ethnic group	Implications for data collection
Biological	Unique variants of human genes, or varying frequencies of such variants (polymorphisms) lead to different biochemistry or physiology	Collect biological data including DNA, blood, and other tissues
Coexisting diseases	One group may have more or less of another disease which raises or reduces the risk of stroke disease, e.g. diabetes	Collect clinical data, including appropriate diagnostic tests
Behavioural	One group may eat more fruits, vegetables, and salads than another, and perhaps smoke less	Collect data on behaviours relating to health
Social	Members of a group may spend less time with friends and family, and other social networks, so increasing psychosocial strain	Collect psychosocial data as potential explanations
Occupational	The pattern of working, including likelihood of employment, the hours worked, and the type of occupations is substantially different	Collect data on employment histories
Economic	Members of a group may earn less than the average or have varying amounts of accumulated family wealth	Collect data on differences in income and wealth and their effect on lifestyles and stress
Health care	Members of a group may be treated differently from the expected standard by health-care professionals	Collect date on quality, quantity and timing of health-care interventions

otherwise, the differences ought to be largely attributed to environmental, behavioural, and social factors. The mortality differences might be partly attributed to excesses or deficits of specific diseases, for which the biology and hence genetic basis is better understood than for ageing. To continue with the example of breast cancer, the mortality rate differs greatly by country of birth group. In England and Wales, as shown by Wild et al. (2006), the rate was comparatively low in South Asian, Chinese and eastern European-born, and high in North and West African-born groups. Since genetic factors are a demonstrated cause of breast cancer, it is important to ask whether such differences are attributable to genetic differences. It is imperative that the question is answered by direct measurement of the presence or absence of the relevant gene variants.

The difference in breast cancer might arise from other factors which vary across the groups, e.g. diet, economic circumstances, environmental pollutants, contraception, and the age at first pregnancy. These are a few of the many social and environmental factors which have biological consequences. Information on such social factors also needs to be collected directly and not assumed.

For causal analysis in this context biological, environmental, and social factors need to be directly measured, both as potential contributors to the causal pathway and as confounding variables. With this theoretical background we can consider the practicalities of research.

9.4 Undertaking research on the health of minorities: getting the basics right

Try Exercise 9.4 before reading on.

Exercise 9.4 Challenges for researchers and balancing ideals with practicalities

♦ What particular challenges do migration, race, ethnicity, and health researchers face when setting research questions, defining concepts, recruiting populations, asking questions, calculating rates, interpreting data, publishing, and acting on the results?

♦ What can researchers do to overcome these challenges?

♦ Which ideals may need to be sacrificed to make research practical and which are sacrosanct?

The ideal research study in a multicultural society would include all migrant, racial, and ethnic groups, have uniformly high response rates, provide data that are comparable across all groups, collect information on all facets of migration status, race, and ethnicity, include data on all potential confounding variables, and be analysed and interpreted in a way that both advances science and develops better health care. No such study exists or is ever likely to. In practice, many ideals are sacrificed to make the study feasible. In making pragmatic choices researchers should, however, make themselves and their audiences aware of the limitations of the work. Research on the health of multicultural societies will not pay dividends either in better services or in yielding insights about the causes of disease if the basic principles of research are breached. These basic principles are reviewed in this section, although many of them have been covered already.

9.4.1 Define the question, aims, purpose, and relevance of the research

Good research starts with clear-cut and unbiased research questions, explicit aims, and specific, measurable, achievable, relevant, and timely—SMART being the acronym—objectives. The way to formulate these is fundamental to guidance on how to do research but readers will need to access general research textbooks (e.g. Bowling and Ebrahim 2006) and those specifically on multi-ethnic population research (e.g. Nazroo 2006). The key point, from this book's perspective, is that the questions, aims, and objectives must be designed to benefit and not harm minority groups (and even better to benefit the entire population). If there is to be a bias, then it should be antiracist and antidiscriminatory to help balance past injustices—there is a strong case for affirmative action even in the research field (positive discrimination). Neutrality, if it can be achieved at all (and most philosophers and social scientists researching the nature of science tend to the view that it cannot be), is, however, the ideal stance for good research.

The underlying purpose of the research beyond benefitting the populations studied, e.g. whether it is for health-care policy or planning or to enhance understanding of the causes of disease, guides the design and detail of the study, data analysis, and the presentation and publication of the results. The twin objectives of better policy/planning and causal understanding are rarely accomplished by one set of data analyses, or even by the one study. When they are, the investigators have been equally interested in achieving both and have planned for this. For example, if the aim is to understand the causes of cancer then listing the SMRs or the incidence rates by migrant, racial, or ethnic group is of limited value. At best this would yield hypotheses for future study. Disease incidence rates and ranks are of value to the health planner, but only if the population studied is representative and the data are presented so as to highlight needs and priorities. Rankings of mortality and morbidity rates and years of life lost serve this purpose admirably, but summary statistics of relative frequency (e.g. the SMR) do not. The principles have been discussed in Chapters 6, 7, and 8 (readers can also consult Bhopal 2008).

Whatever the purpose, the research questions need to be credible to funders (who generally give preference to causal or intervention studies), study populations, journal editors, and readers. Major research projects in the population sciences need to be on the important causes of death, disability, or illness across migrant, racial, and ethnic groups, not on interesting cultural quirks, however tempting these are. It is easy to be side-tracked into the mode of thinking that all differences are interesting and that similarities are boring. My first proper research project in 1984 fell into this trap—I was misled into thinking that traditional medicines were very important in South Asian communities in Glasgow, Scotland. It was very interesting work for me and it led to publications and useful experience. Only later did I realize that I was delving into a minor issue. In the small-scale interview survey I did (100 people selected, 65 interviewed) the importance of diabetes was brought to my attention by several respondents but my mind was unprepared. At about the same time Mather and Keen (1985) published their landmark paper showing that diabetes in UK South Asians was about four times commoner than in the population as a whole. I had been side-tracked! This is a common experience in our field.

9.4.2 **Definition of concepts and precision of terms is essential**

Chapters 1 and 2 provide further information relevant to this section.

Try Exercise 9.5 before reading on.

Exercise 9.5: The need to explain concepts and devise classifications

- ◆ Why do researchers need to specify and explain their use of migration status and the race and ethnicity concepts?
- ◆ Why should they devise their own classifications of migration status, race, and ethnicity? And, why should they not do so?
- ◆ In practice, why are they limited in their inventiveness in devising classifications?

The field of migration, race, and ethnicity is not like chemistry or mathematics which are long-established disciplines where the concepts and vocabulary are agreed, stable, and easily accessed, e.g. in basic textbooks for schoolchildren. Our field is young, controversial, contextual, and complex. Researchers, therefore, need to make explicit how they are using the concepts of migration status, ethnicity, and race, and how they have adapted classifications and methods to the research questions under study. Researchers should not always be constrained by available classifications, usually designed for social purposes. A thoughtful adaptation is likely to be needed. They need to explain in some detail what they are doing and why, and writing as if the reader was in another country and time would probably help. More than ever, research and scholarship are increasingly global affairs so this is good discipline. The kind of terminology used to describe minority ethnic populations (Hispanics, Asians, Blacks, Whites, Chinese, etc.) may suffice for everyday conversation or political exchange within nations but is usually too crude for scientific studies and may not be understood internationally. An internationally agreed vocabulary is the ideal. In its absence researchers should use either existing glossaries such as the one here—based on the one I published in the *Journal of Epidemiology and Community Health* (Bhopal 2004)—or supply their own, if not in their publications then on a website.

This encouragement to inventiveness, e.g. in regard to classifications, should not be seen as an invitation to violate common sense. Researchers should not invent racial or ethnic groups or create irrational labels, e.g. the use of the word Urdu to denote an ethnic group based on the language Urdu, or the phrase Chinese and Asian, both of which can be found in otherwise high-quality research publications. Equally, it is not sensible to try to use the word Indian to include all South Asians, e.g. Bangladeshis, Pakistanis, and Sri Lankans are not Indians (even although they may have been at times in the past). Similarly, researchers have a misleading tendency to treat Africans from Africa and those from the Caribbean as one (sometimes for increased statistical precision). They also have a tendency to treat all Africans as one, which they clearly are not, as they are by far the most heterogeneous peoples of the world. It is not sufficient for researchers to simply inform the readers that they are misusing concepts in these ways! It is disrespectful to the populations studied if terms used by researchers misrepresent them. Wherever possible researchers should use terms that are acceptable to the populations they study. The definition of terms aims to make the work of researchers and practitioners, as well as readers, easier and better. As such, definitions should be agreed in advance of the research, not in retrospect. In multidisciplinary work, especially across national boundaries, agreeing concepts and terminology is a major undertaking. Even having an agreement on paper may not suffice—applying it in practice is difficult.

9.4.3 Denominators and numerators need to match to calculate rates and need to be consistent across population groups

Issues relevant to this section were discussed in Chapters 2, 3, and 5. A census or accurate population register is the essential resource for the denominator required for the calculation of rates for most population-based research, and nearly all work that is based on vital statistic, i.e. births, deaths, fertility, migration, marriage. A census also paints the backdrop for all forms of research that require an understanding of the size and composition of the population. By contrast, population registers usually only have limited background data. However, for minority communities the accuracy of the denominator may be questioned for several reasons, including frequent travel abroad, difficulties in the completion of forms, non-completion, and errors in some details such as age.

Further, the numerator for disease, or other outcome, may also be inappropriate and, in particular, be inflated by the inclusion of visitors (who are not in the denominator).

Very often in migration, race, ethnicity, and health research rates of disease or other health outcome are compared across groups. It is important that these comparisons are valid, i.e. like-for-like. These issues were discussed in Chapter 3 but they are of crucial importance in the interpretation of research so are worth re-emphasizing here. The use of name searching offers a salutary lesson.

Name searching is currently a popular tool among researchers, especially in the early years as the field of work is being developed. This tool is usually applied only to derive the numerator from health status and disease outcome databases. The denominator usually remains that obtained from the census or a population registry without name searching, thus creating a serious mismatch and source of error. The error is an elementary one, but presumably researchers cannot find another solution. Name searching the census or population registry would not be an easy task, mainly because accessing such personal data is problematic, but it is the logical action to derive a comparable denominator that matches the numerator. These kinds of questions about the accuracy and comparability of denominators and numerators are fundamental but are rarely studied in the detail required. Researchers need to be aware of these matters because they are of great importance.

9.4.4 Ensure that there is comparability of populations: tackling confounding

The concept of confounding was discussed in Section 9.3.3. To infer that a disease is commoner in one group compared with another requires, at the very least, that the two groups are comparable in terms of age and sex, because disease patterns are profoundly affected by these factors. To go further and attempt to ascribe the differences to cultural or genetic factors requires that the explanation does not lie in other domains, e.g. socio-economic status. The onus is on the researcher to tease out the reasons for the differences observed. This is not easy, so as a minimum the favoured explanation needs to be set in the context of alternatives. The problem is that researchers usually have a favoured explanation, and that is usually the one that fits with societal norms.

If causal understanding is to result from studies, painstaking attention to the characteristics and comparability of the populations under study will be necessary otherwise confounding is likely to be uncontrolled. Researchers need a high degree of awareness that control of confounding will be incomplete (technically, that there will be residual confounding). Inferences can change radically once interacting and confounding factors are accounted for. For example, Lillie-Blanton et al. (1993) challenged the then established observation that smoking of crack cocaine was more common in African Americans and Hispanic Americans than in White Americans, showing that once social, cultural, and environmental factors were accounted for there were no differences.

9.4.5 Identification of representative populations

Unrepresentative (or biased) population study samples can arise because some of the relevant people have not been identified or have not been recruited. Obviously, this creates problems in data interpretation. The problem is worsened if, as is likely, the degree of sampling bias varies across migrant, racial, or ethnic groups. For example, it is hard to imagine how to avoid unrepresentative samples in studies of undocumented migrants.

Researchers who are knowledgeable about the minority groups under study are more likely to be trusted and more likely to achieve the successful identification of the sample, high response rates, and informed consent that are essential to studying representative populations. Valid recruitment is achievable in relation to most minority groups for most studies, although it would be wrong to imply it is easy. A review of the evidence came to these conclusions:

It is widely believed that racial and ethnic minorities are less willing to participate in health research. Such claims often focus on the US, where it is believed that minority groups' relative unwillingness to participate in health research traces to historic abuses, especially the notorious Tuskegee Syphilis Study. We found that racial and ethnic minorities in the US, particularly African-Americans and Hispanics, are as willing to participate, and in some instances more willing to participate, in health research than non-Hispanic whites, when eligible and invited to participate.

Wendler et al. (2006, p. 8)

An editorial on this review commented:

There are now sufficient examples of studies on marginalised communities that clearly show that it should really be possible to engage with people, irrespective of their ethnic background, and encourage them to participate in research that is ultimately in their and/or their community's best interests. What is now needed is less blame directed at already marginalised people. Instead, those with the power to change the way in which research is conducted should translate the important insights provided by Wendler and colleagues' study into significantly more invitations extended to minority ethnic and racial groups to participate in the research endeavour.

Sheikh (2006, p. 1)

The important message is that the problem does not lie in unwillingness amongst minorities to participate in research but in methodological or logistical matters. Of these, accessing populations easily and at reasonable cost/effort is one of the top-ranking issues. A truly representative migrant, racial, and/or ethnic minority population sample would be nigh impossible to obtain, unless the sampling was linked to the census, which in turn would need to be correct and up to date. Validation studies tend to show modest differences in participation in census, e.g. as in data on completion of census forms by ethnic group in Scotland. Usually, in the absence of valid sampling frames, some convenience sample is recruited.

The validity of the convenience samples we use in practice needs study, and the likely error measured. One common practical decision is to sample from areas where the minority populations tend to live. The work of Ecob and Williams (1991) in the MRC Medical Sociology 'Asian' lifestyle and health study showed that there were substantial differences between people who live in areas where the proportion of the ethnic minority population is high and those who live elsewhere. Such studies of methods are important to help interpret findings. Inner city populations are different from whole population samples, but studies of minorities continue to focus on them for convenience. In a very important, and at the time ground-breaking, Health Education Authority survey the comparison population, unlike the ethnic minority populations, was not an inner city sample but a general population sample, making data interpretation hard (Johnson et al. 2000). Lessons were learned and implemented in the Health Survey for England (1999 and 2004 sweeps) where time- and resource-consuming approaches to also sample from areas with a low concentration of ethnic minorities were used.

There are several ways of sampling (all with drawbacks) depending on the type of information that is required. One can take a random sample of people listed on a population register (e.g. electoral roll, municipal register, health service registration, telephone directory). Alternatively one can sample people who have accessed a service using admission, discharge, or consultation registers. With increasing coding of migrant status, race, and ethnicity in health service data systems these latter approaches are increasingly becoming the preferred practice. More informal networking can be used to find people. The populations assembled in the latter way may be culturally homogeneous, already know each other and therefore comfortable with the situation, and trust the researchers. The commonest method, particularly for small-scale work, is to use, with appropriate permissions in place, the register of a community organization, e.g. the Chinese/Bengali/Indian/Vietnamese Association. Typically, such an organization will not give the data to the researchers but will disseminate information about the research to their members.

Unless the study is set in a place where the minority group of interest is a substantial proportion of the population, a truly random sample might yield few people in that group. The answer here is stratified sampling, i.e. the list of people potentially eligible for study (the sampling frame) is organized by the factor of interest (here migrant, racial, and/or ethnic group) and samples are taken from the relevant sections. Sampling frames that hold information by migration status, race, and/or ethnicity are rare, so such reorganization of lists is problematic. Country of birth is more likely to be on potential sampling frames than race or ethnic group, and in many places using this is the easiest option.

Organizing the list by name is another partial solution—the limitations of this were discussed in Chapter 3. Investigators should ensure their work does not breach data protection laws, e.g. the principle that data should only be used for the purposes for which they were collected. Names are not collected so that race, ethnic group, or migration status can be guessed by researchers and used to study them. Researchers should, therefore, seek appropriate approvals before doing this. Sampling by name works for some groups. The South Asian and Chinese populations do have fairly distinctive names which are being retained across generations. Names have even been used to identify Irish and Polish people. Analysis of names can help define, though far from perfectly, groupings based on religion and language. This technique relies on using the knowledge and skills of trained staff. The characteristic and distinctive nature of the surnames of Urdu, Punjabi, Hindi, and Gujarati speakers permits this approach. Muslim names are similar across the world and many names are also common to Sikhs and Hindus. My name, Raj Bhopal, is recognizably Indian, but most knowledgeable observers would think it to be of a Hindu. My full name is, however, Rajinder Singh Bhopal. The first name identifies me clearly as Punjabi and probably a Sikh, as the ending 'inder' is adopted by Sikhs. The middle name Singh is adopted for Sikh men (women are Kaur), although it is not unique to Sikhs. Bhopal is a rare Indian surname but is immediately recognizable as Indian because there is a city called Bhopal (and formerly there was a state). The region of family origin for this name is, nonetheless, likely to be Punjab because of the first and second names and the language most likely to be associated with it is Punjabi. The religion is almost certainly Sikh. This example illustrates how much information there is in a name. The name Macdonald, alone, tells you the holder has Scottish origins, is likely to be a Protestant Christian and speaks English. Of course, these guesses could well be wrong, but they are a fair starting point. Occasionally, South Asian names, particularly among Christian Indians, are similar (if not identical) to European names. Name analysis is not established as a reliable tool for identifying people of African Caribbean origin as many of the names are similar to European (Christian names).

One major problem with sampling from population registers is that often the addresses (and sometimes names) listed are incorrect. Accuracy of information for minority groups, who are relatively mobile, is usually worse than for the majority population. Addresses on such lists may need to be cross-checked against manual or computerized records, e.g. in the telephone directory or the electoral register (the list of people eligible to vote in local and national elections). Of course, these other sources of information may also be wrong.

Although health services may be required to collect information on migrant status, race, and/or ethnicity of users many do not have accurate data, although the situation is generally improving (see Chapter 3).Another approach, apart from routine coding, is to ask people using a service over a time period to provide their migrant status, race, and/or ethnic group and use this newly collected information to select a sample.

Although it is not currently judged as best practice the investigator can select people on the basis of observation—whether of physical features, clothing, or other markers of race and/or ethnicity. Currently, this would only be justified if asking people was not possible or would interfere with the aims of the study (researchers should take ethical advice). It would be presumptuous for the investigator to assume race and/or ethnicity using these markers. However, as a first step to identify people who can then be asked about themselves this may well be pragmatic and justified.

Where a population group is hard to contact and recruit, and no reasonable lists of contact details exist, the so-called snowball technique can be used. The phrase is a metaphor based on the observation that rolling a snowball down a hill makes it bigger as it accumulates more snow around it. In this method an initial group of people already known to the researchers are asked to start a chain of contacts, i.e. each respondent is asked to give names and addresses of other potential participants. These new people are then approached and invited to take part in the research. They in turn are asked to supply more names.

A mix of pragmatic approaches may be needed to recruit study participants in multi-ethnic studies, and the published experience of recruitment into the Prevention of Diabetes and Obesity in South Asians (PODOSA) trial was fairly typical (Samsudeen et al. 2011).

The possibility that there may be differential response rates across migrant, racial, and ethnic groups to both self-report data (questionnaires or interviews) and other forms of measurement (blood tests) is an obvious consideration. The biases of non-response are difficult to judge. There is evidence that those who participate are different from those who do not, although in some studies the differences have been modest. I am not aware of studies examining response biases by migrant, racial, or ethnic group. It is likely that, as in most studies, non-responders in minority groups are likely to have a different profile from responders.

Response to one aspect of a study may not lead to response to another component. This kind of bias is easier to examine. For example, in the multi-ethnic Health Survey for England 1999, the response rate to the questionnaire was, in relation to other ethnic groups, higher in Bangladeshis, but participation in the physical measures and blood sample components of the study was comparably lower. This also adds to the problem of valid data interpretation.

Rapidly increasing experience shows that minority populations can be recruited into population health studies but usually the effort and cost is higher than for general population samples. Inexpensive passive methods (mail shots) are not very effective, whereas active face-to-face methods tend to be successful but are relatively expensive. Retention into studies, in contrast to recruitment, though often a problem presents no special difficulties in minority groups.

9.4.6 Data collection methods should be valid and cross-culturally equivalent: questionnaires and focus groups

In Chapter 3 the generic principles for maximizing the cross-cultural validity of questionnaires were considered. Here we consider some of the issues in a research study setting.

Health researchers are challenged to rapidly fill huge gaps in knowledge about migrant, racial, and ethnic groups, and their studies are sometimes highly ambitious. Box 9.1 summarizes the span of self-report data and related methods used in a small, cross-sectional study in the late 1980s by Williams and colleagues in Glasgow (Williams et al. 1993).

This kind of all-inclusive approach is not unusual in the field of migration, race, and ethnicity; it is perhaps more common here than in studies of the health of general populations. You may wish to reflect on why this might be so. One explanation is that there is a pressure to fill the gaps in our knowledge. Researchers are also conscious of the complexity of data interpretation and particularly the importance of a solid cultural context, which requires extensive data. Then there

Box 9.1 The span of interview data collected by Williams et al. (1993), and methods

Information was collected by interview-administered questionnaire on current and past health, perceived health, health beliefs, health care, medications, and health-related lifestyle issues including smoking, exercise, drinking and diet, stress and other aspects of mental health. Additionally, details of geographical origins, education, occupation, housing, household organization, child rearing, family support, and religion were collected.

Dietary questions were designed to reveal broad patterns of food choice and frequency of consumption. Stress measures reflected the common division of the field into: (1) structural inequalities, which may or may not give rise to (2); (2) stressors (usually negative events or chronic strains); (3) mediators (usually coping resources or social support); and (4) stress outcomes (usually perceived distress). The focus was on structural inequalities in work, finance, and housing, on possible chronic strains arising, on events involving violence, damage, or perceived racial discrimination, and on social support (as a mediator often compromised by migration). The questionnaires were translated from English into Urdu, Hindi, and Punjabi by an educational psychologist fluent in all four languages. The quality of the translation was tested by the translator and another polylingual interviewer piloting the schedules, and by further discussion with a bilingual doctor (i.e. me) and other bilingual interviewers who between them covered all the languages concerned. Interviewers for the South Asian sample were all literate in English and in at least one of the three South Asian languages concerned, and were given a week's interview training and a further week's close individual supervision.

Source: Data from Williams et al, Health of a Punjabi ethnic minority in Glasgow: a comparison with the general population, *Journal of Epidemiology and Community Health*, Volume 47, Issue 2, pp. 96–102, Copyright ©1992 by the BMJ Publishing Group Ltd. All rights reserved.

are some complex items essential to this kind of inquiry but not needed by others, e.g. migration history, race, ethnic group, racial prejudice, and use of traditional health-care systems and remedies. Finally, whereas in the general research field most people are specialists interested in a particular disease or health issue, in our field people are interested in a population and all their diseases and issues.

The challenges of such a wide span of data collection, and especially of ensuring cross-cultural validity, are self-evident. (These challenges are particularly important for, but not confined to, self-report data; for other types of data, e.g. anthropometric measurements and laboratory tests, there are fewer problems.) The challenges of preparing validated questions are well known, but to ensure they retain their meaning on translation and are suitable for the majority and several minority groups is a formidable if not impossible undertaking, particularly for lengthy questionnaires in several languages such as those used by Williams et al. (1993). While awareness of this has increased, rigorous assessment is still uncommon—in truth, it is an uncomfortable issue to confront. Resources and the time needed to ensure cross-cultural validity are unlikely to be available. Pragmatically, it is a case of proceeding or abandoning the work—and most researchers choose the former. Development of a suite of suitable cross-cultural instruments that can be used off the shelf is part of the work needed to advance our field. As language barriers and indeed illiteracy are common, the self-completion questionnaire may be unsuitable in migration, race, and ethnicity studies. The face-to-face interview, using professional interviewers, is the main alternative, but one has to find and train appropriately qualified staff, which comes at high cost. (Interviews are about 10 times more expensive than self-completion methods.) Other models, e.g. computer, video, and audiotape-based interviews, have promise but have not been widely tested or used (they need to be, as the occasional test shows their promise.)

In preparation for gathering self-report questionnaires (self-completion or interview) focus groups might be used first. Focus groups allow themes to be explored in an interactive way that cannot be achieved using questionnaires alone. Focus group discussions are often a prerequisite for developing questionnaires.

Translation of questionnaires is crucial for the successful collection of information on the health of minority groups, particularly those whose primary language is not English. Issues such as using specific words, phrases, and accents (whether in English or not) tailored to and appropriate for the community under study also need to be taken account of, particularly for interviews. This tailoring may use colloquialisms, and mixing of languages, and may meet the disapproval of official, educated translators. Sometimes translators will find the proper word for an English one, but this may not be one that local people understand. When there is no everyday equivalent for an English word in the target languages it is best to use English rather than an obscure, possibly technical word. This is where your focus group can advise you well. Respondents may not share common assumptions about health and well-being which underlie survey questions, e.g. gardening may be reported as exercise by one group but not another. Minority populations usually comprise a mix in terms of acculturation—some preferring English, others not; and some hold health beliefs very different from the majority, while others have similar ones. In most research on minority health we accept participants' language preferences even though from a methodological perspective we know that this is not ideal. In practice many people will, given a choice, use a mix of English and another language, even when their knowledge of one language is superior. People may well switch during an interview too. For example, I am much more familiar with English than Punjabi. If, however, there was a question on the properties of food described in English as hot/cold (not referring to temperature but to intrinsic properties of the ingredients), I would prefer the Punjabi equivalent words 'garam' (warm/hot) and 'thandha' (cold) because they convey the non-thermal meaning more clearly to me, simply because this variance in meanings is ingrained in the language. So the prior expressed preferences in language may not hold as the interview or focus group proceeds.

In devising questionnaires, researchers should beware of using jargon, colloquialisms, and sayings that are idiosyncratic to the English language, and it may be more appropriate to adopt a simple and descriptive question in order to minimize misinterpretation. The problem is that investigators are reluctant to change the standard English version even when this is sensible (and when it is held in copyright or given on licence this may not be permitted).

It is important for translations to be consistent. Some pointers to translating questions can be found in the *Bristol Black and Ethnic Minorities Health Survey Report* (Pilgrim et al. 1993); an extract is given in Box 9.2.

In devising and translating questions researchers need to be conscious that they may be interpreted quite differently by different migrant, racial, and ethnic groups, either because of subtle problems with translation or underlying concepts. Hanna et al. (2006) have explored this in a detailed study of a questionnaire focusing on tobacco-related behaviours. The difficulties were numerous, and ranged from technical (the written and spoken language is different, as in Cantonese, or there is no written language as in the Sylheti dialect of Bangla, the language of Bangladesh), to conceptual (conveying the idea of a pipe or cigar in languages where there is no culture of using tobacco in these forms), to practical (gaining the involvement of lay members of the community in the process

Box 9.2 Translating the interview schedule—example taken from the *Bristol Black and Ethnic Minorities Health Survey Report*

A variety of difficulties were dealt with in translating the interview schedule into Urdu/Punjabi, including the following.

- There is no equivalent word but the concept is clear, e.g. 'inpatient' is replaced by the Urdu phrase 'a stay in hospital'.

- An equivalent word exists but is obscure or not easily understood by respondents (technical jargon etc.), e.g. 'cervical smear test': interviewers were told to ask initially using the English phrase. Many respondents replied by saying they did not understand. Therefore an explanation was given. 'The passage whereby you have a child, the doctor takes a sample from there to analyse for cancer.'

- There is no equivalent concept in Urdu/Punjabi-speaking culture, e.g. 'social life' is replaced by the Urdu phrase 'meeting and interacting with people'.

- The concept is clear but the expression is culturally inappropriate, e.g. 'female doctor' is translated as 'lady doctor'.

- Both Urdu and English terms are commonly used, e.g. 'dentist', 'optician': here both the English and Urdu terms were used to ensure that there was no misunderstanding.

- The concept is difficult to convey in both English and Urdu, e.g. the concept of 'ethnic identity' is difficult in any language. For the Urdu version it was necessary to be specific and to ask directly if people saw themselves as Pakistani, Asian, Black, etc.

Adapted from Pilgrim S et al, *The Bristol Black and Ethnic Minorities Health Survey Report*, Departments of Sociology and Epidemiology, University of Bristol, Bristol, UK, Copyright © 1993, with permission of the authors.

of establishing the face validity of questions). The resultant modified questionnaires were created in English, Punjabi, Urdu, Sylheti (written in the English alphabet with Sylheti words), and Cantonese (written in the Chinese spoken form). These questionnaires are for use at interview. Simply creating a tobacco use questionnaire with face validity took a year of hard work.

The questionnaires used in ethnicity and health research tend to contain a mix of question types. There are three main types of questions—structured, semi-structured and open-ended—all of which can be asked by self-completion or at interview. The advantage of self-completed questionnaires is that people can consider questions carefully in their own time. They may also be less embarrassed about including details of personal issues. However, these require both familiarity with this format and good reading skills. Interview-based questionnaires allow the interviewer to ask the questions and convey the meanings of questions if they are not fully understood (possibly in an alternative language—something frowned upon by the purist researcher). The interview has great advantages when the study subjects do not read and write the language well. The interviewer must be trained rigorously or major biases can occur. Such biases will be easier to detect if the interview is tape recorded and not simply summarized by the interviewers, but that adds very considerable cost and complexity to an already difficult research task, particularly in large studies. The tapes will need to be transcribed—a very difficult task when the material is in several languages. Minority populations, more so than European-origin majority groups, value face-to-face interaction so interviews tend to work well.

These methods also have fundamental drawbacks, e.g. both interviews and questionnaires are subject to the problem of discrepancy between public and private accounts in that the respondent gives the answer that is perceived as acceptable, possibly desirable, in the circumstances, especially on sensitive or taboo topics. The more honest, but less acceptable, answer may be reserved for private discussions. These private accounts can sometimes be accessed by skilled interviewers over a series of interviews. The answers will also depend on how the respondent interprets the question. For this reason, questions should be kept simple whenever possible.

Researchers must also remember the social aspects of the interview situation, e.g. people from some cultures may find it rude not to be engaged via polite formalities (perhaps over a cup of tea) or to have their own questions, whether about the research or also personal ones about the researchers and their families, ignored. Generally, interviews with minority communities take longer than expected, partly because of this social side. This possibility needs to be included in costings.

In focus groups people are gathered together (perhaps grouped according to sex, ethnic background, etc.) and questions are put to them, e.g. what do you think of local hospital services? The people are then encouraged to talk—in their own language if desired—to discuss issues and exchange experiences. Through these discussions, themes emerge, and often rich and vivid stories of how people have interacted with health services are drawn out. A facilitator is present to keep the discussions relevant to the topic and the group views are collected through open-ended questions. The facilitator uses a topic guide. A questioning route is prepared which will allow for flexibility within the research. Box 9.3 is an example of a questioning route which was used in five focus group meetings held to assess the impact of cardiovascular disease and diabetes in the Chinese and South Asian communities in Newcastle (Elliot 1997).

Box 9.3 Example of a focus group questioning route

The questioning route for focus group on cardiovascular disease and diabetes in minority ethnic groups.

1. Tell us about your diabetes.

   Prompts: previous family history, tests and investigations, hospital admissions, emergencies, treatments, health problems, problems with family diet/cooking arrangements.

2. Tell us about how diabetes has affected your life.

   Prompts: as a mother, as the breadwinner, as a religious person, as a social person.

3. Research shows that the best preventive and rehabilitative care for people with diabetes and heart disease is to lose weight and take more exercise. Tell us about this aspect of your lifestyle.

   Prompts: Do you want to lose weight? Have you tried to lose weight? What makes you put weight on? What makes it difficult to watch your weight? Do you exercise? Do you want to exercise?

Adapted from Elliot et al, *Taking Heart: Reducing diabetes and cardiovascular disease among Newcastle's South Asian and Chinese communities* in *Strategy for commissioning services for coronary heart disease and diabetes for ethnic minority populations in England and Wales: lessons from a four-site pilot study*, Departments of Epidemiology and Public Health and Medicine, University of Newcastle upon Tyne, Copyright © 1998, with permission of the authors.

The focus group gives insight into the attitudes, beliefs, and behaviours of a group. The group is 'focused' in the sense that it involves a collective activity, such as discussing health beliefs. One of the advantages of focus groups is the capacity to exploit group dynamics. By encouraging the participants in the group to interact with one another, the researcher can gain insight into group/social processes. Focus groups and individual interviews elicit different material. Two major problems with focus groups are those of the emergence of group ideology and an opinion leader, both constraining the range and value of opinion.

If the language of the researcher is different from that of the participants, trained interpreters will be needed so that participants may speak in their chosen language and the main issues can then be transmitted back to the facilitator. Facilitators and interpreters then need to agree on the main issues to have emerged. The discussion should be recorded and if possible transcribed. The latter is a difficult and expensive process especially where several languages are used and the transcriber is not expert in all of them. Analysis of data can use theoretically established approaches, and custom-designed computer software. Box 9.4 gives an example of how focus group data can be applied to bring about change, based on the work by Elliot (1997).

I have merely touched on these difficult but vital issues. While many books and papers have been written on the issues of interpretation, translation, and cross-cultural validation, there is not

---

Box 9.4 CHD/diabetes focus group methods and use of data

Focus groups were used in Newcastle to explore CHD and diabetes services for ethnic minorities. Four focus groups were set up: separate male and female South Asian groups, a mixed sex Chinese group, and a minority ethnic health professionals group. The facilitator asked the questions which were interpreted by the community workers and the answers were fed back via the community workers to the facilitator. Immediately after the meeting, there was a group discussion between the facilitator and the community workers (the research group) to go over and clarify the main points raised. This discussion was recorded and the results transcribed. The salient points made were placed under theme headings and discussed and changed until the research group was happy that what was emerging was a true record of what had occurred.

Conclusions were that the minorities knew little about their conditions (as well as preventative strategies) but wanted to know more. All participants had themselves, or knew of people who had, received inadequate health services. The professionals complained that they often did not have the resources to educate the community properly, e.g. materials were not translated and of those that were most were not easily understandable by the community. The professionals were often inundated with calls from people who wanted help with other matters, e.g. filling out social security forms. Some of the health workers had had to change their telephone numbers two or three times.

The results were used in the ethnic health strategy of the local health authority and were influential in gaining funding for a primary care based service for minority ethnic groups with a special focus on diabetes.

Adapted from Elliot et al, *Taking Heart: Reducing diabetes and cardiovascular disease among Newcastle's South Asian and Chinese communities* in *Strategy for commissioning services for coronary heart disease and diabetes for ethnic minority populations in England and Wales: lessons from a four-site pilot study*, Departments of Epidemiology and Public Health and Medicine, University of Newcastle upon Tyne, Copyright © 1998, with permission of the authors.

a standard, feasible, and accepted model of good practice. Hunt and Bhopal (2003) have published guidance on self-report data in multi-ethnic studies in population health settings. That guidance is not easy to apply, and I have had to ignore it myself on several occasions because applying it requires a separate expensive project in its own right. The key process that I have found to be practical, invaluable, and of low cost is to set up a multilingual panel of professional and lay people to examine and discuss materials and questionnaires, comparing and contrasting these in the various language formats. If this were applied, pending the development of a suite of materials in different language formats, we would be moving in the right direction. In addition, it would be worth investigators looking more carefully at what data they collect. For example, is it really worthwhile, given the state of the art, to apply in multi-ethnic studies complex quality of life or mental health questionnaires developed in English? The answer, most probably, is no, because the resulting data will not be comparable across subgroups.

9.4.7 Validity of physical and other measures across all subpopulations needs to be assured

Cross-cultural validity is obviously important in relation to self-report data, but it also matters in other forms of information. Here the difficulty is less with the measurement tool (as for questions) but with the meaning of the result. That said, a measurement method that is generally acceptable to the study participants may not be so across all groups. For example, measurement of hip circumference is quite common in studies examining body shape and especially fat distribution. However, this measurement may not be feasible for reasons of modesty, which is more highly prized in some populations than others. It may be that investigators will need to accept a modification of the usual protocol (normally measured over underwear) to allow measurement over light clothing. Investigators may need to employ staff to permit men to be measured by men and women by women in some groups. As another example, giving blood is not a routine and somewhat trivial matter in all populations. Blood can be prized and its loss may symbolize a loss of strength. Reluctance is likely to vary across populations (and hence different response rates). The issue arising is the comparability of data across subgroups. The larger problem, however, is the interpretation of data, even within a subgroup.

The same value of a physical measure may have differential significance across migrant, racial, and ethnic groups, as illustrated by BMI and waist measurement. BMI is a person's weight in kilograms divided by their height in metres squared, and it has been the most important single measure for studying overweight and obesity in population research for several decades (although it is increasingly under attack in this regard with opponents arguing for waist measures). Based on research linking BMI to adverse health outcomes, the WHO set a BMI ≥ 25 kg/m^2 in adults as overweight, with a BMI ≥ 30 as obese. These cut-offs work well except for sports people and particularly bodybuilders, where a high BMI could reflect a large muscle mass rather than excess fat. For most people, however, a high BMI reflects excess body fat. This is the reason why a high BMI is undesirable. High body fat is a risk factor for many diseases including heart attack, stroke, diabetes, and breast cancer. The studies that generated these WHO cut-off points were mostly in populations of White European origin.

Do these general observations and cut-off points apply across all migrant, racial, and ethnic groups? We would expect on first principles that they would if the BMI accurately reflected fat composition. It turns out that at any BMI, on average, most Asian populations including the Chinese, Malays, and South Asians, have more fat than White populations. (The opposite applies to Polynesians.) The association between BMI and disease probably holds in these populations but the cut-off points for overweight and obesity need to be lower, at least for the prevention and control of some diseases.

The exact cut-off points are under intense discussion with most observers recommending a value of 23 rather than 25 for overweight in most South and Southeast Asian ethnic groups, one exception being Japanese. The difference between a BMI of 23 and 25 for a man of about 1.75 m (5 ft 9 in) weighing 70 kg is about 6 kg or 13 lbs. This is obviously a critically important issue. If the proposed BMI cut-off of 23 (or lower) is accepted—and it already has been by important bodies such as the Indian Society of Cardiologists and a WHO Consultation Committee—it has huge repercussions. For decades Asian people may have been misinformed about their ideal body weight, at least from the perspective of diabetes and heart disease, because the interpretation of the key measure was not valid across racial and ethnic groups. (There are echoes here of the use of IQ scales designed for European population but used across the world, leading to the stigmatizing view that many other populations had a comparatively low IQ.)

Currently there is an emerging view that waist to hip ratio (WHR), or simply the waist measurement, would be a better indicator of excess body fat than the BMI. Several studies suggest this is so for many Asian populations. The WHR requires that a tape measure is passed around the preferably bare or very lightly clad waist and hip. These are difficult measurements to make, especially compared with measuring weight and height. Furthermore, a high WHR may reflect small hips rather than a large waist. There is no doubt there are variations by racial and ethnic group in hip shape and circumference and this matters to cardiovascular and diabetes health outcomes. The waist size also may not reflect the same amount of body fat across groups. There is growing evidence that South Asians have high levels of intra-abdominal fat even at the same waist sizes as White Europeans and that their fat cells are bigger too. The International Diabetes Federation has recommended that in Asian populations the waist size should be less than 90 cm in men (80 cm in women) compared with the recommendation of 94 cm in White men (80 cm in women). Interestingly, in the United States most medical authorities recommend a waist less than 102 cm. There is a growing realization that cross-cultural validity in relation to physical measures requires the adjustment of methods and normal values. The underlying principles are similar to those discussed in relation to self-report data. However, the methods for doing this are even less well developed than for self-report data. The best way to do this is probably to relate the cut-off points to health outcomes in each racial/ethnic group of interest. This requires comparable cohort studies. The data for doing this kind of work are sparse. These arguments are relevant to laboratory measures too, e.g. the effect of a value of 6 mmol/l of LDL cholesterol may not be the same in one racial or ethnic group as in another. One reason would relate to the presence, and the biological interaction, of other risk factors (arguments that are beyond the scope of this introductory book, but are covered in most intermediate-level textbooks of epidemiology). Another reason is that the lifetime burden of measures is likely to differ, especially in those who migrated from developing to developed countries as adults—they probably had low LDL (and BMI) in their country of origin, which rapidly rose after migration.

9.4.8 Choose the right control/standard/reference population

One central issue that arises from these considerations concerns the paradigm of the comparison or standard population, and specifically whether this can or ought to be the White population. We have seen how powerful and how misleading this approach can be. It is powerful because contrasts are often stark and clearly important—and easy to grasp. The idea that one relatively small but extremely rich and powerful segment of the global population—White people of European ancestry—can supply the norms against which all other racial and ethnic groups across the globe are to be judged, however, has been left unchallenged and applied for too long. It is impeding progress. For example, many racial and ethnic groups of non-European origin are currently judged to have an abnormally high prevalence of type 2 diabetes mellitus, as judged by the norms of White populations. Indeed, in any specific environment and given level of body fat people of northern European origin have less type 2 diabetes than virtually all other populations in the world. A better and surely more valid perspective would be to consider the White population to have an abnormally low prevalence. This population (and a few others) can be thought of as unusual or deviant. The question—what protects this population from diabetes even amidst plentiful nutrition—may provide a greater return than why nearly all other human populations have a great tendency to diabetes amidst over-nutrition. The relatively high BMI of populations of European origin with comparatively low body fat, reflecting a high muscle mass, may be one of the explanations.

There is a case for the group with the most favourable health status or risk factor profile to provide the standard population against which others are compared. The standard population would vary from one health outcome to another. This would potentially transform public health, with new and challenging targets.

9.4.9 Interpret data and use the findings to benefit the population studied

Try Exercise 9.6 before reading on.

Exercise 9.6 Publication, dissemination, and impact of research

◆ What problems must researchers in migration status, race, and ethnicity health research plan for in relation to interpretation of data, drawing conclusions, and utilization of research in policy and practice?

◆ How can such research stimulate change to improve the health of minority groups and the majority alike?

Research data do not, in themselves, provide answers. Only researchers and readers of research can do this through their application of the advanced skill of impartial data interpretation. Researchers who know the communities they work with are also more likely to interpret data with minimal error and bias. The researcher and the reader of research need insights into the history, culture, and living conditions of the people studied, particularly to assess the plausibility of the conclusions developed and the acceptability of any recommendations. Such insights, which may be taken for granted, perhaps wrongly so, when the researcher comes from the same migrant, racial, or ethnic group as the study subjects, are not easily acquired. Furthermore, there is limited guidance, training, and expert peer support to assist with interpretation of research on minorities.

Even once armed with insights into data interpretation and the communities under study, the researcher is often left with insufficient and inappropriate data to analyse, because of problems of small sample size, non-response bias, non-comparable groups, and improper ethnic coding, etc. The practical experience of reporting large multiracial multi-ethnic studies is limited worldwide, the main exception being the United States. Normally, such research reports on one minority group contrasted with another population—usually the White majority. Reporting and interpreting data on three or more groups simultaneously is still unusual, but is becoming more common, and using a non-White reference population is still rare. Examining White subgroups is also uncommon. Studies reporting simultaneously on the full range of racial and ethnic groups in a country is Such analysis and reporting is demanding both of intellect and publication space.

In addition to the challenge of the complexity of presenting and analysing data on 10 to 15 groups, in order to interpret them investigators also need to know about all the populations they are presenting data on. Investigators who seek a comprehensive picture may find it difficult to tackle the subject in the required depth. Those who select some population groups are being practical but may be accused of both 'cherry picking' and of inequitable behaviour in relation to groups not selected. These are delicate matters that investigators need to take care over, basing their choices on both scientific rationale and health needs. This said, the primary driver of research is the potential interest and value of gaining an answer to a research question. It behoves us, nonetheless, to check that this approach is not unwittingly worsening inequalities and inequities.

The translation of research into policy and practice is a complex area in any field including, and possibly especially so, for migration, race, ethnicity, and health. Translation of research is under active investigation in itself and minority health researchers need to make contributions to it. The key, perhaps the overriding, principle seems to be that for efficient translation to occur it needs to be anticipated and planned for, i.e. inbuilt into the research process. This requires close liaison throughout the research process between researchers, policy-makers, and those who will ultimately use the research. Such principles are hard to implement in practice because people in all three domains—research, policy, and practice—are busy with their own work, and time and finances are in short supply. The short-term nature of employment contracts is another issue. Research, in particular, is heavily governed by time-limited grants. Unless translation of research and dissemination of research are fully funded (and often they are not) these tasks may not be done well or at all.

I would like to reflect on a few of these issues in relation to one of my special interest—the health of South Asians in Europe.

Over some 40 years in the UK we have witnessed a rapid rise in the number of funded health studies on South Asian populations. This is the largest non-White ethnic group in the UK, and the amount of work is much greater than for other groups even taking population size into account. It cannot be argued that the health of South Asians is particularly poor—it is not. So why is this and what are the generalizable issues arising? UK South Asians are firmly established in the health-care professions, particularly medicine, and in the academic sector. The same is not true of most other ethnic minority groups, e.g. Gypsy travellers, Chinese, East Europeans, Africans. It is natural for minority group researchers to be interested in the health of people from their own group, and they have the background knowledge and motivation to do it. The danger is that over time the research effort grows unevenly and possibly even unjustly so.

A multi-ethnic, multiracial research workforce is needed to generate good research in multicultural societies. The most important of all the tasks in research is to pose the important and imaginative questions and to generate solutions to research challenges. These tasks, surely, need deep insight into the nature of the populations to be studied, and one route to this insight comes from membership of the population. Efforts to develop research capacity among minorities is especially advanced in the United States.

9.4.10 Funding and publishing the research and seeking the generalizations that avoid stereotypes

Try Exercise 9.7 before reading on.

Exercise 9.7 Using research

◆ What problems must researchers in the field of migration status, race, ethnicity, and health foresee and plan for in relation to funding, publication, and dissemination of research?

◆ How can such research stimulate change to improve the health of populations?

In the field of migration status, race, ethnicity, and health very basic information may be needed, e.g. population size or main causes of death. Not all data-gathering exercises, important as they are, are acknowledged as research. Research to be funded through research grants is characterized by the objective of extending the boundaries of knowledge. How can we tell if this might be achieved? Researchers will probably need to go through a rigorous process of review and approval to gain resources and permission to do the work. Many research funding bodies demand external peer review before awarding funding. Peer reviewers are required to assess whether the proposed research will add to existing work and whether the extra knowledge is worth the resources to be spent. The system is far from perfect, but it is the one that has been widely adopted internationally. Typically, 20–30% of grant applications gain funding. Most research also requires approval by ethics committees and some by other bodies too. These bodies will wish to confirm that peer review has taken place, but will look at the proposed work afresh.

Once the work is done the ethics and conventions of research require that it is summarized as a research paper or monograph and submitted for potential publication as a journal article (commonly) or book (rarely). The purpose of this is twofold. First, so that the work can be subjected to peer and editorial scrutiny to check its validity. Second, assuming it is found worthy of publication (usually after much painstaking revision), so that it can be made widely available and placed on the research record for posterity. A huge amount of research is never submitted for publication, and even much that is submitted is never published. Databases abstract and list the contents of thousands of journals (but not all of them). Many research papers are now available throughout the world via the Internet on the day that the final editing takes place and before official publication. Research that is published in this way becomes highly influential. Other scholars, researchers, professionals, and policy-makers will take such published and peer-reviewed findings much more seriously than those in in-house documents or verbal presentations. The published works have a stamp of quality and authority. When review articles are published they are likely to use these works and ignore others. These papers are often given media attention and brought to the attention of the public and their elected representatives. If such papers are to have a lasting impact beyond the place and time of their publication they need to emphasize generalizable findings and draw generalizable conclusions. It is also true that work that draws attention to problems is more likely to be published than work that shows there is no problem. Work that is novel is more attractive to peer reviewers and journal editors and hence more publishable than work that confirms what is already known. Work that has a positive result, i.e. demonstrates an association or that an intervention works, is more likely to be published than other work shows no association or no intervention effects (the outcome is so-called publication bias where the research literature shows positive results whereas in reality this might not be true).

These apparently academic issues pose great challenges to migration status, race, ethnicity, and health researchers. The kind of knowledge they seek to make progress in their country or locality may already be published—even though usually only for the White population. It will be hard to win scarce, competitively granted resources, and to win highly competitive publication space in the top widely read, general journals, for such necessary, but probably not ground-breaking, work. This is not to say such work cannot be published—it can and should be, but it is more likely to be in the specialist journals. (Typically, the general health journals accept 5–10% of papers submitted, specialist journals about 40%.) Even then, specialist journal editors will wish to publish novel findings. The research may be novel in the country in which it was done but not in an international context. Increasingly, research is seen as an international, not a national, endeavour with fewer nationally focused journals. Researchers' career prospects also depend on publishing in the internationally recognized journals. Researchers will need, therefore, to make the work sound exciting—and that usually requires highlighting problems, i.e. minorities are worse off, and giving attention to the positive findings, i.e. differences.

In winning grants, writing up, and publishing the work, however, researchers should have systems to minimize the danger of harm to the minority group studied, particularly the stigma associated with the demonstration of problems, stereotyping, and a fuelling of racism. This is a delicate path to tread. One of my major areas of research at present is cardiovascular disease and diabetes in South Asians in whom disease rates are comparatively high. Lest the population is seen in a negative light I remind audiences that overall mortality rates in South Asians are similar to those of the population as a whole, despite an excess of these specific diseases. The excess is balanced by a deficit of other causes of death, e.g. cancer and accidents.

The great potential benefit of a heavy emphasis on generalizable research is that the work ought to have value beyond the locality and population in which it was done. So research showing the very low rates of cardiovascular disease mortality in the Chinese, for example, in France may have transferable lessons across the Chinese diaspora, and perhaps even in China (Bhopal et al 2011). Equally importantly, this finding may have benefits for the entire French population—why should the entire population not enjoy the low rate of disease seen in the Chinese population in its midst? This argument will be pursued in Chapter 10.

9.5 Conclusions—the challenge of studying migrant, racial, and ethnic groups

The challenge of migration, race, ethnicity and health research includes demonstrating tangible health benefits in addition to satisfying curiosity and extending the boundaries of knowledge. Minority health is a beguiling research theme: it is worthy as it often focuses on underprivileged groups; it is interesting and often unearths unusual results; differences between groups can be demonstrated with ease; and even small studies can yield robust, significant, and relevant results. The full range of research methods in population and medical health science are potentially valuable (see Table 9.1). However, as the research literature has grown, so has criticism about its value.

Try Exercise 9.8 before reading on.

Exercise 9.8 Future research and challenges

- ◆ What challenges will researchers in the field of minority health need to overcome in the future?
- ◆ What, in your opinion, is the future of migration status, race, ethnicity, and health research?

There are numerous challenges in research. Some of these in relation to epidemiology are listed in Box 9.5. There are others relating to other social, population, and medical sciences. One of the greatest overall challenges is to do good work in the light of inherent complexity and amidst criticism. Who are we to believe—those who extol the value of the concepts of race and ethnicity and migration studies or those who criticize them? Researchers are left with the decision to either avoid the controversy and difficulty associated with migration status, race, and ethnicity variables (an action which may be socially, politically, legally, and scientifically unacceptable) or to do their best, with the express intention of continually improving their work. In this book I have demonstrated that even when operationalized with crude classifications, migration status, race, and ethnicity have value in health politics, policy, planning, surveillance, health services, and epidemiological research and in clinical care.

Box 9.5 Some challenges for epidemiological research on ethnicity, race, and health

◆ Inclusion of minorities in research and analysis of data by migrant status, race or ethnicity.

◆ Clarification of the purpose of the research.

◆ Definitions of concepts relating to migration status, ethnicity, and race that are internationally agreed.

◆ Definition and precision of terms, and migrant group/ethnic/racial classifications and classification on how they have been used.

◆ Recognition of heterogeneity within minority and majority groups alike.

◆ Identification of representative populations.

◆ Ensuring comparability of populations that are to be compared, requiring especially socio-economic data over the life-course to show this.

◆ Avoiding misinterpretation of differences that are due to confounding variables.

◆ Accurate measurement of the denominators and numerators in calculating rates.

◆ Ensuring the quality of data, particularly in cross-cultural comparability.

◆ Maximizing the completeness of data collection.

◆ Pinpointing specific genetic basis of genetic hypotheses.

◆ Properly argued interpretation of associations as causal or non-causal.

◆ Maximizing validity and generalizability of the research.

◆ Presentation of research to achieve benefits for the population studied, and avoid stigmatization and racism.

◆ Appropriate action to follow the research that, ideally, benefits the entire population.

Reproduced from Bhopal R, Glossary of terms relating to ethnicity and race for reflection and debate, *Journal of Epidemiological Community Health*, Volume 58, pp. 441–45, Copyright © 2004, with permission from BMJ Publishing Group Ltd.

Both purpose and context are the prime determinants of the way that race and ethnicity concepts are applied, classifications are devised and employed, and data are analysed and presented. Researchers must overcome the many conceptual and technical problems of migration status, race, ethnicity, and health research. One huge task is to achieve a shared, international understanding. We must avoid the mistakes of the past. In Chapter 1 I gave guidelines on how to do this and Box 9.6 (general) and Box 9.7 (refugees) offer some others that were published many years ago but apply as strongly as ever today.

Unfortunately, investigators are not putting such guidelines into practice sufficiently well, as the following euphemistically phrased quote indicates:

Although previous authors who have questioned the value of using race and ethnicity as scientific variables have proposed methodological guidelines aimed at increasing the integrity of these variables, it is clear from our study that researchers have not yet come to a consensus concerning their use.

Comstock et al. (2004, p. 619)

Box 9.6 Recommendations on the use of ethnicity and race in health research (generally)

1. Scientific criteria, based on knowledge from the social, behavioural, and biological sciences, should be used to define the concepts and measurement procedures for categories such as race and ethnicity.

2. Valid and reliable concepts of race, ethnicity, and related notions, such as ancestry or national origin, need to be explored.

3. The concepts of, and language used for, race, ancestry, ethnicity, and related notions need to be assessed among diverse segments of the US population to ensure valid and reliable responses to survey questions.

4. Social, economic, and political forces underlying differences in health status among ethnic and racial populations should be investigated and reported in population studies of health status.

5. When researchers describe differing health status among racial and ethnic populations they should explain (a) why they collected the information, (b) how the information was collected, and (c) what the information means.

6. Active participation of racial and ethnic communities in survey design, application and dissemination should be used to avoid misunderstanding and promote goodwill amongst groups whose health is being assessed.

Adapted from Warren RC et al, The use of race and ethnicity in public health surveillance, *Public Health Reports*, Volume 109, pp. 4–6, Copyright © 1994, US Department of Human Health and Human Services.

Unfortunately that view is still true some 10 years on. In Chapter 10 I will introduce work to create a consensus.

Migrant populations have provided a rich source of striking disease variations which have intrigued the epidemiological imagination. There is still massive potential for causal understanding through the in-depth investigation and explanation of such variations. Cohort and intergenerational effects could sharpen our understanding and prediction of disease frequency, disease causation, and the control of risk factors. Unfortunately, as yet, we have hardly begun to deploy these powerful designs.

The huge potential of research on minorities for service planning and delivery also needs good design and a clear focus, better data, and experience of putting research to use. For future progress we need to recognize that such research should focus on high-priority problems and that the planning of health services needs simple but validated data, different from that for the understanding of disease causes. Improvements will come from conceptual openness and explicit and defined terminology, and imaginative solutions to the fundamental problems of research on minorities, such as matching denominators and numerators, representativeness of the population, comparability of subgroups, and validity of the measurement tools.

The health of diverse minority populations would be served by:

◆ international conferences with the sole purpose of discussing terminology and other methodological issues;

◆ more forums (and perhaps journals) for discussion of the specific problems posed by research on minority groups;

◆ greater emphasis on research on methodological issues;

Box 9.7 Proposed guidelines for research in refugee and internally displaced populations

1. Undertake only those studies that are urgent and vital to the health and welfare of the study population.

2. Restrict studies to those questions that cannot be addressed in any other context.

3. Restrict studies to those that would provide important direct benefit to the individuals recruited to the study or to the population from which the individuals come.

4. Ensure the study design imposes the absolute minimum of additional risk.

5. Select study participants on the basis of scientific principles without bias introduced by issues of accessibility, cost, or malleability.

6. Establish the highest standards for obtaining informed consent from all individual study participants and where necessary and culturally appropriate from heads of household and community leaders (but this consent cannot substitute for individual consent).

7. Institute procedures to assess for, minimize, and monitor the risks to safety and confidentiality for individual subjects, their community, and for their future security.

8. Promote the well-being, dignity, and autonomy of all study participants in all phases of the research study.

Text extracts reprinted from *The Lancet*, Volume 357, Issue 9266, Jennifer Leaning, Ethics of research in refugee populations, pp. 1432–33, Copyright © 2001, with permission from Elsevier.

◆ a focus on the causes and prevention of the major reasons for ill-health;

◆ a greater readiness to research the quality of health care offered to minority groups; and

◆ more research input from minority populations, as investigators, advisers, and participants.

Much research on minority health has been by researchers whose interest is in one (or a group of) disorder(s). They seek a new perspective on that interest and are using the racial and/or ethnic variations model for that primary goal; the health and well-being of the minority population may well be a peripheral secondary interest. More research needs to be done by researchers whose main interest is in minorities and their health, with the disorder, methods, and disciplines being secondary. This requires, among other solutions, a stronger cadre of researchers from minority populations.

Participation by minorities in research, policy-making, and the development of services might be one safeguard against repeating the mistakes of the past. The American College of Epidemiology was one of the early organizations that called for a greater contribution to epidemiology by researchers from minority groups, who are under-represented. The views of the minorities may, however, be interpreted as representing special or vested interests so a partnership of a diverse range of groups is needed.

Wider, constructive debate on the criticisms of migration status, race, and ethnicity research is essential as a step towards agreement on the way forward. This debate is more advanced in the United States than in Europe, but on both sides of the Atlantic, papers intended to stimulate change have had surprisingly little impact. Even scientific journals are largely ignoring their own guidelines on reporting of race and ethnicity research, with most papers still failing to define their concepts and terms, despite editorial requirements to do so.

The perception that the health of minority ethnic groups is poor can augment the belief that immigrants and racial or ethnic minorities are a burden. The perception of poorer health arises from a focus on those differences where the excess of disease is in the minority population. It is naïve to believe that the mere demonstration of inequalities by migration status, race, or ethnicity will narrow them, and it is plausible that such studies can perpetuate and even augment inequalities. It is noteworthy that the concept of race is seldom used to study racism, at least in medicine, but is still frequently applied to infer biological differences between populations. The following quotation from Hilda Parker summarizes this mismatch, although it would be wrong to infer from the quotation that the United States has made great strides (although it has made more than most countries) in studying racism in health care:

> Recent British publications assessing the methods used in studies of ethnicity primarily considered the status of the variables 'ethnicity' and 'race' and advised on the use of appropriate categories. Such scrutiny of ethnicity research is welcomed, yet authors rarely emphasise the importance of racism as a variable. This paper discusses why racism matters as a variable and poses suggestions for its absence from British health services research. Reference is made to USA research to demonstrate that this focus is important and feasible. Health services research that considers ethnicity and excludes the effect of racism may result, at best in an incomplete understanding. At worst, this omission could itself be perceived as a racist practice.
> Parker (1997, p. 256), reproduced with permission from SAGE publications.

Racism, undoubtedly, is a difficult subject to study in the health arena, but there is also a reluctance to take it on.

For many causes, morbidity and mortality rates are lower in minorities, but these gain little attention for reasons discussed earlier. The promise of causal understanding has meant a focus on variation in diseases, as opposed to the quality of services. So there is a gap in the research record on the quality of care received by minority groups (but again the United States has become an exception here in recent years) to the detriment of the services and populations served. Minority populations are seriously under-represented in major studies, especially cohort studies and trials. That health research might be institutionally racist requires study. It would be better that action were taken before the world of research, at least in Europe, is asked to account for itself, either by government, funders, or the law. Europe has something to learn from the United States, although its policy on the inclusion of racial and ethnic minorities (and women) in research has raised difficult questions that need to be resolved. Box 9.8 cites some material that poses these questions.

We should step forward but tread warily, for if we do not, the 22nd century will look no more favourably upon present-day research on migration status, race, ethnicity, and health than we do upon the work of the talented but, in today's light, misguided scientists of the 19th century. Reviewing the principles of minority health research periodically is one way of progressing. In Chapter 10 I will discuss a new consensual approach resulting in 10 guidelines from UK researchers.

Box 9.8 Appropriate representation

The range of possible interpretations of the phrase 'appropriate representation' has left investigators struggling with the practical application of the National Institutes of Health guidelines on the inclusion of minorities in research. At least three goals might be reached by including minorities in clinical research; to test specific hypotheses about differences by race and ethnicity; to generate hypotheses about possible differences by race and ethnicity; and to ensure the just distribution of the benefits and burdens of participation in research, regardless of whether

(Continued)

Box 9.8 (Continued)

there are expected differences in outcome by race or ethnicity. In this paper, we describe possible interpretations of 'appropriate representation' as well as provide a general approach that investigators might use to address this issue. To expand scientific knowledge about the health of minority populations, investigators should be expected to state which goal they have selected and why that goal is appropriate as compared with other possible goals.

Text extracts reprinted from *The American Journal of Medicine*, Volume 116, Issue 4, Corbie-Smith et al, Interpretations of 'appropriate' minority inclusion in clinical research, pp. 249–52, Copyright © 2004, with permission from Elsevier.

9.6 **Summary**

Research is not a value-free activity, particularly when it is on living human beings. Migration status, race, and ethnicity are important to the structure and function of human populations, and it is inevitable that research utilizing these concepts is of interest to, and has influence upon, society and will be interpreted to meet social goals. Just as modern-day work is mostly used to further current goals of social equality and justice, so it was that much research in the past was used to further previous social and political goals such as the continuation of slavery, the justification of Empire, the maintenance of social and material inequality (including apartheid), anti-immigration policies focused on those who were not northern Europeans, eugenics, and the Nazi Final Solution leading to state policies to exterminate Jews, Gypsies, the mentally handicapped, and the psychiatrically ill. The most important lesson from this history is that research on migration status, race, and health needs to be done within an ethical framework emphasizing benefit to the population studied primarily, and to wider society secondarily.

The full range of health sciences and their methodological approaches—literature review, qualitative studies, case histories, case series, laboratory research, analysis of routine statistics, case–control studies, cohort studies, trials—are potentially applicable to migration, race, ethnicity, and health research. It is likely that an explosion of research on the genetic and environmental basis of ethnic/racial variations will occur as virtually all societies become multi-ethnic ones through migration. More cooperation with social scientists is needed to help resolve the social issues that will arise.

Researchers need to make explicit how they are using migration status, ethnicity, and race, and adapting their classifications and methods to the research questions under study. Researchers should not always be constrained by available classifications designed for administrative purposes, though veering from them should be done thoughtfully. Researchers who are knowledgeable about the minority groups under study are more likely to be trusted and more likely to achieve the high response rates and informed consent that are essential, and also to interpret data with minimal error and bias. In writing up and publishing their work, researchers should minimize the danger of harm to the groups studied, particularly the stigma which can ensue from associating them with problems for health-care systems. Over-emphasis of health problems, especially when imbalanced, can lead to for stereotyping and fuel racism.

The ideal population research study would be inclusive of all minority groups, have uniformly high response rates, provide data that are comparable across all groups, collect information on all relevant facets of migration status, race, and ethnicity, include data on all potential confounding variables, and be analysed and interpreted in a way that advances science, improves health status, and develops better health care. In practice, many ideals are sacrificed to make studies feasible. In making pragmatic choices researchers should make themselves and others aware of the limitations of the work. The excitement of this research theme means we can expect a rapid increase of research in this field. The challenge includes demonstrating tangible health benefits in addition to satisfying curiosity and extending knowledge.

References

American College of Epidemiology (1995) Statement of principles: epidemiology and minority populations. *Annals of Epidemiology* 5: 505–8.

Arnold M, Razum O, Coebergh JW (2010) Cancer risk diversity in non-western migrants to Europe: an overview of the literature. European Journal of Cancer 46: 2647–59.

Balarajan R, Bulusu L (1990) Mortality among immigrants in England and Wales, 1979–83. In Britton M (ed.) Mortality and Geography: a review in the mid 1980's, pp. 103–21. London: HMSO.

Barker RM, Baker MR (1990) Incidence of cancer in Bradford Asians. *Journal of Epidemiology and Community Health* 44: 125–9.

Bhopal RS (2004) Glossary of terms relating to ethnicity and race: for reflection and debate. *Journal of Epidemiology and Community Health* 58: 441–5.

Bhopal RS (2008) *Concepts of Epidemiology.* Oxford: Oxford University Press.

Bhopal RS, Donaldson LJ (1998) White, European, Western, Caucasian or what? Inappropriate labelling in research on race ethnicity and health. *American Journal of Public Health* 88: 1303–7.

Bhopal R, Bansal N, Steiner M, Brewster DH, on behalf of the Scottish Health and Ethnicity Linkage Study (2012) Does the 'Scottish effect' apply to all ethnic groups? All cancer, lung, colorectal, breast and prostate cancer in the Scottish Health and Ethnicity Linkage Cohort Study. *BMJ Open* 2: e001957.

Bhopal RS, Rafnsson SB, Agyemang C, Fagot-Campagna A, Giampaoli S, Hammar N, et al. (2011) Mortality from circulatory diseases by specific country of birth across six European countries: test of concept. *European Journal of Public Health* 22: 353–9.

Bowling A, Ebrahim S (2006) *Handbook of Health Research Methods: investigation, measurement and analysis.* Maidenhead: Open University Press.

Cartwright Dr (1851). Africans in America—diseases and peculiarities of the Negro race. *DeBow's Review: Southern and Western States* 11 (http://www.pbs.org/wgbh/aia/part4/4h3106t.html).

Chambers JC, Obeid OA, Refsum H, Ueland P, Hackett D, Hooper J, et al. (2000) Plasma homocysteine concentrations and risk of coronary heart disease in UK Indian Asian and European men. *The Lancet* 355: 523–7.

Comstock RD, Castillo EM, Lindsay SP (2004) Four-year review of the use of race and ethnicity in epidemiologic and public health research. *American Journal of Epidemiology* 159: 611–19.

Cooper R, Rotimi C, Ataman S, McGee D, Osotimehin B, Kadiri S, et al. (1997) The prevalence of hypertension in seven populations of West African origin. *American Journal of Public Health* 87: 160–8.

Corbie-Smith G, Miller WC, Ransohoff DF (2004) Interpretations of 'appropriate' minority inclusion in clinical research. *American Journal of Medicine* 116: 249–52.

Donaldson LJ, Clayton DG (1984) Occurrence of cancer in Asians and non-Asians. *Journal of Epidemiology and Community Health* 38: 203–7.

Donovan JH (1984) Ethnicity and health: a research review. *Social Science and Medicine* 19: 663–70.

Down JLH (1867) *Observations on an Ethnic Classification of Idiots.* (Reprinted in *Mental Retardation*, 1995, 54–7.)

Ecob R, Williams R (1991) Sampling Asian minorities to assess health and welfare. *Journal of Epidemiology and Community Health* 45: 93–101.

Elliot B for the Newcastle Strategy Group (including RSB) (1997) Taking heart: reducing diabetes and cardiovascular disease among Newcastle's South Asian and Chinese communities. In *Strategy for*

Commissioning Services for Coronary Heart Disease and Diabetes for Ethnic Minority Populations in England and Wales: lessons from a four-site pilot study. Newcastle upon Tyne: Departments of Epidemiology and Public Health and Medicine, University of Newcastle upon Tyne.

Ellison GTH, De Wet T (1997) Re-examining the content of the *South African Medical Journal* during the formalisation of 'racial' discrimination under apartheid. Health and Human Rights Project. In *The Final Submission of the HHRP to the Truth and Reconciliation Commission,* pp. 112–31. Cape Town: Health and Human Rights Project.

Gamble V (1993) A legacy of distrust: African Americans and medical research. *American Journal of Preventive Medicine* **9**(6) (Suppl.): 35–7.

Gould SJ (1984) *The Mismeasure of Man.* London: Pelican Books Ltd.

Hahn RA, Stroup DF (1994) Race and ethnicity in public health surveillance: criteria for the scientific use of social categories. *Public Health Reports* **109**: 4–12.

Hanna L, Hunt S, Bhopal R (2006) Cross-cultural adaptation of a tobacco questionnaire for Punjabi, Cantonese, Urdu and Sylheti speakers: qualitative research for better clinical practice, cessation services and research. *Journal of Epidemiology and Community Health* **60**: 1034–9.

Hernstein R, Murray C (1994) *The Bell Curve.* New York: Free Press.

Hunt S, Bhopal R (2003) Self report in clinical and epidemiological studies with non-English speakers: the challenge of language and culture. *Journal of Epidemiology and Community Health* **58**: 618–22.

Johnson MRD, Owen D, Blackburn C, Rehman H, Nazroo J (2000) *Black and Minority Ethnic Groups in England: the second health and lifestyles survey* London: Health Education Authority.

Jones JH (1993) *Bad Blood. The Tuskegee Syphilis Experiment,* 2nd edn. New York: Free Press.

Kaplan JB, Bennett T (2003) Use of race and ethnicity in biomedical publication. *Journal of the American Medical Association* **289**: 2709–16.

Kaufman JS, Cooper RS, McGee DL (1997) Socioeconomic status and health in blacks and whites: the problem of residual confounding and the resiliency of race. *Epidemiology* **8**: 621–8.

Kiple KF, King V (1981) *Another Dimension to the Black Diaspora: diet, disease, and racism.* Cambridge: Cambridge University Press.

Krieger ND, Rowley DL, Herman A (1993) Racism, sexism and social class: implications for studies of health, disease, and wellbeing. *American Journal of Preventive Medicine* **9**(6) (Suppl.): 82–122.

Leaning J (2001) Ethics of research in refugee populations. *The Lancet* **357**: 1432–3.

Lillie-Blanton M, Anthony JC, Schuster CR (1993) Probing the meaning of racial/ethnic group comparisons in crack cocaine smoking. *Journal of the American Medical Association* **269**: 993–7.

Lynn R, Rushton P, Jenson A, Murray C, Brand C, Nyborg H, et al. (2006) Racial IQ research. *Sunday Times* 2 April 2006 (http://www.thephora.net/forum/showthread.php?t=5745).

Marmot MG, Adelstein AM, Bulusu L (1984) *Immigrant Mortality in England and Wales 1970–78: causes of death by country of birth.* Studies on medical and population subjects, no. 47. London, HMSO.

Mather HM, Keen H (1985) The Southall Diabetes Survey: prevalence of known diabetes in Asians and Europeans. *British Medical Journal* **291**: 1081–4.

Matheson LM, Dunnigan MG, Hole D, Gillis CR, et al. (1985) Incidence of colo-rectal, breast and lung cancer in a Scottish Asian population. *Health Bulletin (Edinburgh)* **43**: 245–9.

McKeigue PM (1997) Mapping genes underlying ethnic differences in disease risk by linkage disequilibrium in recently admixed populations. *American Journal of Human Genetics* **60**: 188–96.

Nazroo JY (1997) *The Health of Britain's Ethnic Minorities: findings from a national survey.* London: Policy Studies Institute.

Nazroo JY (ed.) (2006) *Health and Social Research in Multiethnic Societies.* Abingdon: Routledge.

Office of Management and Budget (1977) Race and Ethnic Standards for Federal Statistics and Administrative Reporting. Directive No. 15. Washington, DC: Office of Management and Budget.

Osborne NG, Feit MD (1992) The use of race in medical research. *Journal of the American Medical Association* **267**: 275–9.

Parker H (1997) Beyond ethnic categories: why racism should be a variable in ethnicity and health research. *Journal of Health Service Research and Policy* **2**: 256–9.

Pilgrim S, Fenton S, Hughes A, Hine C, Tibbs N (1993) *The Bristol Black and Ethnic Minorities Health Survey Report*. Bristol: Departments of Sociology and Epidemiology, University of Bristol.

Ranganathan M, Bhopal R (2006) Exclusion and inclusion of nonwhite ethnic minority groups in 72 North American and European cardiovascular cohort studies. *PLoS Medicine* **3**: 1–8.

Rothschild H (ed.) (1981) *Biocultural Aspects of Disease*. London: Academic Press.

Samsudeen BS, Douglas A, Bhopal RS (2011) Challenges in recruiting South Asians into prevention trials: Health professional and community recruiters' perceptions on the PODOSA trial. *Public Health* **125**: 201–9.

Sheikh A (2006) Why are ethnic minorities under-represented in US research studies? *PLoS Medicine* **3**: e49.

Skrabanek P (1994) The emptiness of the black box. *Epidemiology* **5**: 553–5.

Taylor AL, Ziesche S, Yancy C, Carson P, D'Agostino R Jr, Ferdinand K, et al. (2004) Combination of isosorbide dinitrate and hydralazine in blacks with heart failure. *New England Journal of Medicine* **351**: 2049–57.

Warren RC, Hahn RA, Bristow L, Yu ESH (1994) The use of race and ethnicity in public health surveillance. *Public Health Reports* **109**: 4–6.

Wendler D, Kington R, Madans J, Van Wye G, Christ-Schmidt H, Pratt LA, et al. (2006) Are racial and ethnic minorities less willing to participate in health research? *PLoS Medicine* **3**: e19.

Whitridge Williams J (1926) *A Text-Book for the Use of Students and Practitioners*. New York: D Appleton & Co.

Wild SH, Fischbacher CM, Brock A, Griffiths C, Bhopal R (2006) Mortality from all cancers and lung, colorectal, breast and prostate cancer by country of birth in England and Wales, 2001–2003. *British Journal of Cancer* **94**: 1079–85.

Williams R, Bhopal R, Hunt K (1993) Health of a Punjabi ethnic minority in Glasgow: a comparison with the general population. *Journal of Epidemiology and Community Health* **47**: 96.

Woywodt A, Haubitz, Haller, Matteson EL (2006) Wegener's granulomatosis. *The Lancet* **367**: 1362–6.

Other sources and further reading

Allmark P (2004) Should research samples reflect the diversity of the population? *Journal of Medical Ethics* **30**: 185–9.

Barker J (1984) Black and Asian old people in Britain. *Research Perspectives on Ageing*, pp. 1–53 Surrey. Age Concern Research Unit.

Bhopal RS (1986a). The interrelationship of folk, traditional and western medicine within an Asian community in Britain. *Social Science and Medicine* **22**: 99–105.

Bhopal RS (1986b). Bhye Bhaddi: a food and health concept of Punjabi Asians. *Social Science and Medicine* **23**: 687–8.

Bhopal RS (1990) Future research on the health of ethnic minorities: back to basics. A personal view. *Ethnic Minorities Health. A Current Awareness Bulletin* **1**(3): 1–3.

Bhopal RS (1997) Is research into ethnicity and health racist, unsound, or important science? *British Medical Journal* **314**: 1751–6.

Bhopal RS (2000) Race and ethnicity as epidemiological variables. Centrality of purpose and context. In Macbeth H (ed.) *Ethnicity and Health*, pp. 21–40. London: Taylor and Francis.

Bhopal RS, Donaldson LJ (1988) Health education for ethnic minorities—current provision and future directions. *Health Education Journal* **47**: 137–40.

Bhopal R., Vettini A, Hunt S, Wiebe S, Hanna L, Amos A (2004) Review of prevalence data in, and evaluation of methods for cross cultural adaptation of, UK surveys on tobacco and alcohol in ethnic minority groups. *British Medical Journal* 328: 76–80.

Bhopal RS, Bansal N, Fischbacher CM, Brown H, Capewell S (2012a) Ethnic variations in the incidence and mortality of stroke in the Scottish Health and Ethnicity Linkage Study of 4.65 million people. *European Journal of Preventive Cardiology* 19: 1503–8.

Bhopal RS, Bansal N, Fischbacher C, Brown H, Capewell S (2012b) Ethnic variations in chest pain and angina in men and women: Scottish Ethnicity and Health Linkage Study of 4.65 million people. *European Journal of Preventive Cardiology* 19: 1250–7.

Bhopal RS, Bansal N, Fischbacher CM, Brown H, Capewell S (2012c) Ethnic variations in heart failure: Scottish Health and Ethnicity Linkage Study (SHELS). *Heart* 98: 468–73.

Black N (1987) Migration and health. *British Medical Journal* 295: 566.

British Medical Journal (1996) Ethnicity, race and culture: guidelines for research, audit and publication. *British Medical Journal* 312: 1094.

Chiu M, Austin PC, Manuel DG, Shah BR, Tu JV (2011) Deriving ethnic-specific BMI cutoff points for assessing diabetes risk. *Diabetes Care* 34: 1741–8.

Erens B, Primatesta P, Prior G (2001) *Health Survey for England: the health of minority ethnic groups '99.* London: The Stationery Office.

Kaufman JS, Hall SA (2003) The slavery hypertension hypothesis: dissemination and appeal of a modern race theory. *Epidemiology* 14: 111–26.

Krieger N (2002) Shades of difference: theoretical underpinnings of the medical controversy on black–white differences in the United States, 1830–70. In LaVeist TA (ed.) Race, Ethnicity and Health, pp. 11–33. San Francisco: Jossey-Bass.

Krieger N, Sidney S (1996) Racial discrimination and blood pressure: the CARDIA study of young black and white adults. *American Journal of Public Health* 86: 1370–8.

Leslie C (1990) Scientific racism: reflections on peer review, science and ideology. *Social Science and Medicine* 31: 891–912.

London Chinese Health Resource in partnership with Kensington, Chelsea and Westminster Health Authority, London (1995) *Needs Assessment: a study of the family planning and sexual health needs of the Chinese Community in Kensington, Chelsea and Westminster.* London: London Chinese Health Resource Centre.

Marquez MA, Muhs JM, Tosomeen A, Riggs BL, Melton LJ III (2003) Costs and strategies in minority recruitment for osteoporosis research. *Journal of Bone and Mineral Research* 18: 3–8.

Mason S, Hussain-Gambles M, Leese B, Atkin K, Brown J (2003) Representation of South Asian people in randomised clinical trials: analysis of trials' data. *British Medical Journal* 326: 1244–5.

McKeigue PM (1989) Diet and fecal steroid profile in a South Asian population with a low colon-cancer rate. *American Journal of Clinical Nutrition* 50: 151–4.

McKeigue PM, Marmot, MG, Syndercombe-Court YD, Cottier DE, Rahman S, Riemersma RA (1991) Relation of central obesity and insulin resistance with high diabetes prevalence and cardiovascular risk in South Asians. *The Lancet* 337: 382–6.

McKenzie K, Crowcroft NS (1996) Describing race, ethnicity and culture in medical research. *British Medical Journal* 312: 1054.

Muntaner C, Nieto J, O'Campo P (1996) The bell curve: on race, social class, and epidemiologic research. *American Journal of Epidemiology* 144: 531–6.

Patel S, Unwin N, Bhopal R, White M, Harland J, Ayis SA, et al. (1999) A comparison of proxy measures of abdominal obesity in Chinese, European and South Asian adults. *Diabetic Medicine* 16: 853–60.

Rahemtulla T, Bhopal R (2005) Pharmacogenetics and ethnically targeted therapies. *British Medical Journal* 330: 1036–7.

Rotimi CN (2004) Are medical and nonmedical uses of large-scale genomic markers conflating genetics and 'race'? *Nature Genetics* **36**: S43–S47.

Salomon JA, Tandon A, Murray CJL (2004) Comparability of self-rated health: cross sectional multi-country survey using anchoring vignettes. *British Medical Journal* **328**: 258–62.

Salway SM, Higginbottom G, Reime B, Bharj KK, Chowbey P, Foster C, et al. (2011) Contributions and challenges of cross-national comparative research in migration, ethnicity and health: insights from a preliminary study of maternal health in Germany, Canada and the UK. *BMC Public Health* **11**: 514.

Savitz DA (1994) In defense of black box epidemiology. *Epidemiology* **5**: 550–2.

Terry PB, Condie RG, Mathew PM, Bissenden JG (1983) Ethnic differences in the distribution of congenital malformations. *Postgraduate Medical Journal* **59**: 657–8.

Chapter 10

Theoretical, ethical, and future-orientated perspectives on health, migration status, race, and ethnicity

Objectives

After reading this chapter you should be able to:

- Consider the theories and principles learnt earlier in an ethical, enquiring and future-orientated way to improve the health of minority groups.

- Analyse and articulate the future potential of migration status, race, and ethnicity in a number of health settings—clinical care to individuals, public health initiatives, health-care planning, research, and policy-making.

- Understand that minority health research is not simply for the benefit of minorities but of the entire population, including the majority.

10.1 Introduction: theory

Before reading on try Exercise 10.1.

Exercise 10.1 Theories

- What is a scientific theory?

- What theories, if any, can you discern as underlying the use of migration status, race, and ethnicity in the health field?

- What theories about the influence of migration status, race, and ethnicity on health status have lost favour and which are currently in favour?

- What theoretical ideas about health and disease, migration status, race, and ethnicity hold up?

- Why is the use of migration status, race, and ethnicity growing in importance?

A scientific theory is a rational exposition, based on general principles, that explains apparently disparate (but actually interconnected) observations, ideas, and mechanisms about the natural world and allows predictions to be made and empirically tested. Although many theories about race and ethnicity have been developed, in both the biological and the social sciences, it seems to me that currently none command wide acceptance. There is, however, a steady stream of articles and books that are re-examining basic concepts. We also have the increasing production of diagrams illustrating possible cause and effect relationships underlying the relationship between race, ethnicity, migration status, and health status (see Section 10.6 for my example). As there are no widely accepted theories underpinning our subject, the result is a trend towards a largely empirical approach where the results are interpreted in themselves without reference to a broader framework of theoretical knowledge. There is also a fragmented approach to the subject with disparate concepts, methods, terminology, and interpretation. Advancement and maturity of disciplines is characterized by good theory. Good theory makes work easier to do, interpret, and generalize. We need more and better theories, and much more time spent on discussing these, as the quotations here testify:

> *Many epidemiologists continue to use the variable race uncritically and with little attention to theory. That is, they fail to consider possible social determinants of racial inequalities in health, including mechanisms originating from exposure to multiple forms of racial discrimination.*
>
> Muntaner et al. (1996, p. 535)

> *In generally trying to explain why some people are more susceptible to disease, health researchers propose that one clear, essential set of characteristics is shared by everyone in a category. This essentialism assumes we each have a 'true' identity inherent in us, and that we carry it from the moment of conception, or at least from the cradle to the grave.*
>
> *Essentialism can be social as well as biological.*
>
> Pfeffer (1998, p. 1382), reproduced with permission from BMJ Publishing Group Ltd.

One or more overarching theories might also help to unite the currently somewhat separate fields of indigenous health, asylum/refugee/undocumented migrant health, and ethnicity/race health. It may be that theories will be embedded within the larger field of inequalities in health. Recently, for example, Lorent and Bhopal (2011) explored the relevance to ethnicity and health of Tilly's theory of durable inequality, which aims to explain why inequalities arise and are sustained in societies.

Biological theories based on species and subspecies, and in modern day understanding on gene variants, have almost certainly had their 'moment of glory', although they are still part of the core dialogue in the field of minority health. This is another reminder that widespread acceptance of a theory does not make it right—race as difference in biology was deemed self-evident and even now commands attention despite its demonstrated flaws.

Hopefully, we will never return to the kind of thinking considered by Michael Banton in this quotation:

> *Consider the remarks of Gilbert Murray (1900: 156) the classical scholar, humanitarian and devoted supporter of the League of Nations:*
>
> 'There is a world hierarchy of races... those nations which eat more, claim more, and get higher wages, will direct and rule the others, and the lower work of the world will tend in the long-run to be done by the lower breeds of men. This much we of the ruling colour will no doubt accept as obvious.'
>
> *In these remarks nations, as political units, are equated with race, as biological units. The position of white people at the top of the hierarchy is attributed to their racial character and the future division of labour throughout the world is represented as an expression of this hierarchy. So the statements reflect a theory that is simultaneously biological and sociological.*
>
> Banton (1987, p. vii), reproduced with permission of Cambridge University Press.

Although genetic research continues to examine the global distribution of genetic variants, and to match the findings to racial and ethnic groupings, a renaissance of biology in the race and ethnicity fields seems improbable. The theory that all humans evolved in one place (monogeny)—probably Africa—and migrated from there fairly recently in evolutionary terms (60 000–70 000 years ago) is the key to understanding this viewpoint. While it stands—and at present it is firmly rooted despite continuing scientific scrutiny—it is hard to envisage how the concept of race as clearly separable subspecies can work. The contrary theory (perhaps fitting with common sense) that the human species *Homo sapiens* evolved in several places has been relegated to the fringes of scientific study. Should it ever return to centre stage then the concept of races as ancient and separate species/subspecies (polygeny) that have converged over long time periods might return. At present the unequivocal demonstration of the continuum of genetic variation across the globe, and hence among human populations internationally, means that a genetically based classification of races is not feasible. This does not mean that genetically based factors do not contribute, but they cannot hold centre stage in the great drama of migrant group, racial, and ethnic variations in human health. These ideas have been firmly established by population genetics and have been reaffirmed by modern genetic studies of DNA samples from across the world (see also discussions in Chapters 6 and 9).

Population sciences such as demography and epidemiology have made only modest contributions to theoretical debates on health status and migration status, race, and ethnicity (in contrast to general theories about health and disease where the contributions have been considerable). Theories tend to be superficial, e.g. over time there is convergence of disease risk factors and disease patterns, without a deep-level explanation of why this happens and why there are exceptions. Rather, these disciplines have used theories and concepts primarily from biology, anthropology, and sociology. The contribution of demography and epidemiology has been more at practical levels, e.g. the development of classifications and comparison of the value of different means of assessing and assigning migration status, race, and ethnicity.

Population sciences and the professions and disciplines that use them have, however, stimulated theoretical work by continuing to demonstrate the importance of variations by migrant, racial, and ethnic group in health and disease, and hence to public health and health care. In the absence of this empirical work it is likely that this subject would wither given the theoretical criticisms and methodological difficulties. The concepts of race and ethnicity, however, fit very well into the more general theories of health and disease developed by demographers and epidemiologists. This type of pragmatic, and apparently atheoretical, approach is common in these disciplines, e.g. in the equivalent lack of well-developed theories on sex, gender, age, education, and class-based variations in health and disease. While the approach may be pragmatic as scholars have correctly stated, it is underpinned, nonetheless, by theories, albeit poorly articulated and possibly superficial ones.

To quote James Nazroo:

> ... it is a mistake to assume that the process of identifying 'ethnic' groups is theoretically neutral (hence my use of the term 'un-theorised' rather than atheoretical).
>
> Theory is brought in surreptitiously—ethnicity, however measured, equals genetic or cultural heritage. This then leads to a form of victim blaming where the **inherent** characteristics of the ethnic (minority) group are seen to be at fault and in need of rectifying.
>
> Nazroo (1998, pp. 715–16), reproduced with permission from John Wiley and Sons.

These points on ethnicity apply equally to work examining the health of migrants, indigenous peoples, Roma/Gypsy traveller populations, and of course racial groups. 'Un-theorized' is a useful word—it indicates that the discipline has not yet paid attention to theory building. It is no surprise that journals specializing in race, ethnicity, migration, and health, e.g. *Ethnicity and Health*, the one recently edited by Nazroo, are placing special emphasis on putting research into a theoretical context.

In all these areas—and more—demographers and epidemiologists look to the biological or social sciences for theories. Collaborations between social, epidemiological, and biological scientists in theoretical work are needed (as already happens so successfully in empirical research).

Since the Second World War the social sciences have dominated theoretical discussions on migration, race, and ethnicity. Social historians have also produced important insights. Clearly, this is wholly appropriate as these concepts shape societies and social interactions between populations, population subgroups, and individuals. The contribution of the social sciences, however, goes much deeper than merely describing the impact of migration, race, and ethnicity on society, and two profound insights have emerged that seem evident, in retrospect.

First, the insight, indeed theory, that societies have created concepts such as race and ethnicity to meet their own social purposes, i.e. the concepts are socially constructed. The same, obviously, would apply to various kinds of classifications of migrants, e.g. asylum seekers or economic migrants. If so, migrant, racial, and ethnic groups do not actually exist in any biological or external way. (According to social constructivism all labels and values are also social constructs—a perspective that I largely accept.) Leaving aside philosophical debates on the existence or not of objects and ideas outside one's mind, this is a powerful and provocative idea. If it is correct then we could also envisage societies that have no concepts of this kind. We could envisage societies that socially construct in radically different ways, e.g. thinking of African-origin and European-origin populations as one race or ethnic group and Indians and Pacific Islanders as another. Many medical scientists concur, generally, with this view as the following quotation, where 'racial' is used to mean biologically determined race, shows:

> National, religious, geographic, linguistic and cultural groups do not necessarily coincide with racial groups: and the cultural traits of such groups have no demonstrated genetic connection with racial traits.
> UNESCO statement on race, 1950 (in Kuper *et al.* 1975, p. 344)

This view implies that our current concepts and classifications have no secure long-term foundation, and certainly not one based on nature. It is a much needed correction to the biological ideas that preceded it but in my view it goes a little too far. The social construction of migrant groups, races, and ethnic groups, whatever groupings are chosen, needs to be based on information to permit such social construction. What is this information? Is it not the biological, ancestral, and cultural factors that underpin the concepts of race (colour, hair texture, physiognomy, etc.), migration status (place of birth of self and ancestors), and ethnicity (language, ancestral origins, clothing, traditions, and so on)? Is this kind of information not processed by humans to make important social decisions? The neurological research studying humans' responses to faces indicates that it is so (Golby et al. 2001). No doubt, some of this processing is innate and some of it is socially conditioned. Astonishing recent research shows that babies of about 6 months of age process information about 'same race' faces differently from 'other race' faces. While it is just conceivable that babies are already socially conditioned by that age it seems equally plausible the brain is hard-wired to process such information—just as it is in the case of language. This is a rapidly developing field of enquiry. A clean separation of the social and the biological is often impossible in the human species, which is characterized by its socialization, which must itself have a biological foundation.

Armed with these social constructs we gain deeper understanding of the importance of migration status, race, and ethnicity to human societies and accept that the practical issues like group categories and labels will be subject to both local context and change over time. This perspective gives us a social lens to understand why matters are as they are.

The second huge contribution from the social sciences is encapsulated by the terms racialization and reification. Racialization is the process whereby for individuals, groups, and institutions, perceiving the social world in terms of racial and ethnic groups becomes an ingrained habit, one that seems normal and necessary. The same applies to migration research—better to use racialization, though migrationization would be the equivalent word (perhaps invented here). Population research in the United States is racialized to see health problems, especially, in terms of Black and White populations.

Once this happens it is a small step to perceiving these racial and ethnic divisions as real, perhaps even inviolable. This latter step is called reification—making real something that does not deserve that status. A complex and somewhat nebulous concept, race, and a crude classification, the Black/White division, becomes over time a natural way of thinking and in due course the classification arising becomes routine, rigid, and unchanging. While internationally, research on White/Black and even White/non-White is seen as crude, in the United States it is sufficiently normal to be commonplace.

Habits and routines are an ingredient of our social worlds, and sometimes they can be helpful. Eating is natural, but eating three meals a day is not. Other routines are possible and possibly even better. In the same way, I believe, perceiving humans as comprising different subgroups using the cues underlying migration, race, and ethnicity is natural but the divisions (subgroups) we create are not. Other divisions (subgroups) are possible. Is it possible to have no divisions at all? Difference does not necessarily need to be enshrined in divisions at societal level, even though humans will perceive differences. The choice is ours, and we should do what is best for human society—this is a task for all of us, led by our politicians. It is difficult to work out what is best. It depends on viewpoints and goals. France is a multicultural country that has purposively avoided the use of ethnicity and race in modern times. There is even a widespread myth that doing so is illegal (but it is no more so than in other European countries—all are bound by the same overarching data protection and human rights laws). It would be hard to argue that France has gained any benefits from this stance and the approach seems to be creating difficulties for minorities, but difficulties which are obscured for lack of data. France is certainly not a country without divisions on the lines of migrant status, race, or ethnicity notwithstanding its policy. Here are two world views, one from Carleton Coon, who published an extensive classification of the races of humanity in 1962, perhaps the last work of its kind. The other is from the Bikhu Parekh, one of the leading UK academics in race relations.

> If the races of man stay where they are best adapted, it creates much less trouble than when they move into each other's territories.
>
> Do the minds of all races work in the same fashion, do not their emotions differ with differences in their hormonal peculiarities, and is it not possible that cultures vary to a certain extent in terms of these variations? These questions require research, and the results may mar the vision of a single world culture.
>
> If the world is to become united, the union must be a loose confederation of very different units, or it will not long endure.
>
> Coon (1963, pp. 130–1), reproduced with permission from Elsevier.

A multicultural society should be based on equal citizenship, and five areas have been identified for consideration, and commitment for change:

1. elimination of discrimination
2. equality of opportunity
3. equal respect
4. acceptance of immigrants as a legitimate and valued part of society
5. the opportunity to preserve and transmit their cultural identities including their languages, cultures, religions, histories and ethnic affiliations.

> Parapharased from Parekh (in Modood et al. 1997, p. ix), with permission
> from Policy Studies Institute.

Theoretical work is needed both to understand and to reconcile such different viewpoints. It is time for a new and hopefully more integrated theory. When scientists in a field of endeavour cannot agree on basic concepts, according to Thomas Kuhn, a major shift in thinking is under way, and if it is not, it is overdue. In his words, it is time for a paradigm shift (Kuhn 1996). Pending developments of new paradigms, people using migration status, race, and ethnicity need to be thoughtful and aware, and be ready to contribute their own views to ongoing and forthcoming debates. At present, the flexible approach to application of concepts, and the development and evolution of classifications, indicates that our field is following a social constructivist and non-reifying approach.

10.2 Ethics of migration, ethnicity, race, and health policy, practice and research

Before reading on try Exercise 10.2.

Exercise 10.2 Ethics

◆ Why is an ethical code so important in the migration, race, ethnicity, and health arena?

◆ In the context of minority health reflect on the ethical codes that require professionals to: (1) do no harm; (2) do good; (3) offer autonomy; (4) be just.

◆ How can these codes prevent the return of misuses of race science?

An ethical code is a code of correct behaviour. Such codes must, necessarily, change with time and differ to some extent from place to place. Ethical codes are not rigid and incontestable, even although they may be given stability by fundamental principles (sometimes enshrined in religion and laws). Furthermore, they are different for different disciplines. Ethical codes are highly developed in medicine, and these codes have deeply influenced public health—not least because public health is often dominated or strongly influenced by medicine. Adaptations of these codes for epidemiology and for medical and public health are available (e.g. see the website of the International Epidemiological Association, http://ieaweb.org/). As discussed in Chapter 8, there are codes for undertaking research with ethnic minorities that are strong on ethics. To my knowledge, however, no such codes are obligatory, as the ethical code of the medical profession is. Ethical codes are, nonetheless, vital to the minority health field. While it would be wasteful and possibly even harmful to create separate and new ethical codes for migration, ethnicity, and race research and practice, we do need to consider the potential influences that might require a change of emphasis or application of general existing codes as we now consider.

10.2.1 Do no harm (non-maleficence)

'Do no harm' is the immemorial requirement of doctors, who have the power of life or death in their hands. In my view this is the most important ethical pillar in the migration, race, ethnicity, and health field. Articulating the concepts of race or ethnicity and migration status draws attention to differences, potentially magnifying their importance. These differences can be used in damaging ways, as emphasized throughout this book. The way that data are put to use depends on the social circumstances, and these may change rapidly, especially as the economy changes.

Researchers and practitioners need to be sensitive to wider events. At the time of writing, the continuing repercussions of the suicide missions that destroyed the Twin Towers in New York, the wars in Iraq and Afghanistan, the furore over the proposal by Iran to develop nuclear energy, the turmoil in the Middle East, and the backlash as people either defend or refute the right to freedom of speech, are a few of the background issues that matter. The economic consequences of the banking crisis in 2008 are undermining race relations, and progress in policy and service development. It is a difficult time, even with the best of intentions, to release research or make proposals relating to improving the health of minorities—especially Muslims given the obvious Islamophobia—or even to publish the ideas in this book. These proposals, and particularly research data, could be used to drive wedges between population subgroups, especially between followers of Islam and of other religions. A headline and front page article in a Scottish newspaper on 31 January 2013 argued that the special efforts made to improve services for minorities in an area in south Glasgow were damaging the health prospects of the general population (an improbable claim). This is not to advocate self-censorship or to suggest that no change should be proposed—but that researchers should have awareness of the primary goal of health improvement in relation to the possible harm that could take them further from it. The health researcher in the field of migration, race, and ethnicity has a secondary duty that is a companion to the primary one of gaining and using knowledge—to foster a milieu of equality, justice, tolerance, and sensitivity, and to counter harmful tendencies to the contrary. Only then, I propose, can benefits occur, as discussed next.

10.2.2 Beneficence—doing good

Doing good—beneficence—lies at the heart of public health, medicine, and all health professions. Unfortunately, the intention to do good often, and perhaps even mostly, does not lead to good. As is so often the case, a historical analysis gives clarity. It is worth reflecting upon the harm done by the extensive use in medicine of enemas, bloodletting, heavy toxic metals, electroconvulsive treatment (ECT) for many disorders, thalidomide, hormone replacement therapy (for heart disease prevention), and a multiplicity of drug and other interventions. All of these were used on a mass scale to do good but they did harm. Health and health-care interventions are not implemented in a climate of undiluted beneficence—there are additional social, political, commercial, and other motives. As discussed in some detail in this book, beneficence towards migrants and racial or ethnic minorities is by no means universal, either across time or place. Indeed, with a few exceptions, the record is of antipathy and sometimes hostility by the majority to such minorities.

Doing good in this context requires a special effort of will, and is a struggle against lack of knowledge, information, expertise, leaders, finances, and competing priorities. Nonetheless, the general imperative of medical ethics to do good also provides the specific imperative to ensure that some populations, migrant, racial, and ethnic minorities being an example, are not excluded from acts of beneficence. This general ethic is, in the long term, more powerful than even legislation and policy, for it is an ingrained part of every health professional's training and mental make-up. Doing good is also the governing value of health institutions, including those responsible for training and education. In exceptional circumstances, however, even this ethic can be overridden as we have already considered, e.g. as in the case of Nazi Germany. Without the ethic of beneficence in place it is better not to draw attention to differences among migrant, racial, and ethnic groups. With it the interesting though sometimes daunting challenges are worth tackling.

To do good in professional settings needs competency in a variety of attitudes and skills. Competency is moving to the core of clinical education. It is achieved through education, training, research, and an understanding and respect for both the individuals and the groups that comprise the population to be served. Respect is a key word, and it may develop in a variety of ways. Education, research, or training does not always engender respect for others, and sometimes the opposite happens. Nonetheless, widespread education must be the starting point, and that requires the inclusion of minority health in the curriculum. It is proving rather difficult to integrate ethnicity and race into medical curricula in a rigorous and solid way, but we must keep trying, as Joe Kai and colleagues attest:

> As learning to value ethnic diversity begins to feature more consistently in medical training it will inevitably include 'token' approaches that lack coherence. However, even imperfect first steps can provide useful lessons and create momentum for change. In an increasingly diverse society, which serves to enrich our lives and experiences, doctors must learn to value ethnic diversity to deliver effective health care. In doing so, they will bring mutual benefits for their patients and themselves.
>
> Kai et al. (1999, p. 622)

While one can respect the autonomy and differences of others without understanding them, the current view is that increasing the knowledge base of professionals is a necessary prerequisite. A professional culture that requires respect for everyone, irrespective of migrant status, or racial or ethnic group, is the goal. Admittedly, it seems sad that such a goal needs to be set. (Undoubtedly, the most vigorous, rigorous, and demanding work in this field is taking place in the United States, driven by explicit policy and standards, as considered in Chapter 8.)

10.2.3 Respect and autonomy

Respecting and understanding others is not easy. At the minimum it requires a tolerance of others, but it also needs an interest in others, a wish to learn about them, and an active effort to perceive their world view in a positive light. Clearly, minority groups need to do this, if only to adjust to living in multicultural societies. The majority population has no such immediate need, but in the interest of a better society they should reciprocate. The idea that the process of learning should be two-way lies at the heart of multiculturalism. Multiculturalism seems to me to be the only possible direction for the modern world, and hence for modern health-care systems, yet it is coming under attack (see Chapter 4, particularly Section 4.2.5 on The Netherlands). I think that these attacks misrepresent multiculturalism as a society of many distinct and separate cultures—which is surely the opposite of the truth. The alternative to multiculturalism, that the dominant culture remains wholly or largely unchanged while the minority ones integrate, assimilate, and conform to the norms of the majority is, in my view, both impossible and highly undesirable.

Just as with the force of gravity, where each object in the universe exerts a force on surrounding objects, so it is with individuals and social subgroups. (Unlike gravity and inanimate objects, the mutual social influence is not subject to simple, formulaic assessment.) The correct response, I propose, is for active but sensitive debate to seek and nurture those changes that benefit society. By respecting and understanding minority populations we might learn of the cultural and other forces that are leading, e.g. in the UK, to superb educational achievements among British Chinese children, the low levels of psychological stress in Bangladeshis in East London despite economic deprivation, low divorce rates, the continuing low prevalence of smoking amongst Sikhs (men and women) and other South Asian women, the low rates of alcoholic liver disease in most minority groups, and the low levels of CHD in men of African origin. There are also other values that may exist in minority communities but which are not promoted although they may bring many health benefits, e.g. practising religion on a daily basis, close-knit families, traditional health care, herbal remedies, and systems of health such as yoga. There may be something to be learned from practices that are portrayed negatively by the media, e.g. arranged marriages. There is also much to learn from the majority population that can benefit minorities, e.g. the generally greater attention given to physical activity, preventative health services such as screening for cancer, work–life balance, flexibility in gender roles in marriage and the workplace, and individual freedom. These are only a small sample of the potential benefits of multiculturalism in public health.

Respect is the pre-condition for autonomy. In medical ethics the competent patient (hence excluding, e.g., young children and the mentally impaired) must give informed consent for all procedures and for research. Autonomy is a pre-eminent medical ethic in current times. It overrides beneficence. The classic example of this is the Jehovah's Witness patient who refuses a life-saving blood transfusion against medical advice. The competent person has the right to refuse treatment.

Minorities are sometimes subtly, but sometimes crudely, coerced into changing their way of life in their new society. Autonomy of minority populations to live in their own preferred, perhaps traditional, way is not easy to achieve. Compromises are essential. Tensions have arisen on matters such as Sikhs refusing to wear crash helmets while motorcycling, the lack of organ donations from some minority populations, the larger family sizes of some minority groups because of positive attitudes to children and negative ones to contraception, female circumcision (usually called genital mutilation), pressure exerted on young people by the family in favour of arranged marriages, and so-called honour killings where people going against the tradition are murdered. These are a few examples of issues that relate to culture, health care, and public health. A common complaint expressed by politicians and in the media is that minority groups are resistant to change and integration. By contrast, within minority communities, the pace of change can seem bewilderingly and frighteningly fast as centuries-old traditions are wiped out in a few years or decades. These are very difficult issues that require sensitive consideration to create a sense of fairness and to handle justly. Justice requires that such issues are properly considered and appropriate laws and policies are framed that balance the needs of the individual, the group, and society as a whole.

10.2.4 Justice, fairness, and equality

Justice is the core value that underpins equity. Justice is fairness—fairness that is built into social structures. Justice also underpins law. The importance of justice to the migration, race, ethnicity, and health agenda is great.

Justice changes when human values on right and wrong change, and therefore it varies in time and place, for change does not occur at a constant rate everywhere. In the modern era in many countries justice requires that individuals are treated equally. Amazingly, this very new idea has become almost the norm—as if any other situation is inconceivable. Yet it was not true in many places until recently, and is still not true in so many respects. Moreover, justice also requires that social groups are also treated equally. Perhaps most remarkably of all, justice may include compensation for historical injustices. In this special circumstance, everyone may not be treated equally, and there may be positive action in favour of some individuals and groups. Such affirmative action can create great tensions, not only between groups but also within groups, around ethnic and racial identities. Genetics has been used to resolve these, as indicated in the quotation below. Mostly, these tensions revolve around the right to access resources.

> Genetics can affect questions of ethnic identity (such as who counts as Cherokee or Maori), religious identity (who counts as Parsee or Jewish), family identity (who counts as a descendant of Thomas Jefferson), or caste (who counts as Brahman or Dalit). These identities overlap in various ways, and genetic evidence will not affect them all equally. But clearly confusion looms when genetic markers conflict with other kinds of markers of group membership, such as a shared culture or historical narrative. Does it make you any more English, or Sioux, or Jefferson if your identity has been corroborated by a genetic marker?

> *Two years ago, after a bitter monetary dispute, the Seminole Nation of Oklahoma passed a resolution that will effectively expel most black Seminoles, or Seminole Freedmen. The Freedmen are the descendants of former slaves who fought alongside the Seminoles in the Seminole Wars and who have been officially recognised as members of the Seminole Nation of Oklahoma since 1966. The new constitution says that to be part of the tribe, a person must show that he or she has one eighth Seminole blood.*
>
> Elliot and Brodwin (2002, pp. 1469–70), reproduced with permission
> from BMJ Publishing Group Ltd.

This viewpoint, that equality and equity are part of social justice, is now enshrined in constitutions, treaties, international conventions, and laws (whether local, national, or international).

The full consequences of a social justice stance are never easy to grasp or implement, and this applies in the field of migration, race, ethnicity, and health. It is, in most modern societies, unfair, unjust, and in some places illegal to deliver a service, knowingly or unknowingly, to one migrant, racial, or ethnic group that is either superior or inferior to that delivered to another group. It is acceptable, and perhaps even mandatory, however, to target resources and expertise to redress historical wrongs, so creating temporary conditions that favour the population that was previously unfavourably discriminated against. There are many examples of positive discrimination including the Indian Health Service in the United States that was set up to meet the specific needs of Native Americans, the reservation of jobs and university places for scheduled castes in India, and the reservation of lands for Australian Aborigines. This is a deep paradox—to promote equality, we may need to treat people and groups unequally, a point well captured by the phrase 'fair discrimination'. It is very difficult to know when fair discrimination is justified and when it is no longer needed, especially as it is very difficult to withdraw a privilege. In principle, fair discrimination is important in the field of minority health: indigenous minorities, Roma/Gypsy and Traveller populations, previously discriminated racial or ethnic groups, and disadvantaged migrant groups may all merit consideration.

The Scottish Executive's 2002 strategy for minority ethnic health is aptly called *Fair for All*, a title that is now used for the wider diversity agenda to include inequalities by sex, sexual orientation, disability, and other grounds for potential discrimination (see Chapter 8). Indeed, the phrase is now used widely in the UK. Fairness is something that is intuitively right and something virtually all agree with, at least in theory.

Justice is important not only to the allocation of resources and setting of priorities, but also to autonomy and human rights. Competition between varying ethical principles, or even within a principle, is inevitable. For example, justice requires proper and effective use of resources—it is not right to waste resources when there are unmet needs. It would be fair and just, at least in an ideal world where all needs could be met, to translate hospital information in the hundred or so languages read in a typical metropolitan area such as London, Amsterdam, New York, or Sydney. Then the public could exercise its choice and equity would be achieved. The cost of simply developing this (and not even distributing it) would, however, be very high—at present perhaps £100 000 for a typical two- to four-page pamphlet translated into 100 languages. If there were 500 such pamphlets, a reasonable estimate considering the complexity of health care, that would come to £50 million. The materials would need updating every couple of years, perhaps more often. The printing, storage, and distribution costs would be additional. Materials in many languages would probably not be read for lack of demand, interest, illiteracy, and the fact that people are often able to read several languages including English. This apparent ideal of meeting every group's needs for information conflicts with the inherent injustice in wasting scarce resources, an act that deprives people with other equally or more pressing needs. The need for delicate judgements cannot be escaped and a balance needs to be found. Some principles for finding such a balance were discussed in Chapter 7 on priority-setting.

On a larger scale than the delivery of health care, laws against racism and for equality may infringe other deeply held values, ethics and laws, for example, those promoting freedom of speech and action. Currently, in most countries, freedom of speech is curtailed but this will be constantly challenged. These clashes usually require resolution on a grand scale—by parliamentarians or the law courts, not only nationally but internationally. The ethics of medical research are, indeed, governed by truly international codes.

10.2.5 **Research ethics**

This is a big topic that I touched on in Chapters 8 and 9. As is often the case, it is safe to conclude that the ethics of research generally are largely applicable to minority groups. The principles enshrined in the Nuremberg Code, e.g. those emphasizing informed consent, are excellent starting points. Indeed, such codes are usually written following the abuse of minorities—and this one was designed to prevent a repetition of the abuses by Nazi scientists (see Chapter 6).

Yet some modifications may be necessary. Ethical codes may need to be modified to emphasize the importance of including minority populations in research and not bypassing them on non-scientific grounds such as researchers' unfamiliarity with them, increased heterogeneity of research samples, real or perceived communication barriers, and extra costs. This may require purposive strategies, policies, and even laws, as has already happened in the United States (see Chapter 8). Above all, it will require that researchers have the necessary awareness, expertise, and resources to achieve inclusivity. In recent years we have seen these points being raised in guidance issued by research ethics committees and research funders, but they have not been incorporated in a formal or binding way.

Ethical codes on confidentiality and informed consent may also need modifications to optimize these for use in minority health research. For example, if a person from a minority group is not able to read it is unethical, surely, on the grounds of waste of resources to send written information about a project. It may even alienate such people by pointing to their illiteracy, and hence belittling them. To recruit such people into research may require access to personal information including telephone numbers. It may be ethical to telephone or even call at the doorstep of such a person, a behaviour that ethical committees usually frown upon, because it is considered a greater infringement of privacy than a letter. The right to be invited in an appropriate manner needs to be balanced against the right to privacy of personal data such as a telephone number. To take another example, informed consent may not be easy to gain or to record in writing. Some small leap of imagination may be needed, such as recording of the consent on a video or audio recorder. Where this is not possible, a witness may need to confirm oral consent. A thumbprint might be considered as a time-honoured alternative to a signature. Ethical codes should also consider research in cultures where it is most common for the head of the household or the whole family, or even a whole village or community to decide on participation. Thus individual informed consent is not always the only or best way forward.

The point of research is to learn and apply that knowledge. It is important that we can see the effects—and that requires research on outcomes, i.e. evaluation. In Chapter 8 I discussed the evaluation of policies, with a focus on checking they were being implemented, and in Chapter 9, I discussed briefly some research methods including trials (the gold standard for evaluation). I now discuss the broader issue of the need for evaluation.

10.3 **Evaluating interventions in ethnicity and health**

Before reading on try Exercise 10.3.

Exercise 10.3 Evaluation

- ◆ Why is it necessary to evaluate at all?
- ◆ How can we demonstrate the benefits of working with indicators of migration status, race, and ethnicity?
- ◆ Why are our endeavours in the health field difficult to evaluate?

Evaluation is difficult, even for specific effects of circumscribed actions such as giving a drug to treat pneumonia or other such easily definable conditions. Even this type of intervention usually requires the complexities and expense of a randomized, double-blind, placebo-controlled trial so that biases and confounding factors can be taken into account. Common sense has repeatedly been shown to be misleading in assessing the value of such technologies. Evaluation of the combined effects of laws, policies, strategies, and interventions on minority health poses challenges of a higher order. Nonetheless, it is important for us to ask the question, 'Is this activity benefiting our society as a whole, and the minority populations within it, and are the costs in line with the benefits?'. Posing the question is valuable, even though it may be almost impossible to answer it in a definitive way. The question needs to be tackled by a mix of approaches including political, historical, and social policy analysis; monitoring of health and related states; and both observational and experimental research on specific interventions. Societies need to be ready to change direction if necessary.

The underlying premise of this book is that variations in health care, health and disease by migrant status, race, and ethnicity are too large to be ignored, and that acknowledging and acting upon them is better than ignoring them. I have acknowledged one price to be paid—highlighting differences may widen divisions in society. If the discovery and study of such variations does no good, or does harm, then it would be better to retrace our steps, dismantling research policies, monitoring programmes, and research projects. In the first edition of this book I made what in retrospect seems an extraordinary statement, i.e. 'It is largely a matter of faith, and inference from general observations, that currently the benefits exceed the harms'. (This was not to deny the sheer intrinsic interest of the topic from a scholarly, research point of view.) Six years later, I am able to say that the view that the benefits exceed the harms has spread. Overall, it seems to be so, but clear-cut evidence of effectiveness and especially cost-effectiveness is still sparse.

International comparisons hold one, admittedly difficult, approach to analysis and evaluation. The period since 2005 has been fraught with racial tensions, as witnessed by examples such as riots across France and in both London, UK and Sydney, Australia, and great unhappiness at the possible role of racism in the weak response of the US authorities to the flooding of New Orleans. There has been disorder in England, The Netherlands, and Denmark over a number of matters that have been linked to socio-economic deprivation and social segregation. Greece is one of the European states where racism has become open, with the rise of the far right. The plight of the Roma and indigenous populations has worsened, despite policy and strategy advances. Across the world, surveys report a negative attitude to immigration even as it accelerates. On the other hand, it is clear that multicultural societies and cities (with high rates of immigration) are flourishing, e.g. London, New York, Paris, Amsterdam, and Vancouver (almost always at the top or near the top of the UN league table of the finest places to live). The excitement of a multicultural society came to the fore at the London Olympics where so many athletes from Britain's minorities made the UK proud.

It is not apparent that racial disharmony is less in multi-ethnic countries which proclaim themselves as single-identity nations having no place for race-based policies or data. France is such a country. For many years France either was, or was perceived to be, a haven for people suffering from racism. Now problems have come to the fore. It is likely, in my view, that these problems have existed for a long time and have not been tackled openly, because of ostensibly race-free policies. Since 1999, by contrast, Scotland has openly declared a social justice agenda with equality in race and ethnicity as one of several core components. To date we have seen no social backlash, and the accrual of small but noticeable benefits to the health care of minority and majority populations alike (e.g. areas for prayer and meditation in hospitals that are suitable for people of any religion, or none, alike; more choice in the type of food in hospitals; and more choice in the gender of the health professional treating you). It is becoming clear that in attending to the needs of disadvantaged groups, the spin-off benefits are enjoyed by the whole population.

On the smaller scale, beneficial impacts of interventions to better manage and control numerous health problems in minority groups, including diabetes, heart disease, and tuberculosis, have been demonstrable. The methodology of controlled trials is increasingly being applied to evaluate specific interventions targeted at minority populations in relation to their costs. The most important principle is that the benefits, harms, and costs of working in the area of migration status, race, and ethnicity need to be kept under close scrutiny. The scrutiny should be international and continuing. However, at this point there is every reason to be optimistic that our faith in this approach is well founded.

10.4 **Continuing education in migration, ethnicity, race, and health**

The study of race as, primarily, a biological indicator is outdated and no longer trusted. Nonetheless, a resurgence of interest in biological variation across human populations, and the genetic basis of disease variation, is under way with the new gene mapping technologies. The net, long-term effect of this work is unclear at present so readers should keep abreast of it. The modern approach whereby race is perceived as a socially constructed concept encapsulating the social history of a group, and ethnicity is seen as a complex variable that combines cultural, social, and biological features is still under development. Adding to this is the complexity of migration histories and acculturation. Clarity on how best to work within this complex environment is slow in coming, at least partly because scholars and researchers generally favour one of three concepts—race, migration status, or ethnicity. In recognition of the limitations of such selectivity (my own preference being ethnicity) this edition is pointing to the complementary and overlapping nature of these three perspectives. Readers would do well to incorporate all three into their work.

The embedding of this perspective on inequalities and inequities within the broader social determinants of the health agenda is overdue, but is clearly coming. Also, minority health issues are being more closely aligned with other equality work (gender, disability, etc.). Learning about these other fields and how they relate to (or intersect with) minority health is necessary. (This is the subject of the growing field of intersectionality.)

The perspective that these variables are of greatest value for pinpointing and tackling inequalities, rather than exploring the causes (aetiology) of disease, is becoming established. This work of migration status, race, and ethnic coding became much easier and of higher priority when it was embedded in the wider equalities agenda, itself promoted by law. The wider agenda is politically important and obviously relevant to everyone, and hence commands the attention of leaders. The number of people trained formally in ethnicity and health, either for research or health-care practice, is small, and opportunities for attending courses are limited. There are few textbooks designed to teach the concepts and principles of the subject in the health context in a comprehensive way, though several have been published recently. There are, however, numerous textbooks on specific topics as listed in the Bibliography and excellent online overviews of the subject (see Ethnicity and health websites: A selection).

It is hard to predict how history will judge current efforts to make use of migration status, race, and ethnicity. As a minimum we should show our successors that we were conscious of our need to probe and question our subject matter, to learn, and to do better.

Learning in this field will come largely from peers who are grappling with problems that have no easy answers. How are we to move from theory and concepts to classifications, to data systems, to information, to policy, to plans, to projects, to routine health care, and to show such actions are effective and, even better, cost-effective? The concrete and generalizable answers to these questions do not exist, and may never exist because the world is rapidly changing. Perhaps all we can hope for are general principles and experiences that we can apply to specific circumstances using our judgement. We particularly need good examples of practical benefits that have demonstrably improved health or health care in a cost-effective way.

We are seeing a rapid rise in the number of websites, academic journals, e-mail lists, conferences, research projects, newspaper and newsletter articles, and student and research staff projects on migration, race, and ethnicity. Networking to a regional, national, and even international community offers a route to more efficient management of tough challenges. Some of the numerous portals to web-based knowledge, books, and articles are given at the end of this book (Ethnicity and health websites: A selection).

Ultimately, in multicultural nations and continents virtually everyone will need to know more, and that requires foundational education in schools, colleges, and universities. For health professionals and health researchers—at least those in the population sciences—a solid and comprehensive knowledge base will be necessary. The current largely ad hoc approach to migration, race, ethnicity, and health education, sometimes based on a few introductory lectures or seminars, will need to be substituted with both core and integrated teaching spanning the subject.

In this field there are relatively few exemplars (classic works illustrating success), but as compensation, we have the excitement of now developing them and creating a better future.

10.5 Predicting a future for migration, race, ethnicity, and health: a peek into the crystal ball

Try Exercise 10.4 before reading on.

Exercise 10.4 The future

- What would a good (but realistic) future for migrant and racial and ethnic minority health be like?

- Imagine this from the point of view of a clinical practitioner, public health practitioner, a health planner, a policy-maker and a researcher.

- Now, imagine this from the point of view of a member of a minority population, and separately, a member of the majority population.

Gazing into the crystal ball is a hazardous action for a writer—it is far safer to pontificate in the impermanent form of a lecture, seminar, and discussion over coffee. The written word can be held to account, with no chance of obfuscation, and rare opportunities for retraction, clarification, or modification. This second edition, however, is such an opportunity and I now repeat my lightly edited previous text with an update.

Some predictions, however, seem absolutely safe. Unless a global catastrophe occurs that leads to retrenchment and mass repatriation, probably itself leading to or resulting from a third world war, there will be an inexorable mixing of nations and their peoples that has already been accelerated by migration, international trading, exploration, colonization, and the rise of tourism in the last 600 years. (In the last 6 years, despite a recession, this prediction held.) In a hundred years from now the idea of a nation founded on a single (or a few) racial or ethnic groups bound by one skin colour, language, or religion will seem quaint. Rather, the global problems of climate change, energy needs, and shortages of essentials such as water will bring people into close contact to generate solutions or share in tragedies (as tens, perhaps hundreds, of millions of people are probably going to be displaced by rising sea levels and other natural disasters). The multiracial/ethnic nation will be the norm and people who claim mixed ancestry will be common and, unlike in the past, glad to be so. The creative power of such societies, already so obvious in places such as London, New York, Sydney, and Vancouver, will be unquestioned.

What is less easy to predict is the effect of these changes on ethnic and race relations. If solutions to cultural clashes are not found we could find ourselves in a world at war, whether between or within countries. Given solutions we could be immensely enriched by sharing cultures. To continue with this particular point, the teachings of a Prophet who can win the hearts and minds of hundreds of millions of Muslim people across the globe and unite them so strongly to a common purpose—such as the defence of his respect—surely deserve a worldwide audience. Perhaps in these teachings there are solutions to the myriad of problems we face, the greatest of these being poverty. The Prophet Muhammed requested all his followers to give 10% of their earnings as charity. Perhaps this teaching holds the solution to poverty. The many who convert to Islam, even in this era of anti-Islamic tendency, report benefits. Equally, perhaps radical Muslims can also find the solution to the problems that trouble them through peaceful means that would have won the approval of the Prophet and will win widespread respect. How do we move from the clashing of cultures to their cross-pollination and mutual enrichment? (In the last 6 years, no advances in this front have occurred so I leave the question open.)

In a future world of violent clashes, the content of this book and its focus on health and health care will become irrelevant and even derisory. In a world where clashes are handled in constructive ways, the approaches discussed here may offer great opportunities to entire populations, minorities and majorities alike, by applying the best in health that each culture has to offer. Let us strive for the better future, illustrated by the imaginary health-setting scenarios below.

10.5.1 **Clinical care scenario: a 10-year look into the crystal ball**

The health professional of 2024 has the concepts of migration status, race, and ethnicity ingrained in her through her direct exposure to multicultural societies. While at school she learned about the unity yet amazing diversity of humanity. This foundation was essential to her medical studies where the importance of race, ethnicity, and related concepts such as migration, religion, and language were emphasized not only in the formal curriculum (teaching was both in a module and integrated through the course), but also at the bedside by the teaching staff, who themselves typified a multicultural society. Her class comprised of students from 20 countries, and 16 ethnic groups from her own country. Curricular activities fostered opportunities for learning about all the diversity represented in the class, with a strong focus on how people maintain their health in different cultures. The teaching and work was embedded in the context of human rights, equality laws, and the social determinants of disease.

She did a project in one of the local minority community organizations, both learning about and earning the respect of, the people she served. Her elective was in a village overseas, where she enjoyed her immersion in a foreign setting. Her postgraduate studies and work encouraged her to apply and extend her learning. She took a special interest in the health beliefs and attitudes of the Chinese population (the longest-lived population in her country), and took a lot of pride in integrating their good ideas into the advice on healthy living she gave to all her patients. She made a special study of traditional Chinese medicine, which she found to be effective for several conditions that were difficult to manage.

By the end of her training she was comfortable with her own ethnicity, and that of her patients, and ready to teach the next generation of health professionals. She always made a point of emphasizing the limitations of the unthinking, routine, and simplistic use of race and ethnic group labels at the bedside and set an example by making sure that there was a good clinical reason for mentioning her patient's ethnic group, and if there was, explaining it and then exploring all the relevant facets. She taught her students to avoid superficiality and routine using the following quotation:

> In regions of the United States such as ours, where the population is predominantly of European-American or African-American descent, the description of race is often distilled down to 'black' or 'white'. Thus, in our institution and in those with similar demographics, the fourth spoken word of many case presentations broadly describes the patient as black or white.

Caldwell and Popenhoe (1995, p. 614)

She took special pride in her work in helping to train interpreters on medical matters, and the fact that the health service's policy-makers and her peers turned to her for advice on improving services for minorities in her locality. Her roles and skills and services beyond her clinical role were appropriately recognized in the awards and promotions committees. This, together with excellent clinical results and good patient feedback, meant she was a role model for other clinicians in the hospital. (I think there has been incremental progress on these issues in recent years.)

10.5.2 Public health scenario: 2024

The public health practitioner of 2024 knew, as his predecessors did, that information is the key to success in health improvement. The difference is that he has it at his fingertips. In 2014 the WHO convened an International Working Group that prepared a handbook defining and operationalizing migration status and the concepts of race and ethnicity and health. (My prediction this would happen in 2012 was wrong. To date the WHO has not moved beyond the stage of making recommendations.) The handbook was revised every 2 years with an ongoing online commentary on potential improvements. The handbook, despite controversy, led to sharing of ideas and information, particularly on terminology and classifications, such that everyone could now access these, together with an interpretation, online. Moreover, the accompanying active electronic discussion allows global sharing of ideas and practice.

The public health practitioner works with the national coding systems which ensure that every existing and all new databases have a common approach and one that itself maps onto the census and population registration classifications. Commonality in numerators and denominators, and opportunity for international comparison, means that he can produce data and a cogent commentary including international, national, regional, and local comparisons. All the problems of small numbers are still present, but the ability to aggregate data for 5, 10, and even 15 years is a boon.

Primary research also now pays attention to meticulous description of the migration history, racial, and ethnic composition of study populations so that aggregation of data by systematic review and meta-analysis is possible. The health authority, hospitals, primary care services, and individual health professionals are very interested in these data and as a result work hard to ensure the information they supply is accurate. The most satisfying aspect of the work is that the data are used to help both modify and evaluate the local health strategy. For several years, no one has questioned the worth of these data and it seems amazing that there was a time when strategy and plans on migration status, race, and ethnicity and health were made largely by guesswork. So many examples of beneficial changes exist (at low cost) that cynicism about the value of such data has evaporated.

The public health practitioner took special pride when Waqar Ahmad (see the quotation) spoke to him at a conference and said that his reports were not racialized, but helpful to minority populations. Rather, his reports pinpointed both similarities and differences and extracted the key messages for health improvement, paying particular attention to those conditions where minority populations were doing well and how the whole population could benefit from the knowledge:

> For black people this focus (racialization) is almost exclusively on cultures and ethnicities, genetics and metabolisms, being different and therefore inferior.
>
> Ahmad (1993, p. 22)

Everyone realizes that the indicators of migration status, race, and ethnicity are contextual and need regular modification. The categories are not reified here! (Again, incremental but accelerating progress has been made on these fronts.)

10.5.3 Health-care planning: 2024

The Director of Health Care Planning, responsible for implementing policy for 6 million people, had found it very hard in 2014 to meet competing demands, and in particular to persuade the Director of Finance to set aside extra funds to develop the service to meet the needs of minority populations. One particular problem was that short-term funding increases from the period 1997–2007 led to developments that could not be sustained when funding was extremely tight (most of the time since 2008). There have been some improvements recently, resulting from the implementation of important policy and strategic principles developed in the years 2000–10. The Director, of course, knows that it takes a long time to bring about lasting changes.

Change really took off when the policy and strategic documents on minority health were firmly integrated into the region's overall strategy on health and health-care improvement and linked to the challenge of reducing inequalities, the top political priority for the last 20 years. Emphasis on the quality and effectiveness of services, and particularly the resources saved by getting the services right first time for minority populations, has resulted in huge satisfaction among patients, staff, and managers. In particular, the use of accident and emergency services has declined and become more appropriate, attendance at medical care has improved with fewer missed appointments, and readmission rates have declined.

The merging of the business case with the ethical one, accelerated once funding became tight in 2008, has been powerful. The funding formula for our population's share of health-care resources has been changed to make explicit, and take into account, two important points that generally hold: (1) that most of the minority groups are younger so they use fewer resources for diseases of old age, e.g. dementia and cancers (even though it is clear that the age structure is converging); (2) some patients from minority groups do use more resources in relation to time spent in consultations, services for children and women, diabetes, and cardiovascular diseases.

Readjustment of the formulae for components of health care has made it possible to meet demands within specific services without altering the overall budget. Even the finance director was happy with these changes. Finally, we have solved the problem of mainstreaming. No project is now funded for less than 3 years; rules for what will happen after this time are established at the outset and an evaluation is done before decisions are taken to mainstream and these are based on demonstrable success in health outcomes and costs. The decision to mainstream is heavily influenced by our Equality and Equity Health Forum, a committee comprising professionals and members of the public representing a range of communities. Then, we have a 3-year time-frame for mainstreaming of successful projects, i.e. a time-frame of at least 6 years in total. Mainstreaming is a responsibility of a senior manager and a senior clinician working together. The Director of Planning's satisfaction has been in having made some inroads into a really tough assignment. She can hold her head high and say her department has conformed to the spirit of national policy and, of course, the law. Not surprisingly, as some people knew even in the 20th century, many of the changes have benefited everyone. For example, the Caribbean-style menus are very popular, cheap, and healthy, and the signs around the hospital based on symbols are really appreciated by all our older patients, not just the minority patients. (The last few years have seen much turmoil in health-care systems, with financial restraints being widespread such that progress has been slow on these matters and sometimes ground has been lost.)

10.5.4 Policy-making: 2024

The policy-maker of 2024 frames his ideas in the light of widespread experience of what does and does not work. Of course, politics isn't primarily about evidence, but about ideas and visions, which can be moulded, shaped, and improved by experience and evidence. So when the Minister for Health asked for a speech on where the nation was going in relation to the health of minority groups his office was able to summarize the successes and failures of the last 10 years and compare approaches with those of other nations. Of course, this would not be possible without the superb information supplied by our information and public health departments. Even now, however, evidence tends to be sparse. In particular, randomized controlled trials that can supply information for the local migrant, racial, and ethnic groups are not available. However, usually there is some relevant information somewhere in the world that can be interpreted in the light of local descriptive data and qualitative studies. The initiatives of the WHO and IOH in 2013–18 spurred on new work internationally to augment and follow the contribution of the United States, and equally importantly provided a means for synthesis and dissemination of information. Then, working quickly with the ideas of the National Equality, Equity and Diversity Health Forum, that had themselves been shaped in debates over the preceding few years, he was able to come up with realistic proposals that would gain wide support, help the country stay in the vanguard, and not exceed available budgets.

Policy-making became easier because for several reasons: cross-party political consensus that international migration and resultant ethnic diversity is essential to our nation's development; an increase in participation in the political processes by minority groups that resulted in sharing of responsibility in decision-making and implementation; national information systems that produced data by migration status, race, and ethnic group; and, sad to say, since a health authority was taken to court under the race relations laws. Thankfully, the case was withdrawn by mutual consent when the health department agreed to review all policies once again and set up systems to do a diversity check on all relevant policies and more importantly on their implementation. On this occasion the health authorities implemented their equality policies fully. The policy-maker's greatest satisfaction is from the observation that the policy-making is generic—the principles that work for one disadvantaged group seem to work for others too, even new groups arriving as refugees. Finally, the policies are getting the best out of people by creating a healthy and participating population and environment. The struggles in policy-making of the previous 50 years now seem to be over, at least as long as the political consensus remains. (Remarkably, I judge that we have seen huge progress in policy across numerous countries in the last 6–8 years.)

10.5.5 Research: 2024

The researcher of 2024 takes it for granted that a range of variables on migration, race, and ethnicity are a core if not essential feature of population-based research, and that minority groups are also both invited and expected to participate in other kinds of research based on tissues and organs and done mainly in the laboratory. The research community does not simply do this from a sense of what is right, or even because of the intrinsic interest, but to maintain the long-term health of the research infrastructure. If researchers did not do this, in some parts of the country where the minorities are present in large numbers there would be insufficient people to participate in research and insufficient people to train as researchers.

The turning point was a binding statement (so-called concordat) to a large extent inspired by the leadership of the NIH in the United States, on required good practice in research issued jointly by the research councils, the Department of Health, the major research charities, and some key leaders of minority organizations in several countries. This stated that research funding was contingent upon, and would meet the associated costs of, attention to issues of population diversity. The aim was both to fill a deep hole in the research databases relating to the health and health care of minorities and create an extensive infrastructure that would make the research possible. One big job was education for researchers and the public alike about the limits and potential of this kind of research.

Everyone was pleasantly surprised by how much cooperation and interest there was. The recruitment and training of a cadre of researchers from a wide range of minority populations was also pivotal. There were many talented people to recruit from, especially among the refugees, where highly qualified people were doing manual jobs. A strategic and proactive approach was taken to finding, training, and retaining in long-term careers people from previously under-represented groups. We now have people from most minority groups and a network that allows sharing of expertise. Ethical committees have been instrumental in monitoring how well the research concordat has been implemented, and to be frank, forcing the recalcitrant to comply. We have more equity in research. The academic journals are brimming with good-quality migrant, race, ethnicity, and health research. The press, and particularly the sector catering to minority populations, has shown a real appetite for this work with better balance in the reporting. Research has helped to identify and reduce racism. Luckily, an emergent opinion in the early 21st century that the research establishment itself might be institutionally racist was quickly deflected by decisive action. Finally, the controversy about the relative value of measures of migration status, race, and ethnicity died down when most researchers followed the WHO/IOH guidance published in 2018. Effectively, Oppenheimer's view (see quotation) prevails and Huxley and Haddon's recommendation of 1935 is implemented. The third edition of Raj Bhopal's book in 2020, rather than having one paragraph on race as predicted in the 2007 first edition, no longer had to use much space to explain basic concepts, and was equally at ease with migration status, race, and ethnicity. Both race and ethnic group are widely understood as a social construct. Ethnicity has become the dominant concept worldwide. Its flexibility and breadth, as outlined by Oppenheimer (2001), once seen as weaknesses, were its strength:

> *As a social construct, each ethnic group contains a history...and alters over time; the use of ethnic group should make the researcher sensitive to the effects of generation, changing economic status, social class, relations with other groups, discrimination, and relative political power.*
>
> Oppenheimer (2001, p. 1053)

(Judging on progress, I think that there has been much good work, but this will only truly flourish once NIH-type policies are widespread, whether backed by law or not.)

10.5.6 **The public's perspectives**

The public in 2024 is no longer a little confused by why migration status, race, and ethnicity data are important to improve health and health care because there are so many good examples of benefits that are plain to see and understand. Also, information is only entered once at registration with the health service in a simple online form that can be completed either in writing or by speaking into the telephone or pocket computer. Of course, the health service staff will help you complete it if necessary and you are free to update it any time. The information is shared on a need to know basis and linked automatically to the full range of health and social services.

It is very helpful and interesting to be able to see, at a touch of a button, how our people are faring. The reasons why the disease patterns are so different have been well understood and are providing food for thought. Information about health and disease and health care is also available easily at the touch of a keypad. The public can choose the language and level of complexity, with automatic computerized translation of information that can be read or heard.

The public are invited to comment and feed into health plans as well as research projects. Mostly, this is inbuilt into the system with representative patient panels rather than 'ad hoc' consultation exercises with community groups.

In the patient encounter, if interpreting is required it is done by video link, which is much more efficient than transporting interpreters to health premises.

It would be wrong to pretend all challenges have been solved—they have not. The big change is that there is a common purpose—we seem to have agreed the way forward. The stop–start–reverse approach to service development of the 1980s, 1990s, and early 2000s is over. (I made no predictions in relation to the public in the 1st edition.)

10.6 **Conclusions**

The concepts of race and ethnicity are constructed on factors that are pivotal in the lives of humans, and to the way humans organize their societies. Migration is the driving force here—if there was no migration *Homo sapiens* would comprise one much more homogeneous population in East Africa. As societies have become more complex and spread, and the typical size of human settlements has risen, these concepts have become more important. Fundamentally, race and ethnicity reflect some of the factors, or strictly conglomerates of factors, that allow humans to differentiate, albeit over long periods of time, their social groups from the social groups of others. This is not to deny that similarities far outweigh differences whether we examine things at the individual or group level. Equally this does not imply that race or ethnicity are features of nature. They are not. They are created from fundamental factors, some of which are natural and some social. The composite of factors that are considered to comprise race and ethnicity is subject to change over time and may vary by place. Try Exercise 10.5 before reading on.

Exercise 10.5 The changing nature of race and ethnicity in a migrant population over time

Imagine a small group of immigrants—perhaps asylum seekers given refugee status from a war zone in Africa. They are settled according to national policy in a small town in an industrialised, wealthy nation.

◆ What will happen to them in terms of their race and or ethnicity over time, and over one, two, five, and ten generations?

Consider two scenarios. First, they freely and usually, interbreed with the wider society. Second, they mostly interbreed within their own national group—whether within the town, or finding partners of the same racial/ethnic group from elsewhere. The first scenario is easy to predict. This population will rapidly become assimilated, and over a few generations, apart from a few physical signs (perhaps in hair texture or facial features and swarthy skin), there will be little else left though the DNA of the population will record this absorption for posterity. There may be other superficial but long-lasting signs of the existence of this group of people—perhaps in the names, family folklore and memorabilia. The traditional language, foods, and customs are likely to be lost, except those closely tied to religion, if it is preserved. The second scenario may lead to long term preservation even over hundreds, perhaps thousands, of years as witnessed by the Roma in eastern Europe (migrants from India) and the Parsees in India (from Persia, now Iran). There can be a remarkable preservation not only of biology but also culture in these circumstances. In most migrant groups we see an intermediate form of change. How the society modifies its response over time will vary according to which scenario unfolds.

The theoretical basis of work on migration, ethnicity, race, and health is not easy to define. This does not make it atheoretical just, to echo Nazroo, untheorized. It is difficult, if not impossible, to think about complex matters without a theory, even although the theory cannot be articulated easily, at least in a valid way that is easy to grasp. Achieving a stronger and more explicit theoretical base is a continuing challenge. This book has pointed to some of the theories that have informed discussion of race and ethnicity in epidemiology, public health, and health care, and in the wider spheres of health, science and society.

Epidemiology is based on finding and explaining population differences, and migration status, race, and ethnicity variables are among the most powerful available, though they are better at finding than explaining. Explaining needs better theories and models based on these. Scholars of race, ethnicity, and health have created a number of potentially explanatory models that explore how the associations between these concepts and health appear. In the first edition of this book four such models showed these associations, with no comment from me, but with encouragement to readers to study the original publications. These models attempt to explain why inequalities by migrant status, race, and/or ethnicity arise and are sustained. Models are designed to help simplify complex subjects. I believe our subject is too complex to be captured in any valuable explanatory way by causal diagram-type approaches. At best, such illustrations can provide a way of organizing our thoughts, but when they become complex (and closer to reality) this function can also be lost. In addition, I think there is more to be gained in producing a causal diagram for specific issues, e.g. variation in colorectal cancer. Building on my evolutionary model in Figure 6.1, I have extended the thinking to modern times in Figure 10.1. The left half of the diagram shows how migration from and indeed within Africa some 60 000–70 000 years ago over many millennia led to differentiation among human populations. The genetic differences arising have been closely aligned in modern times with the concept of race, and cultural ones with ethnicity, but as we have seen these are merely issues of emphasis. There would have been differentiation in many other ways but I have limited these to socio-economic and technological. The time period of 60 000–70 000 years was enough to cause differentiation but not enough to create new human species. In modern times, especially in the last 1000 years or so, new migrations have created multicultural societies. In these new societies immigrants come with variations in health status from their place of origin (whether effectively permanent as in genetic ones or highly changeable, e.g. low blood pressure). The effects of the migration process (e.g. selection effects), the journey, the new life circumstances, and discrimination at the new settlement, all influence the health status of migrants. The complexity of the process is self-evident.

This should not, however, inhibit us from applying this general thinking to help us understand specific diseases and health problems. Based on a review of the literature and examination of complex causal diagrams I proposed a relatively simple four-stage causal model (Figure 10.2) to help explain the high rate of type 2 diabetes mellitus in South Asians compared with European origin populations (Bhopal 2013). The development of this kind of model is important to make progress in causal understanding in our field.

Public health and medical care are humanitarian disciplines that are focused on the most needy (the sick) who are often also the most economically disadvantaged. Migration status, race, and ethnicity are good at pinpointing need and economic disadvantage (though there are exceptions, e.g. rich immigrants allowed entry to the country on economic grounds). For this and other reasons,, notwithstanding the potential to harm that is inherent in the work, migration status, race, and ethnicity will remain important. It is imperative for us to improve our work so that the benefits substantially outweigh the harms.

I have argued that the key to doing good in this field is a social and cultural milieu of equality/non-discrimination. Given this, the thoughtful application of the approaches of social and population health sciences to migration, race, and ethnicity should yield workable classifications and data that can be interpreted using epidemiological frameworks for analysis. These frameworks are good for assessing error and bias (misclassification, mis-measurement, information bias, selection bias, confounding) and interpreting cause and effect (see Chapter 9). The analysis arising can feed into needs assessment (Chapter 5), priority-setting (Chapter 7), the inequalities debate (Chapter 6), policy and strategy-making (Chapter 8), and scholarship and research (Chapter 9). There is a virtuous cycle around data—the more they are used the more the enthusiasm for their collection and for improvement in data systems (Chapters 2, 3, and 5). Data also improve services both directly (through better decisions) and through the Hawthorne effect, whereby awareness of being monitored is a motivator for better performance.

This age of equality of humans, enshrined in international legislation, has coincided with, or perhaps has been caused by, the intermingling of the inhabitants of the globe. The mixing of the world's populations is not without its problems, but the benefits probably outweigh these. The response of the health-care system in each country is shaped by local circumstances, and yet in broad historical terms there are many features in common (Chapter 4). The intermingling through migration has brought, in the wake of slavery, colonialism, and scientific racism, a freer exchange of ideas, labour, art, culture, business, science, and technologies. Who can deny that, notwithstanding tensions and setbacks, increasing mutual respect and opportunity has accompanied this intermingling? I was born in India in 1953, 6 years after the end of the British Raj (rule), to parents who were governed by the British. My parents had, in this 'jewel of the British Empire', 4 years of schooling between them, before they emigrated to Glasgow, one of the great cities of the motherland. I was raised by them in Scotland from the age of 2. That I have penned this book while holding the Chair of Public Health at the University of Edinburgh testifies to the power of

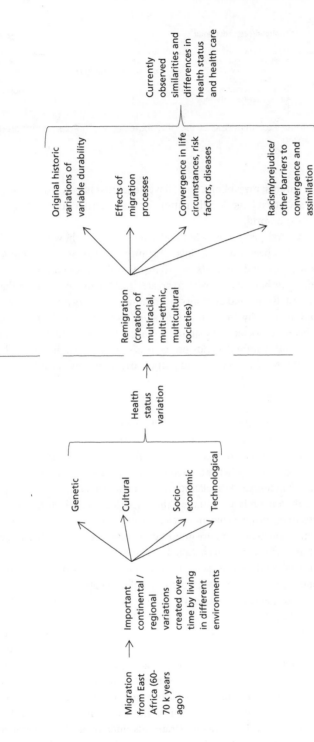

Fig. 10.1 A model linking evolutionary and present-day forces to produce variations in health status and health care by migration status, race, and ethnicity.

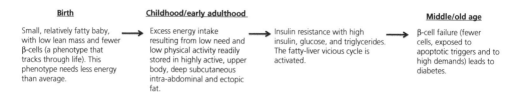

Birth	Childhood/early adulthood		Middle/old age
Small, relatively fatty baby, with low lean mass and fewer β-cells (a phenotype that tracks through life). This phenotype needs less energy than average.	Excess energy intake resulting from low need and low physical activity readily stored in highly active, upper body, deep subcutaneous intra-abdominal and ectopic fat.	Insulin resistance with high insulin, glucose, and triglycerides. The fatty-liver vicious cycle is activated.	β-cell failure (fewer cells, exposed to apoptotic triggers and to high demands) leads to diabetes.

Fig. 10.2 A four-stage model explaining the excess of diabetes in South Asians compared with Europeans (see Bhopal 2013).

such intermingling. My parents, my siblings, and I have benefitted hugely from this cross-cultural opportunity, but so has society at large, locally, nationally, and internationally. My family's story is repeated endlessly across the world.

The combination of cultural perspectives is an advantage. This is shown *par excellence* in the world of literature. Travel has been extolled, since time immemorial, as a core component of the experience of life. The benefits, and the costs, are shared by minorities and the majority alike. It behoves us all to maximize the benefits. There is no greater goal for any society than that its citizens should be long-lived, free of disease and disability, brimming with energy, creative and full of ideas. In other words, that they are healthy. In so far as migration status, race, and ethnicity can contribute to the creation of a healthier society they should be coveted. As with children, so it is with such ideas. How they develop and mature depends on us. It is our responsibility to work together to agree how to use these ideas to bring benefit, and particularly to improve health (Mir et al 2013).

10.7 **Summary**

There is no single theory (or group of theories) on migration, race, ethnicity, and health that is widely accepted or applied. Biological theories based on species and subspecies have not withstood testing, and social theories have not yet been articulated in a way that has made a major impact in medical sciences. Advances in the science of genetics are reopening old debates on the biological underpinnings of racial and ethnic differences. Articulating coherent and useful theories on migration, race, and ethnicity in the health domain is a continuing challenge. Migration status, race, and ethnicity conform, and contribute, to the general epidemiological theories on the forces that shape population differences in health status, and hence they are important in public health and health care.

International migration and greater international exchange through tourism and communication are creating multiracial, multi-ethnic societies, demanding clarity of understanding around both the similarities and differences between subgroups of populations. Used wisely, the indicators of migration status, race, and ethnicity have the potential to improve public health, health care, clinical care, and medical science, but used unwisely they can do immense damage. Stringent attention to the principles of ethics and justice is essential as the primary safeguard against harm.

A rational, analytic approach to the interpretation of data, set within broader epidemiological theories of health, is needed. Interventions utilizing migration status, race, and ethnicity need to be carefully evaluated to judge the likely balance of benefits to costs. In a political environment where anti-immigration sentiment is high and encouraged, the use of indicators of migration status, race, and ethnicity may be counterproductive. There is an imperative to achieve benefits in terms of health improvement and to demonstrate this unequivocally. This imperative mandates that we continue to learn. A realistic 10-year vision for better clinical practice, health-care planning, health policy, and research is offered. Scholarship and research to advance theoretical understanding as well as underpin practical advances is accelerating. In the future, historians and health scholars and researchers will subject our work to scrutiny. We should ensure that they conclude that not only did we do our best with our limited knowledge, but we built well on our legacy, and learned the painful lessons of the past.

Acknowledgments

Text extract reproduced from Banton M, *Racial Theories*, Cambridge University Press, Cambridge, UK, Copyright © 1987 by permission of Cambridge University Press.

References

Ahmad WIU (ed.) (1993) *Race and Health in Contemporary Britain.* Milton Keynes: Open University Press.

Banton M (1987) *Racial Theories.* Cambridge: Cambridge University Press.

Bhopal RS (2013) A four-stage model explaining the higher risk of Type 2 diabetes mellitus in South Asians compared with European populations. *Diabetic Medicine* 30: 35–42.

Caldwell SH, Popenhoe R (1995) Perception and misperceptions of skin colour. *Annals of Internal Medicine* 122: 614–17.

Coon CS (1963) Growth and development of social groups. In **Wolstenholm G** (ed.) *Man and his Future,* pp. 120–31. London: J and A Churchill Ltd.

Elliot C, Brodwin P (2002) Identity and genetic ancestry tracing. *British Medical Journal* 325: 1469–71.

Golby AJ, Gabrieli JDE, Chiao JY, Eberhardt JL (2001) Differential responses in the fusiform region to same-race and other-race faces. *Nature Neuroscience* 4: 845–50.

Kai J, Spencer J, Wilkes M, Gill PS (1999) Learning to value ethnic diversity—what, why and how? *Medical Education* 33: 616–23.

Kuhn TS (1996) *The Structure of Scientific Revolutions,* 3rd edn. Chicago, IL: University of Chicago Press.

Kuper L (ed.) (1975) *Race, Science and Society.* London: Allen and Unwin.

Lorant V, Bhopal RS (2011) Ethnicity, socio-economic status and health research: insights from and implications of Charles Tilly's theory of durable inequality. *Journal of Epidemiology and Community Health* 65: 671–5.

Mir G, Salway S, Kai J, Karlsen S, Bhopal R, Ellison GT, et al. (2013) Principles for research on ethnicity and health: the Leeds Consensus Statement. *European Journal of Public Health* 23: 504–10.

Modood T, Berthoud R, Lakey J, Nazroo J, Smith P, Virdee SBS (1997) *Ethnic Minorities in Britain: diversity and disadvantage.* London: Policy Studies Institute.

Muntaner C, Nieto J, O'Campo P (1996) The bell curve: on race, social class, and epidemiologic research. *American Journal of Epidemiology* 144: 531–6.

Nazroo JY (1998) Genetic, cultural or socio-economic vulnerability? Explaining ethnic inequalities in health. *Sociology of Health and Illness* 20: 710–30.

Oppenheimer GM (2001) Paradigm lost: race, ethnicity, and the search for a new population taxonomy. *American Journal of Public Health* 91: 1049–55.

Pfeffer N (1998) Theories of race, ethnicity and culture. *British Medical Journal* 317: 1381–4.

Other sources and further reading

Bhopal RS (1997) Ethnicity. In **Boyd KM** *et al.* (eds) The New Dictionary of Medical Ethics, pp 89–90. London: BMJ Books.

Bhopal R (2009) Chronic diseases in Europe's migrant and ethnic minorities: challenges, solutions and a vision. *European Journal of Public Health* 19: 140–3.

Bhopal RS (2012) The quest for culturally sensitive health-care systems in Scotland: insights for a multi-ethnic Europe. *Journal of Public Health* 34: 5–11.

Cooper RS, Kaufman JS (1999) Is there an absence of theory in social epidemiology? The authors respond to Muntaner. *American Journal of Epidemiology* **150**: 127–8.

Duster T (2005) Medicine. Race and reification in science. *Science* **307**: 1050–1.

Lynn R, Rushton P, Jenson A, Murray C, Brand C, Nyborg H, et al. (2006) Racial IQ research. *Sunday Times* 2 April [letters].

Ruffin J (2010) The science of eliminating health disparities: embracing a new paradigm. *American Journal of Public Health* **100** (Suppl. 1): S8–S9.

Schoenbach VJ, Reynolds GH, Kumanyika SK (1994) Racial and ethnic distribution of faculty, students, and fellows in US epidemiology degree programs, 1992. Committee on Minority Affairs of the American College of Epidemiology. *Annals of Epidemiology* **4**: 259–65.

Shields AE, Crown WH (2012) Looking to the future: incorporating genomic information into disparities research to reduce measurement error and selection bias. *Health Services Research* **47**: 1387–410.

Appendix

Terminology, categories, and censuses in Canada, Brazil, India, Australia, Fiji, Mauritius, South Africa, and Singapore

Canada

The first census in what is now Canada took place in 1666. Data on ethnic or racial origins have been collected in all but one (1891) of the national censuses. In the 1901 census information was collected under four colour categories—white, red, black, and yellow. Mixed coloured children were designated as non-White which is typical of racial categorization in many countries. It is illogical, but fitted with and perpetuated the racial theory of White superiority in the hierarchy of races.

In 1981, 'Black' was not listed on the census questionnaire, though respondents could specify 'Black ethnic origin' in the write-in box. The mark-in response 'Black' was added to the 1986 census questionnaire and included again in 1991. Some respondents objected to the presence of 'Black' as an ethnic group in the 1991 census questionnaire. (The same kind of objections occurred in Scotland after the 2001 census.) The removal of the 'Black' check-off entry in 1996 resulted in the decreased reporting of 'Black' and the increased reporting of African and Caribbean origins. This is one example of how political considerations are important in influencing classifications, and subsequently the interpretation and presentation of the statistics.

The idea of multiple ethnicities has been tackled since 1986. Since 1986, an instruction to specify as many ethnic groups as applicable has been included in the question on ethnic origin.

With ethnicity, religion, and language data, Canada has a rich data set to provide information that is required under the Multiculturalism Act, the Canadian Charter of Rights and Freedoms, and other legislation. The amount of information has increased greatly, partly to meet the demand for information arising from federal government policy on multiculturalism, and this trend can be seen even between 1991 and 2001. Information on ethnicity in the 2001 census is in the section headed socio-cultural information. The key question on ethnicity relates to the person's ancestors, with exemplars based on countries. In addition there is a list of ethnic groups (question 19) that is justified by the need to promote equal opportunity. Several questions relate to original inhabitant/aboriginal status. In 2001, the 25 ethnic categories and subcategories used to classify individual ethnic origins included:

1. British Isles origins

2. Aboriginal origins

3. Caribbean origins

4. Latin, Central, and South American origins

5. African origins

6. Arab origins

7. West Asian origins

8. South Asian origins.

In 2006 facets of ethnicity were captured as in 2001. The structure of the census changed in 2011, with internet-based acquisition of base information supplemented by sample surveys (e.g. the Household Survey, which does include a great deal on various facets of ethnicity). Ethnicity was not included in the 2011 short form but language was. Many countries, like Canada, are moving to new kinds of census taking with more emphasis on record linkage (as The Netherlands did some time ago). It will be interesting to see the effect of this on data on migration status, race, and ethnicity.

The Canadian experience provides an excellent example of how complex race and ethnicity are, and how difficult it is to devise classifications in a scientifically objective, rational, and consistent way.

Brazil

The Brazilian approach is unusual in modern times in being based predominantly on colour. The census is held every 10 years and it asks the question, 'what is your colour or race?'. There are tick boxes for responses with no space for written responses. The response categories are white, black, brown, mixed, yellow, and indigenous (referring to the indigenous Indian population). There is also a question 'what is your nationality?' with three tick box options: Natural Brazilian, Brazilian Citizenship, and Foreigner. There are three related questions: 'In which Brazilian state or foreign country were you born?' a question regarding uninterrupted stay in Brazil, and 'In which state or foreign country was your previous residence?'. The centrality of migration, race, and ethnicity in censuses is well shown in Brazil. In 2008 the first survey of the ethno-racial characteristics of the population took place. The results of the 2010 census showed the non-White groups had formed a majority in the country (the census website is in Portuguese so I have not been able to extract the details).

India

The 2001 census was the sixth since independence from Britain in 1947. No questions were asked regarding race or ethnicity as we are discussing them but there are questions for mother tongue and other languages and birthplace, specifying the state/country. There were two questions relating to caste and tribe. The 2011 census asked about nationality (as declared) and country of birth.

Australia

Since 1961, the Census of Population and Housing has been held every 5 years. The census is collected from householders and is self-completed. Ethnicity has not been collected, although a question about ancestry was asked in 1986. A number of variables from 1996 may be used to derive ethnicity. Questions for 2001 asked for citizenship, country of birth, year of arrival, Australian or overseas birthplace of father and mother, language most often spoken at home, Australian indigenous origin, and ancestry. The question that is closest to ethnicity is 'what is the person's ancestry?' The examples given include: Vietnamese, Hmong, Dutch, Kurdish, Australian South Sea Islander, Maori, Lebanese; and there is scope to provide more than one ancestry if necessary. Australia analyses the variables ancestry, birthplace, and parents' birthplace—Australia or overseas—as an indicator for the ethnic background of first- and second-generation, Australians. The inextricable intermixing of migration and ethnicity is well exemplified here. The 2011 census continued this approach of using geographical origins and social/cultural characteristics to assess the ethnic composition of the nation. The 2011 census, in addition to the variables already mentioned, collected information on religion. The Australian Bureau of Statistics has published detailed guidance on the classification of cultural and ethnic groups, the latest in 2011.

The 2011 census asks whether the person is of Aboriginal or Torres Strait Islander origin, citizenship, birthplace of person and parents, arrival in Australia, language, ancestry, and religion. While the guidance emphasizes that ethnicity is a matter for self-identification, there is no ethnicity question per se in the census.

Fiji

A census has been held since 1881. In the 1996 census questions relating to ethnicity were place of birth and an ethnic group question. One response was accepted for ethnicity. The enumerator was instructed to 'record the group or race to which the person considers he or she belongs. If there is any doubt as to the person's racial origin, record the father' (Fiji Census 1996, p. 281). (In most countries the mother's ethnic group gets priority over the father's.) Enumerators used the following classification codes:

1. Fijians

2. Indians

3. Chinese and part-Chinese

4. European

5. Part-European

6. Rotuman

7. Other Pacific Islanders

8. All others

9. Not stated.

The 2007 census had only three ethnic groups—Fijian, Indian, and Others—in the classification. It also collected data on religion and language.

Mauritius

Mauritius has held a decennial census since 1846, and its last census was in 2011. Information is collected on citizenship and linguistic group in the population censuses. According to the constitution, the Mauritian population includes a Hindu community, a Muslim community, a Sino-Mauritian community, and the general population. The last time a question was asked on the ethnic composition of the community at a population census was in 1972. The question was: 'To which of the following communities does this person claim to belong? Hindu, Muslim, Sino-Mauritian (Sino is a descriptor for Chinese), General Population'. The 2011 census asks about the language of forefathers, i.e. ancestors, as well as current languages spoken and read. These questions are good proxies for ethnic composition of the population.

South Africa

The census takes place every 5 years and it uses categories that arise from the apartheid era. Traditionally, the enumerator or the household member completing the questionnaire is asked to judge how each member of the household would describe themselves, i.e. there is no requirement to ask them.

Now, interviewers are instructed to accept the response that is given even if they don't agree with it. In 1996, there was no reference to the nature of the question but in 2001 the categorization was described as population group. In 1996 only four options were available with no 'other' category, which became available in 2001. A range of related questions—religion, country of birth, and languages spoken in the home—allow a fairly detailed analysis of ethnicity. In the 2011 census the question 'How would the person describe him/herself' was asked with the choices Black African, Coloured, Indian or Asian, White or Other. Language, birthplace, and citizenship were also included.

Singapore

The definition used by Statistics Singapore was that 'ethnic group refers to a person's race as declared by that person. For those of mixed parentage, they are usually declared under the ethnic group of their fathers'. Ethnic group data came from the household register and were pre-printed on the census forms in 2000 for verification with the respondent. The Singapore government and statistical departments classify the population under four main ethnic groups: Chinese, Malay, Indian, and Others, with many subcategories falling under each main category.

The Chinese category lists 22 subcategories, including Hokkien, Teochew, Cantonese, Hakka, Hainanese, Hockchia, Foochow, Henghua, Shanghainese, plus 'other Chinese'. The Malay category refers to persons of Malay or Indonesian origin and contains 18 subcategories, listing Javanese, Boyanese, Bugi, and 'other Malays'. The Indian category contains groups that have origins in India, Pakistan, Bangladesh, and Sri Lanka. It lists 24 subcategories: Tamils, Malayali, Punjabi, Bengali, Singhalese, plus 'other Indians'. 'Other' refers to all other groups not already listed including Eurasian, Caucasian, Arab, and Japanese. In 2010 a register-based approach was taken with a sample answering questions. Ethnic/dialect group was declared by the respondent.

Glossary

The major sources for the Glossary are:
Bhopal R (2003) Glossary of terms relating to ethnicity and race: for reflection and debate. *Journal of Epidemiology and Community Health* **58**: 441–5.
Bhopal RS (2008) *Concepts of Epidemiology*. Oxford: Oxford University Press.

Aboriginal Relating to the original inhabitants of a land.

Aborigine While it has a general meaning referring to the original inhabitants of a land (*see* **Native** and **Indigenous**), and is used that way, it is most often associated with the original inhabitants of Australia, and unless qualified would probably be interpreted in that way.

Absolute risk The actual amount, usually expressed as a rate, of a disease/illness event occurring in a population under study, i.e. without comparison with another population.

Acute An adjective commonly applied to diseases that have a short time course, as opposed to a long one (*see* **Chronic**).

African A person with African ancestral origins who self-identifies, or is identified*, as African, but usually excluding those of other ancestry, e.g. European and South Asian. This term is the currently preferred prefix for more specific categories, as in African American. (In terms of racial classifications, this population approximates to the group historically known as Negroid or similar terms.) In practice, northern Africans from Algeria, Morocco, and such countries are excluded from this category and it is used for sub-Saharan Africans (*see also* **Black**)

Afro-Caribbean/African Caribbean A person of African ancestral origins whose family settled in the Caribbean before emigrating and who self-identifies, or is identified, as Afro-Caribbean (in terms of racial classifications, this population approximates to the group known as Negroid or similar terms) (*see also* **Black**).

Alien A foreigner from another place, usually another nation. This term is not much used in our field but it is used in official texts and rules on immigration.

Allele *See* **Gene**.

American Indian *See* **Native American**.

Asian Indian A term currently used synonymously with **South Asian**, but with the important limitation that major South Asian populations such as Pakistani and Bangladeshi may not identify with it. This term is being used in North America to distinguish this population from Native Americans, previously known as American Indians.

Asian Strictly, this label applies to anyone originating from the Asian continent. In practice, this term is often used in the UK to mean people with ancestry in the Indian subcontinent. In the United States the term has broader meaning, but is mostly used to denote people of Far Eastern origins, e.g. Chinese, Japanese, and Filipinos. More specific terms should be used whenever possible.

Association A statistical link between one risk or exposure factor and an outcome of interest (usually a disease or death). In this context the risk factor is migration status, race, or ethnicity and the variable links to health outcomes.

[*A person can be identified in ways including by country of birth of self, parents, and grandparents; ancestral language or origins; name; some religions; or by observation.]

Asylum seeker A person seeking asylum, i.e. leave to stay in a foreign country, on the grounds of fear of persecution or actual persecution.

Bangladeshi A person whose ancestry lies in the Indian subcontinent who self-identifies, or is identified, as Bangladeshi (*see also* **South Asian**). Between 1947 and 1971 the land known as Bangladesh was East Pakistan and before that India. There is no clear-cut equivalent in terms of racial classifications, though historically northern Indians have been classified as Caucasian, and some Indian tribes as aboriginal. (The racial term Malayan, coined by Blumenbach, is forgotten.)

Black A person with African ancestral origins, who self-identifies, or is identified, as Black, African, or Afro-Caribbean (*see* **African** and **Afro-Caribbean**). The word is often capitalized to signify its specific use in this way. In some circumstances the word Black signifies all non-White minority populations, and in this usage serves political purposes. While this term was widely supported, including by the populations so described, in the late 20th century there are signs that such support is diminishing.

Blood pressure Usually refers to the pressure in the arteries supplying the body except for the lungs (i.e. not veins and pulmonary arteries) as measured by a **sphygmomanometer**.

Case A person with the disease or problem under investigation.

Case–control study A study where cases are compared with **controls**, people who are drawn from the same population. These comparisons help to test hypotheses about the causes of disease.

Caucasian An Indo-European. This is Blumenbach's 18th-century term for the White race of humankind, which he named after the people who lived in the Caucasus. This term is usually used synonymously with Caucasoid, European, or White. Alone amongst terms derived from traditional racial classification, Caucasian remains popular in both science and everyday language.

Cause Something which has an effect, in the case of epidemiology this effect being (primarily) a change in the frequency of risk factors or adverse health outcomes.

Chinese A person with ancestral origins in China, who self-identifies, or is identified, as Chinese. (In terms of historical racial classifications, Chinese would be included in the group known as Mongolian or Mongoloid.)

Cholesterol A lipid (fatty substance) that is essential to many bodily functions. It is transported in the blood via lipoproteins. Cholesterol and other lipids carried by low density lipoproteins (LDL/VLDL) are a risk factor for coronary heart disease (and vascular diseases), while those carried by high density lipoproteins (HDL) seem to be protective.

Chromosome *See* **Gene**.

Chronic An adjective commonly applied to diseases that have a long-lasting time course, and usually applied to diseases that are not caused by infectious agents, accidents, or poisons.

Cohort study A study where people with a risk factor or health problem of interest are followed up to observe the outcomes, e.g. new cases of disease. It is also known as a prospective or longitudinal study.

Competing causes A concept where alternative causes of disease, usually as causes of death, are in competition with each other, e.g. one explanation of the comparatively low rates of coronary heart disease in the Afro-Caribbean population is that the atherosclerotic process kills people from stroke. If this were to be controlled, it may be that coronary heart disease would become more common.

Confounding The distortion of an association between the risk factor under study and an outcome by other (confounding) factors that influence both the outcome and the risk factor under study.

Congenital A health problem present at birth.

Control/control group A comparison population that is used in a number of study designs so as to permit inferences about the pattern of risk factors, health outcomes, or treatment effects in the study population of interest.

Coronary heart disease A group of diseases resulting from reduced blood supply to the heart, most often caused by narrowing or blockage of the coronary arteries that supply blood to the heart.

Cot death A synonym for the sudden infant death syndrome, which is unexplained death in infancy.

Creole An uncommon word used to describe people of mixed European and African ancestry living or originating from the West Indies and parts of South America. The main use of this term in ethnicity and health research is in Dutch studies of the Surinamese, who are divided mainly into Creole and Hindu (*see also* **Hindu**). Creole is also a language.

Dementia *See* **Senile dementia**.

Demography The scientific study of population, particularly the factors that determine its size and shape.

Denominator The bottom half of a fraction, and in the context of this book the population at risk of disease.

Diabetes (mellitus) A disease characterized by high levels of glucose in the blood caused by either lack of or ineffectiveness of the hormone insulin.

Disease A bodily dysfunction, usually one that can be described by a diagnostic label. (For simplicity, this book concentrates on discussing diseases and uses this word as a general term also including other health problems, e.g. death, disability, illness, etc.)

Distribution The frequency with which each value (or category) occurs in the study population. The distribution of many variables takes on a characteristic shape. *See* **Normal distribution**.

Down's syndrome A congenital, genetic disorder, leading to mental retardation and a characteristic face, caused by the presence of three chromosomes instead of two at the site of the 21st chromosome.

Effect modification The phenomenon whereby the relative risk associated with a risk factor is altered by the presence of another characteristic. The classic example is that the risk of lung cancer is much greater in smokers who were also exposed to asbestos. In our context, the question is whether the effects of risk factors such as smoking vary by migrant status, race, or ethnic group (as for asbestos).

Environment A broad conception, sometimes taken to mean everything except genetic and biological factors, and sometimes qualified and narrowed, e.g. the physical environment.

Epidemiology The science and craft that studies the pattern of diseases (and health, though usually indirectly) in populations to help understand both their causes and the burden they impose. This information is applied to prevent, control, or manage the problems under study.

Ethnic minority group Usually, but not always, this phrase is used to refer to a non-White population. Alternatively, it may be used to describe a specific identifiable group, e.g. Gypsy Travellers and less commonly Irish in the UK. Some people consider the phrase inaccurate and prefer minority ethnic group, but the two phrases are used synonymously.

Ethnicity The social group a person belongs to, and either identifies with or is identified with by others, as a result of a mix of cultural and other factors including one or more of language, diet, religion, ancestry, and physical features traditionally associated with race (*see* **Race**). Increasingly, the concept is being used synonymously with race but the trend is pragmatic rather than scientific.

Ethnocentrism The tendency to perceive and interpret the world from the standpoint of one's own culture. In epidemiology the tendency is reflected in the practice of using the White population as the norm or standard (*see* **White**).

European An inhabitant of Europe, or one with ancestral origins in Europe. Commonly, this is used in epidemiology and public health as a synonym for White or as qualifying the term White, e.g. European White. White Europeans are placed in the racial classification Caucasian, also known as Europid (the latter has not proven popular).

Exposure A general term to indicate contact with the postulated causal factors (or agents of diseases) used in a way similar to risk factor.

Fetal origins of disease hypothesis The phrase encapsulating the idea that early life circumstances, particularly *in utero*, have an important and lasting effect in determining health and disease in later life.

Foreign/foreigner From another place, and usually another country.

Gene The discrete basic unit (made of DNA or deoxyribonucleic acid) of the chromosome, which itself consists of numerous genes and other DNA material. Genes carry information coding for specific functions, e.g. making proteins. There are two genes (one from the father and one from the mother) at a particular location on a chromosome—both for the same function. Variants of the same gene on a particular location are called alleles. There are 23 pairs of chromosomes in each cell in human beings (46 in total), and the number of genes is estimated at about 24 000.

General population Everyone in the population being studied, irrespective of race or ethnicity.

Genetic drift Genetic evolution, characteristically observable in small populations, arising from random variations in gene frequency.

Gypsy *See* **Roma**.

Halal A word meaning something that is permitted in the Muslim faith, most usually relating to food as in Halal meat, where some forms of flesh are forbidden (Haram).

HDL *See* **Cholesterol**.

Health-care needs Effective preventative or medical interventions which improve health in its broadest sense.

Health needs Factors needed to improve the health of individuals and populations.

Health A desired ideal, that includes being free of disease, disability, and infirmity, that is characterized by well-being and functioning in society.

Hindu Strictly, anyone who practices the religion of Hinduism. An old, now seldom used, term for Indians. A term occasionally used more or less synonymously with South Asian. In some countries such as The Netherlands the term is used to describe the ethnicity of Surinamese of Indian subcontinent ancestry.

Hispanic A person of Latin American descent (with some degree of Spanish or Portuguese ancestral origins), who self-identifies, or is identified, as Hispanic irrespective of other racial or ethnic considerations. In the United States this term, often used interchangeably with Latino, is considered an indicator of ethnic origin.

Hypertension A condition of having blood pressure above an arbitrarily defined level (usually set at 140/90 mmHg). Hypertension is associated with many adverse outcomes, particularly atherosclerotic diseases.

Hypothesis A proposition that is amenable to test by scientific methods (*see* **Null hypotheses**).

Illegal migrant *See* **Undocumented migrant**.

Illness The state of being unwell, often due to disease.

Immigrant *See* **Migrant**.

Incidence/incidence rate The number of new cases of a disease or other condition in a defined population within a specified period of time. When this number is divided by the numbers of people in the relevant population we have the incidence rate.

Indian A person whose ancestry lies in the Indian subcontinent who self-identifies, or is identified, as Indian (*see* **South Asian**). (There were major changes to India's geographical boundaries in 1947 when Pakistan was created.) The term may also be used to refer to North American Indians.

Indigenous This term means a person who belongs naturally to a place in the sense of long-term family origins (*see* **Aboriginal** and **Native**). This term is sometimes used to identify the majority population, e.g. in the UK as an alternative to the word White. In some parts of the world, e.g. Australia, the word indigenous is used specifically to refer to aboriginal populations (*see* **Aborigine**). When a specific aboriginal population is specified the term is capitalized, e.g. Australian Aborigine.

Institutional racism *See* **Racism**.

Interaction The concept is that of effect modification. The term is used in statistical analysis to see whether effect modification exists. *See* **Effect modification**.

Irish A person whose ancestry lies in Ireland who self-identifies as, or is identified by others as Irish, but generally restricted to the White population (*see* **White**).

LDL/VLDL *See* **Cholesterol**.

Longitudinal study *See* **Cohort**.

Majority population When used in race/ethnicity studies this phrase is usually used as a synonym for White or European.

Maori A person who self-identifies, or is identified, as a member of the indigenous peoples of New Zealand—Polynesian by ancestry.

Migrant A person who moves from one place to another, but most commonly used for people who move from one country to another to live there on a permanent or semi-permanent basis. The term is sometimes, wrongly, applied to the offspring of migrants born in the country of settlement. An error of the opposite kind is made when people born abroad, but with ancestry in the country of settlement, are not referred to as migrants. This is one illustration of how migration is intertwined with ancestry, race, and ethnicity.

Minority ethnic group *See* **Ethnic minority group**.

Mixed race or ethnic group A group of people identifying themselves as offspring of parents (or more distant ancestors) of different ethnic or racial groups. Such people may be identified by others as such through birth records. The increasing importance of the category mixed (ethnicity or race) is self-evident. The increasing acceptance of sexual unions that cross ethnic and racial boundaries is adding both richness and complexity to most societies. The way to categorize people born of such unions is unclear and the current approaches are inadequate, partly because the number of potential categories is huge. The solution is, most probably, to offer space for free-text responses for individuals to describe themselves. These responses, however, need to be coded, analysed, summarized, quantified, and published. Without this, individually small but collectively large populations remain hidden.

Mulatto The offspring of a White person and a Negro (*see* **Negro**), although the term has been more generally applied to mixed race. Outdated race concept, now interpreted as pejorative. Not recommended.

Native Usually, this word is used to refer to populations born, or with family origins, in a place (*see* **Indigenous**). This was, in the recent past, also a pejorative term meaning populations belonging to a non-European and imperfectly civilized or savage race, so writers need to take care.

Native American A person who belongs to, and is perceived to belong to, one of a large number of indigenous (aboriginal) peoples of North America. Native American is the umbrella term used in the US census. Many other terms are used for indigenous populations of South America and Canada.

Negro A person of Black African ancestry. Traditionally one of the major classes of races. Though the word is still in use (e.g. in the 2010 US census) as a race category, it is becoming outdated. It is pejorative except when used by Black Africans themselves, or in historical or scientific contexts. Use with care.

Non-Asian/non-Chinese, etc. This type of term is rarely defined but self-evidently implies those not belonging to the group under study. This degree of non-specificity is not usually recommended, but is used where there is little or no alternative.

Normal distribution A statistical distribution that describes well a great many biological variables. The mean, median, and mode values are identical, the distribution is symmetrical around this value, and one standard deviation (a measure of the spread of values) encapsulates 68% of the population. It is known as, and described well by, the phrase 'bell curve'.

Numerator The top half of a fraction, and in the context of this book the number of cases of disease.

Occidental This is a very rarely used term meaning a native or inhabitant of the Occident (West), and effectively a synonym for European, but readers need to be aware of it as the antonym of Oriental. It is too general to be useful.

Octoroon The offspring of a White person and a quadroon (*see* **Quadroon**). Outdated race concept.

Oriental A term meaning a native or inhabitant of the Orient (East). This term is in occasional use in epidemiology, usually referring to Far Eastern populations. It is too general to be useful.

Pacific Islander A umbrella term used in the US census to describe a large diversity of people of Polynesian or Melanesian ancestry, who perceived themselves, and/or are perceived, to be so.

Pakistani A person whose ancestry lies in the Indian subcontinent who self-identifies, or is identified, as Pakistani (*see* **South Asian**). Some Pakistanis may have birth or ancestral roots in the current territory of India but identify with Pakistan, a country created in 1947.

Participant The word that is replacing (study) subject, as in study participant.

Placebo An inactive substance or procedure used as a medicine for psychological effect; and commonly used in the control group in a trial.

Population A complex concept with a multitude of meanings, but crucially for our purposes the people in whom the problem under study occurs, and in whom the results of the research are to be applied.

Population attributable risk The fraction of the disease risk that results from a particular risk factor that can be calculated by a formula that uses prevalence of the risk factor and relative risk.

Prevalence/prevalence rate The number of cases of a disease or other condition in a given population at a designated time. When this number is divided by the number of people in the relevant population we have the prevalence proportion, also commonly called the rate.

Proportional mortality (or morbidity) ratio (PMR) A summary measure of the proportion of deaths/disease due to a specific cause in the study population compared with either all causes or another cause. These numbers, when taken from two populations, can be divided for comparison to create a ratio.

Public health An activity to which many contribute, most usually defined as the science and art of prolonging life, preventing disease, and promoting health through the organized efforts of society.

Quadroon The offspring of a White person and a mulatto, i.e. one quarter non-White (*see* **Mulatto**). An outdated race concept.

Race By historical and common usage the group (subspecies in traditional scientific usage) a person belongs to as a result of a mix of physical features such as skin colour and hair texture, which reflect ancestry and geographical origins, historically as identified by others or, increasingly, as self-identified. The importance of social factors in the creation and perpetuation of racial categories has led to the concept broadening to include a common social and political heritage, making its usage similar to ethnicity. Race and ethnicity are increasingly used as synonyms, causing some confusion and leading to the hybrid terms race/ethnicity (*see* **Ethnicity**).

Racial prejudice Negative beliefs, perceptions, or attitudes towards one or more ethnic or racial groups.

Racialize/racialization The process by which societies become organized by racial (or ethnic or migrant) group because of the use of racial group concepts and classifications. The idea underlying this concept is that there is some imposition that creates something that does not naturally exist.

Racism/institutional racism A belief that some races are superior to others, used to devise and justify individual and collective actions which create and sustain inequality among racial and ethnic groups. Individual racism is usually manifested in decisions and behaviours that disadvantage small numbers of people. Institutional racism, whereby policies and traditions, sometimes unwittingly, favour a particular racial or ethnic group, may be less obvious but may disadvantage large populations. Racism is against international law.

Randomized controlled trial (RCT) A high-level method of evaluating the effects of an intervention. A randomly selected subgroup of study participants get the intervention, while the remainder do not (these form the control group). The control group may get a placebo. The groups are followed up to ascertain outcomes. If the participants do not know whether they are in the study intervention or placebo group the trial is said to be a blinded RCT.

Rate In this book this refers to the calculation of the amount of disease (or equivalent) in a defined population. *See* **Incidence, Prevalence, Numerator, Denominator**.

Reference/control/comparison This refers to the standard against which a population that is being studied can be compared to permit an analysis of similarities and differences. The concept is fundamental to epidemiology, and this terminology is preferable to non-specific ethnic or racial terms such as non-Asian, or general, or even White population.

Refugee A person who has been granted asylum, i.e. leave to stay, usually because of persecution or well-grounded fears of persecution in the land of origin.

Reification The bringing into reality of something that does not exist. The idea, like racialization, is that use of race, ethnicity, and migration status might lead to a sense of real subgroups of a population in ways that are rigid where that is not so.

Relative risk The ratio of the incidence of disease in one population (the study population) compared with another (the control population).

Risk factor A factor associated with an increased probability of an adverse outcome, but not necessarily a causal factor.

Roma/Romany Roma is the preferred name for the people of nomadic inclination who left India variously 500–1000 years ago and settled in various parts of Europe. Romany is one of their traditional languages. They are also known as Gypsies, and in some places that is the norm, but unfortunately there are now negative overtones to that word.

Senile dementia Brain disease characterized by loss of intellect, usually irreversible and caused by degenerative processes usually associated with old age.

Sexually transmitted diseases (STDs) The group of diseases mainly transmitted during sexual behaviour, e.g. syphilis. Some STDs may be transmitted in other ways too, e.g. HIV by blood transfusion.

Sickle cell disease/anaemia A genetic disorder whereby the haemoglobin, the oxygen-carrying molecule in red blood cells, crystallizes and distorts the blood cell into a sickle shape when oxygen in the cell is low. The result is anaemia and other health problems.

Sickness The state of being unwell or dysfunctional, often as a result of disease.

SMR (standardized mortality/morbidity ratio) The ratio of the number of events observed in the study population divided by the number that would be expected if it had the same age-specific rates as the standard population (usually the fraction is multiplied by 100). A figure of more than 100 reflects an excess of disease, less than 100 a deficit. The SMR takes into account age differences between populations.

South Asian A person whose ancestry is in the countries of the Indian subcontinent, including India, Pakistan, Bangladesh, and Sri Lanka and sometimes also other surrounding countries (in terms of racial classifications, most people in this group probably fit best into Caucasian or Caucasoid but this is confusing and is not recommended). This label is usually assigned, for individuals rarely identify with it. *See also* **Indian, Asian Indian, Asian, Pakistani, Bangladeshi.**

Standardized mortality (or morbidity) ratio *See* **SMR.**

Stratified sample The people selected for (or participating in) a study where the sampling frame is organized by subgroups, e.g. men and women, or age groups. Then random samples are chosen within each subgroup.

Subject A person who is studied, i.e. a member of the population under study (*see* **Participant**).

Theory A system of ideas offered to explain and connect observed factors or conjectures. A statement of general principles or laws underlying a subject.

Trafficking/trafficked person In this context this is about trade in humans who are moved, often against their will or full knowledge and consent, from one place to another. Such people may be moved for enforced labour, domestic servitude, prostitution, and other such reasons.

Traveller A member of a number of traditional groups of people who live a nomadic lifestyle, including, for example, Irish Travellers. Gypsies are also sometimes known as Gypsy Travellers. *See* **Gypsy** and **Roma.**

Trisomy 21 *See* **Down's syndrome.**

Tuberculosis A multisystem infection caused by the bacterium *Mycobacterium tuberculosis.*

Undocumented migrant A person who is living in a country without permission from the appropriate authorities. Such people include those brought into the country against their permission (e.g. trafficked persons), people entering the country aiming to claim asylum, those who claim asylum but were not successful and did not leave the country, and student, tourists, and temporary workers who remain after their permission to stay permit expires.

Western A person or populations with ancestry in a region conventionally known as the West, effectively European countries, as distinguished from Eastern or Oriental populations. This loose term is not recommended, especially as some authors include industrialized countries such as Japan as 'Western'.

White The term usually used to describe people with European ancestral origins who self-identify, or are identified, as White (sometimes called European, or in terms of racial classifications, the group usually known as Caucasian or Caucasoid). The word may be capitalized to highlight its specific use. The label is widely acceptable to the populations so described. The term has served to distinguish these groups from those groups with skin of other colours (black, yellow, etc.), and hence derives from the concept of race but is used increasingly as an indicator of ethnicity. There are problems of poverty and excess disease in subgroups of the White population, which cannot be unearthed and tackled by solely using the label White. A breakdown of the category is recommended e.g. Polish White.

Bibliography

This is a small selection, given the ease with which readings can be found using the internet. I have severely trimmed the lists to make space for extra writing. A longer bibliography is given in the first edition. Books and reports are given here and references at the end of each chapter.

Bahl V, Hopkins A (1993) *Access to Health Care for People from Black and Ethnic Minorities*. London: The Royal College of Physicians of London.

Barkan E (1992) *The Retreat of Scientific Racism*. London: Cambridge University Press.

Barnett A (1950) *The Human Species*. Bungay: The Chaucer Press Ltd.

Bhopal RS (2008) *Concepts of Epidemiology*. Oxford: Oxford University Press.

Bhugra D, Bahl V (eds) (1999) *Ethnicity: an agenda for mental health*. London: Gaskell.

Biddiss MD (ed.) (1970) *Gobineau: selected political writings*. London: Jonathan Cape.

Biddiss MD (1979) *Images of Race*. Leicester: Leicester University Press.

Blumenbach JF (1865) *The Anthropological Treatises of Johann Friedrich Blumenbach*. London: Anthropological Society.

Bolt C (1970) *Victorian Attitudes to Race*. London: Routledge and Kegan Paul.

Bowling A, Ebrahim S (2006) *Handbook of Health Research Methods: investigation, measurement and analysis*. Maidenhead: Open University Press.

Cashmore E (1996) *Dictionary of Race and Ethnic Relations*, 4th edn. London: Routledge.

Chadwick J, Mann WN (1950) *The Medical Works of Hippocrates*. London: Blackwell Scientific Publications Ltd.

Coker NE (2001) *Racism in Britain. An Agenda for Change*. London: King's Fund.

College M, van Geuns HA, Svensson PG (1986) *Migration and Health: towards an understanding of the health care needs of ethnic minorities. Proceedings of the Consultative Group on Ethnic Minorities, The Hague, Netherlands, 28–30 November*. Copenhagen: World Health Organization, Regional Office for Europe.

Cruickshank JK, Beevers G (1990) *Ethnic Factors in Health and Disease*. Oxford: Butterworth.

Department of Health (1992) *Annual Report of the Chief Medical Officer on the State of Public Health 1991*. London: HMSO.

Diamond J (1998) *Guns, Germs and Steel*. London: Vintage.

Directorate of Health [Norway] (2009) *Migration and Health—challenges and trends*. Oslo: Directorate of Health Publication Office.

Dreachslin JL, Gilbert MJ, Malone B (2012) *Diversity and Cultural Competence in Health Care: a systems approach*. San Francisco: Jossey-Bass.

Ebling FJ (ed.) (1974) *Racial Variation in Man*. London: Institute of Biology.

Ellison E, Goodman AH (2006) *The Nature of Difference—science, society and human biology*. Boca Raton, FL: CRC Press.

Fernandes A, Miguel JP (2009) *Health and Migration in the European Union: better health for all in an inclusive society*. Lisbon: Instituto Nacional de Saude Doutor Ricardo Jorge.

Gomez LE, Lopez N (eds) (2013) *Mapping 'Race': critical approaches to health disparities research*. New Brunswick, NJ: Rutgers University Press.

Gunaratnam Y (1993) *Checklist. Health and Race: a starting point for managers on improving services for black populations*. London: King's Fund.

Health Education Authority (1994) *Health and Lifestyles: black and minority ethnic groups in England*. London: HEA.

International Organization for Migration (IOM) (2009) *International Migration Law No. 19—Migration and the Right to Health: a review of international law.* Geneva: IOM.

International Organization for Migration (IOM) (2009) *Migration Health: better health for all in Europe—final report.* Brussels: IOM Migration Health Department.

Kai J (2003) *Ethnicity, Health and Primary Care.* Oxford: Oxford University Press.

Kelleher D, Hillier S (1996) *Researching Cultural Differences in Health.* London: Routledge.

Kohn M (1996) *The Race Gallery: the return of racial science.* London: Cape.

LaVeist TA (2005) Minority Populations and Health: an introduction to health disparities in the United States, 1st edn. San Francisco, Jossey-Bass.

LaVeist TA, Isaac LA (eds) (2013) *Race, Ethnicity, and Health: a public health reader,* 2nd edn. San Francisco, Jossey-Bass.

Linnaeus C (1806) *A General System of Nature Through the Three Grand Kingdoms of Animals, Vegetables, and Minerals [Systema Naturae].* London: Lackington Allen & Co.

Loue S (1998) *Handbook of Immigrant Health.* New York: Plenum Press.

Macbeth H, Shetty P (eds) (2000) *Ethnicity and Health.* London: Taylor and Francis.

Malik K (2008) *Strange Fruit—Why Both Sides are Wrong in the Race Debate.* Oxford: Oneworld Publications.

NHS Health Scotland (2012) *Review of Equality Health Data Needs in Scotland 2012.* Edinburgh: NHS Health Scotland.

Olumide J (2002) *Raiding the Gene Pool: the social construction of mixed race.* London: Pluto Press.

Panayi P (2010) *An Immigration History of Britain: multicultural racism since 1800.* Harlow: Pearson Longman.

Polednak AP (1989) *Racial and Ethnic Differences in Disease.* Oxford: Oxford University Press.

Rawaf S, Bahl V (eds) (1998) *Assessing Health Needs of People from Minority Ethnic Groups.* London: Royal Colleges of Physicians of the United Kingdom, Faculty of Public Health Medicine.

Razum O, Spallek J, Reeske A, Arnold M (2011) *Migration-sensitive Cancer Registration in Europe. Challenges and Potentials.* Frankfurt: Peter Lang International Academic Publishers.

Robinson M (2002) *Communication and Health in a Multi-ethnic Society.* Bristol: Policy Press.

Royal College of General Practitioners (North London Faculty) (1967) *A Symposium on the Medical and Social Problems of an Immigrant Population in Britain.* London: Royal College of General Practitioners.

Salway S, Barley R, Allmark P, Gerrish K, Higginbottom G, Ellison G (2011) *Ethnic Diversity and Inequality: ethical and scientific rigour in social research.* York: Joseph Rowntree Foundation.

Scottish Ethnicity and Health Research Strategy Working Group (2009) *Health in our Multi-ethnic Scotland: future research priorities.* Edinburgh: NHS Health Scotland.

Segal UA, Elliott D, Mayadas NS (2010) *Immigration Worldwide: policies, practices, and trends.* Oxford: Oxford University Press.

Stepan N (1982) *The Idea of Race in Science.* London: Macmillan.

Temple B, Moran R (eds) (2006) *Doing Research With Refugees—Issues and Guidelines.* Bristol: Policy Press.

US Department of Health and Human Services (1985) *Report of the Secretary's Task Force on Black and Minority Health.* Washington, DC: US Government Printing Office.

US Department of Health and Human Services (2001) *National Standards for Culturallyand Linguistically Appropriate Services in Health Care—Executive Summary.* Washington, DC: Office of Minority Health.

World Health Organization (2010) *Health of Migrants—the way forward: report of a global consultation.* Geneva: WHO.

World Health Organization Regional Office for Europe (2010) *How Health Systems can Address Health Inequities Linked to Migration and Ethnicity.* Copenhagen: WHO Regional Office for Europe.

Williams C, Johnston MRD (2010) *Race and Ethnicity in a Welfare Society,* 2nd edn. Maidenhead: Open University Press.

Ethnicity and health websites: A selection

All website addresses were checked for access in June 2013. (It is perhaps reflective of the changing and unstable nature of our field that very many websites listed in the first edition had become inactive.)

Organizations' websites relating to migration, ethnicity, and race

American Public Health Association—on minority health: http://www.apha.org/about/Public+Health+Links/LinksMinorityHealth.htm

Asian American Health—an information portal to issues affecting the health and well-being of Asian Americans in the United States: http://asianamericanhealth.nlm.nih.gov/

Australian Government National Health and Medical Research Council—Australian government's policy on aboriginal and Torres Strait Islander health: http://www.nhmrc.gov.au/guidelines/publications/e52

California Healthline—Creating a culturally competent health care system: http://www.californiahealthline.org/think-tank/2012/creating-a-culturally-competent-health-care-system.aspx#

CILT, the National Centre for Languages: http://www.cilt.org.uk/

Council of Europe—guidelines on migration and healthcare: https://wcd.coe.int/ViewDoc.jsp?Ref=CM/Rec(2011)13&Language=lanEnglish&Ver=original&Site=CM&BackColorInternet=C3C3C3&BackColorIntranet=EDB021&BackColorLogged=F5D383

Equality and Human Rights Commission (UK): http://www.equalityhumanrights.com/

Equality Impact Assessment—Department of Health guidelines: http://webarchive.nationalarchives.gov.uk/20130107105354/http://www.dh.gov.uk/en/Publicationsandstatistics/Publications/PublicationsPolicyAndGuidance/DH_090396

Institute of Medicine (USA): http://www.iom.edu/About-IOM.aspx

Institute of Race Relations (IRR): http://www.irr.org.uk/about/

International Epidemiological Association: http://ieaweb.org/

NHS Health Scotland—Advancing equality in health: http://www.healthscotland.com/equalities/index.aspx

Pan American Health Organization (PAHO)—Mainstreaming ethnic equity in health policies: http://www.paho.org/English/AD/GE/Ethnicity.htm

Race for Health—a UK Department of Health-funded, NHS-based programme that works with PCTs and Trusts to drive forward improvements in health for people from black, and minority ethnic backgrounds: http://www.raceforhealth.org

Royal College of Nursing—Transcultural Health Care Practice: an educational resource for nurses and health care practitioners web-based educational materials on ethnicity and health: http://www.rcn.org.uk/development/learning/transcultural_health/transcultural

South Asian Health Foundation (UK): http://www.sahf.org.uk/

Stormfront—example of a racist website: http://www.stormfront.org/forum/t538924/

UNC Gillings School of Global Public Health Minority Health Project to eliminate health disparities: http://www.minority.unc.edu/reports/

US Department of Health and Human Services—Office for Civil Rights: http://www.hhs.gov/ocr/

US Department of Health and Human Services, Agency for Healthcare Research and Quality—Excellence centres to eliminate ethnic/racial disparities (EXCEED): http://www.ahrq.gov/research/exceed.htm

United States Holocaust Memorial Museum: http://www.ushmm.org/

World Health Organization (WHO): http://www.who.int/en/

Reports and general information on specific topics

Adolf Hitler—Wikipedia entry: http://www.en.wikipedia.org/wiki/Adolf_Hitler

Adolf Hitler—*Mein Kampf*: http://www.hitler.org/writings/Mein_Kampf/index.html

Adversity.net—Racial Privacy Initiative: http://www.adversity.net/RPI/rpi_mainframe.htm

American Anthropological Association—Response to OMB Directive 15: Race and Ethnic Standards for Federal Statistics and Administrative Reporting: http://www.aaanet.org/gvt/ombdraft.htm

Australian Government National Health and Medical research Council—guidelines on improving aboriginal health through research: http://www.nhmrc.gov.au/guidelines/publications/r47

Deadly Medicine. Creating the Master Race—United States Holocaust Memorial Museum exhibition: http://www.ushmm.org/museum/exhibit/online/deadlymedicine/overview/index.php?content=overview_300k

Department of Health—Heart disease and South Asians: delivering the National Service Framework for Coronary Heart Disease: http://webarchive.nationalarchives.gov.uk/+/www.dh.gov.uk/en/Publicationsandstatistics/Publications/PublicationsPolicyAndGuidance/DH_4098586

Department of Health—Ten-point plan of the Chief Executive http://webarchive.nationalarchives.gov.uk/+/www.dh.gov.uk/en/Publicationsandstatistics/Bulletins/DH_4072494

Department of Health—Emergency multilingual phrasebook: http://webarchive.nationalarchives.gov.uk/20130107105354/http://www.dh.gov.uk/PublicationsAndStatistics/Publications/PublicationsPolicyAndGuidance/PublicationsPolicyAndGuidanceArticle/fs/en?CONTENT_ID=4073230&chk=8XboAN

Department of Health—Practical guide to ethnic monitoring in the NHS and social care: http://webarchive.nationalarchives.gov.uk/20130107105354/http://dh.gov.uk/en/publicationsandstatistics/publications/publicationspolicyandguidance/dh_4116839

Disparities/inequalities calculator: http://seer.cancer.gov/hdcalc/index.html

Health-care Needs Assessment—Black and minority ethnic groups: http://www.birmingham.ac.uk/Documents/college-mds/haps/projects/HCNA/04HCNA3D4.pdf

Health Survey for England 1999—The Health of Minority Ethnic Groups '99: http://www.archive.official-documents.co.uk/document/doh/survey99/hse99-00.htm

Health Survey for England 2004—Health of Ethnic Minorities: http://www.ic.nhs.uk/pubs/hse04ethnic

International Organization for Migration—Migration law database: http://www.imldb.iom.int/section.do

National Institute on Minority Health and Disparities (NIMHD)—NIH strategic plan for reducing disparities: http://www.nimhd.nih.gov/about_ncmhd/index2.asp

neurodiversity.com—History of scientific racism: http://www.neurodiversity.com/racism.html

New Zealand History Online—Treaty of Waitangi: http://www.nzhistory.net.nz/taxonomy/term/133

NHS Lothian—updated race equality scheme 2008–11: http://www.nhslothian.scot.nhs.uk/OurOrganisation/KeyDocuments/Documents/race_equality_scheme_updated2008-2011.pdf

NHS Health Scotland—Scottish Health and Ethnicity Research Strategy Steering (SHERSS) group: http://www.healthscotland.com/resources/networks/SHERRS.aspx

Peggy McIntosh: White Privilege: Unpacking the Invisible Knapsack—Daily effects of white privilege in a racist society: http://www.amptoons.com/blog/files/mcintosh.html#daily

Stephen Lawrence Inquiry—Recommendations: http://www.archive.official-documents.co.uk/document/cm42/4262/sli-47.htm

The Scottish Government—Fair for All (summary). http://www.scotland.gov.uk/Publications/2001/12/10395/File-1

The Scottish Government—One Scotland—Many Cultures. Working Together for Race Equality. The Scottish Executive's Race Equality Scheme: http://www.scotland.gov.uk/Publications/2002/11/15866/14287

United Nations Permanent Forum on Indigenous Issues—Declaration on the Rights of Indigenous Peoples: http://social.un.org/index/IndigenousPeoples/DeclarationontheRightsofIndigenousPeoples.aspx

US Centers for Disease Control and Prevention—Tuskegee syphilis study: http://www.cdc.gov/tuskegee/

US Department of Health and Human Services, Agency for Healthcare Research and Quality—National Healthcare Disparities Report, 2005 http://www.ahrq.gov/qual/nhdr05/nhdr05.htm

US Department of Health and Human Services Office of Minority Health—the National CLAS Standards: http://minorityhealth.hhs.gov/templates/browse.aspx?lvl=2&lvlID=15

World Health Organization—publications on ethnicity and migration: http://www.googlesyndi-catedsearch.com/u/who?q=ethnicity&sa=OK&sitesearch=who.int&domains=who.int

Statistics and census (these and other national agency websites were used in Chapter 2)

Australian Bureau of Statistics—Census Dictionary 2011: http://www.abs.gov.au/ausstats/abs@.nsf/mf/2901.0

Brazil's Statistical Agency (IBGE)—Demographic Census: http://www1.ibge.gov.br/english/estatistica/populacao/censo2010/calendario.shtm

CensusInfo—census information worldwide: http://www.censusinfo.net/worldwide.html

Centers for Disease Control and Prevention—FastStats, health statistics: http://www.cdc.gov/nchs/fastats/Default.htm

Department of Statistics Singapore: http://www.singstat.gov.sg/

General Register Office for Scotland—Information about Scotland's people: http://www.gro-scotland.gov.uk/

Infoplease—ethnicity and races by countries: http://www.infoplease.com/ipa/A0855617.html

Office for National Statistics—Census 2011, England and Wales: http://www.statistics.gov.uk/census2001/profiles/commentaries/ethnicity.asp

Statistics Canada: http://www12.statcan.ca/census-recensement/index-eng.cfm

Statistics South Africa: http://www.statssa.gov.za/

United Nations Economic Commission for Europe—2010 population census round: http://www1.unece.org/stat/platform/display/censuses/2010+Population+Census+Round

United Nations Statistics Division—population and housing census dates: http://www.un.org/depts/unsd/demog/cendate/index.html

United States Census Bureau: http://www.census.gov/

Some journals specializing in ethnicity and health

Cultural Diversity and Ethnic Minority Psychology: http://www.apa.org/pubs/journals/cdp/index.aspx

Ethnicity and Inequalities in Health and Social Care: http://www.emeraldinsight.com/products/journals/journals.htm?id=eihsc

Ethnicity and Disease: http://www.ishib.org/wordpress/?page_id=39

Ethnicity and Health: http://www.tandfonline.com/toc/ceth20/current

Journal of Immigrant and Minority Health: http://www.springer.com/uk/home/generic/search/results?SGWID=3-40109-70-35544009-0

Journal of Transcultural Nursing: http://www.sagepub.com/journalsProdDesc.nav?prodId=Journal200814

Transcultural Psychiatry: http://tps.sagepub.com/

Some networks

AEN—Aotearoa Ethnic Health Network: http://lists.aen.org.nz/listinfo.cgi/aen-aen.org.nz

British Sociological Association Race and Ethnicity Study Group: http://www.britsoc.co.uk/specialisms/RaceandEthnicitySG

DiversityRx (USA): http://www.diversityRx.org

Ethnic Health List: minority_ethnic_health@mail.ac.uk

MIGHEALTHNET—Information network on good practice in health care for migrants and minorities in Europe: http://mighealth.net/uk/index.php/Main_Page

Minority Health e-network: https://www.jiscmail.ac.uk/cgi-bin/webadmin?A0=minority-ethnic-health

Muslim Health Network: http://www.muslimhealthnetwork.org/

Index

Note: page numbers in *italics* refer to figures, tables, and boxes. Those in **bold** refer to glossary entries.